Concussion in Sports

Guest Editors

WILLIAM P. MEEHAN III, MD
LYLE J. MICHELI, MD

CLINICS IN SPORTS MEDICINE

www.sportsmed.theclinics.com

Consulting Editor
MARK D. MILLER, MD

January 2011 • Volume 30 • Number 1

SAUNDERS an imprint of ELSEVIER, Inc.

W.B. SAUNDERS COMPANY

A Division of Elsevier Inc.

1600 John F. Kennedy Blvd. ● Suite 1800 ● Philadelphia, Pennsylvania 19103

http://www.theclinics.com

CLINICS IN SPORTS MEDICINE Volume 30, Number 1
January 2011 ISSN 0278-5919, ISBN-13: 978-1-4557-0506-1

Editor: Ruth Malwitz
Developmental Editor: Donald Mumford

Clinics in Sports Medicine (ISSN 0278-5919) is published quarterly by Elsevier Inc., 360 Park Avenue South, New York, NY 10010-1710. Months of issue are January, April, July, and October. Business and Editorial Offices: 1600 John F. Kennedy Blvd., Ste. 1800, Philadelphia, PA 19103-2899. Customer Service Office: 3251 Riverport Lane, Maryland Heights, MO 63043. Periodicals postage paid at New York, NY and additional mailing offices. Subscription prices are $297.00 per year (US individuals), $466.00 per year (US institutions), $147.00 per year (US students), $337.00 per year (Canadian individuals), $563.00 per year (Canadian institutions), $205.00 (Canadian students), $408.00 per year (foreign individuals), $563.00 per year (foreign institutions), and $205.00 per year (foreign students). Foreign air speed delivery is included in all *Clinics* subscription prices. All prices are subject to change without notice. **POSTMASTER:** Send address changes to *Clinics in Sports Medicine*, Elsevier Health Sciences Division, Subscription Customer Service, 3251 Riverport Lane, Maryland Heights, MO 63043. Customer Service (orders, claims, online, change of address): Elsevier Health Sciences Division, Subscription Customer Service, 3251 Riverport Lane, Maryland Heights, MO 63043. Tel: 1-800-654-2452 (U.S. and Canada); 314-447-8871 (outside U.S. and Canada). Fax: 314-447-8029. E-mail: journalscustomerservice-usa@elsevier.com (for print support); journalsonlinesupport-usa@elsevier.com (for online support).

Reprints. For copies of 100 or more of articles in this publication, please contact the Commercial Reprints Department, Elsevier Inc., 360 Park Avenue South, New York, NY 10010-1710. Tel.: 212-633-3812; Fax: 212-462-1935; E-mail: reprints@elsevier.com.

Clinics in Sports Medicine is covered in *MEDLINE/PubMed (Index Medicus) Current Contents/Clinical Medicine, Excerpta Medica,* and *ISI/Biomed.*

Printed and bound by CPI Group (UK) Ltd, Croydon, CR0 4YY

Transferred to Digital Print 2011

Contributors

CONSULTING EDITOR

MARK D. MILLER, MD
S. Ward Casscells Professor of Orthopaedic Surgery, University of Virginia, Charlottesville;
Team Physician, James Madison University, Harrisonburg, Virginia

GUEST EDITORS

WILLIAM P. MEEHAN III, MD
Director, Sports Concussion Clinic, Division of Sports Medicine, Department
of Orthopedics; Division of Emergency Medicine, Department of Medicine,
Children's Hospital Boston, Boston, Massachusetts

LYLE J. MICHELI, MD
Director, Division of Sports Medicine, Children's Hospital Boston, Harvard Medical
School, Boston, Massachusetts

AUTHORS

JULIAN E. BAILES, MD
Professor and Chairman, Department of Neurosurgery, West Virginia University,
Robert C. Byrd Health Sciences Center, Morgantown, West Virginia

GARNI BARKHOUDARIAN, MD
Department of Neurosurgery, David Geffen School of Medicine at UCLA, Los Angeles,
California

CHRISTINE M. BAUGH, AB
Research Coordinator, Center for the Study of Traumatic Encephalopathy, Boston
University School of Medicine, Boston, Massachusetts

ROBERT C. CANTU, MD
Co-Director, Center for the Study of Traumatic Encephalopathy, Department of
Neurology, Boston; Associate Professor of Neurology and Pathology, Sports Legacy
Institute, Waltham; Clinical Professor, Department of Neurosurgery, Boston University
School of Medicine, Boston; Chief of Neurosurgery Service, Director of Sports Medicine,
Department of Neurosurgery, Emerson Hospital; Chairman, Department of Surgery,
Emerson Hospital, Concord; Co-Director, Neurologic Sports Injury Center, Department
of Neurosurgery, Brigham and Women's Hospital, Boston, Massachusetts

MICHAEL W. COLLINS, PhD
Assistant Director, Sports Concussion Program; Associate Professor, Department of
Orthopaedic Surgery and Neurological Surgery, University of Pittsburgh Medical Center,
Pittsburgh, Pennsylvania

TRACEY COVASSIN, PhD, ATC
Assistant Professor, Department of Kinesiology, Michigan State University, East Lansing, Michigan

DANIEL H. DANESHVAR, MA
MD/PhD Graduate Student, Center for the Study of Traumatic Encephalopathy, Department of Neurology, Boston University School of Medicine, Boston, Massachusetts

PIERRE D'HEMECOURT, MD
Director, Primary Care Sports Medicine Fellowship, Division of Sports Medicine, Children's Hospital, Boston, Massachusetts

RJ ELBIN, PhD
Assistant Professor, Department of Kinesiology, Leisure and Sport Science, East Tennessee State University, Johnson City, Tennessee

BRANDON E. GAVETT, PhD
Instructor of Neurology, Director of Neuropsychology, Center for the Study of Traumatic Encephalopathy and Alzheimer's Disease Center, Boston University; Department of Neurology, Boston University School of Medicine, Boston, Massachusetts

CHRISTOPHER C. GIZA, MD
Associate Professor-In-Residence, Department of Neurosurgery; Division of Pediatric Neurology, Department of Pediatrics; Interdepartmental Programs for Neuroscience and Biomedical Engineering, UCLA Brain Injury Research Center, Semel Institute, David Geffen School of Medicine at UCLA, Mattel Children's Hospital–UCLA, Los Angeles, California

KEVIN M. GUSKIEWICZ, PhD, ATC
Kenan Distinguished Professor and Chair; Director, Matthew Alan Gfeller Sport-Related Traumatic Brain Injury Research Center, Department of Exercise and Sport Science, University of North Carolina at Chapel Hill, Chapel Hill, North Carolina

DAVID A. HOVDA, PhD
Professor, Departments of Neurosurgery and Medical and Molecular Pharmacology; Interdepartmental Program for Neuroscience, UCLA Brain Injury Research Center, Semel Institute, David Geffen School of Medicine at UCLA, Los Angeles, California

ERIC W. JOHNSON, PsyD
Instructor, Neuropsychology Fellow, Department of Orthopaedic Surgery, Sports Concussion Program, University of Pittsburgh Medical Center, Pittsburgh, Pennsylvania

NATHAN E. KEGEL, MSEd
Department of Orthopaedic Surgery, Sports Concussion Program, University of Pittsburgh Medical Center, Pittsburgh, Pennsylvania

MARK R. LOVELL, PhD
Professor, Department of Orthopaedic Surgery; Director, Sports Concussion Program, University of Pittsburgh Medical Center, Pittsburgh, Pennsylvania

PAUL MCCRORY, MBBS, PhD, FRACP, FACSP, FACSM, FFSEM, GradDipEpidBiostats
Associate Professor, Centre for Health, Exercise and Sports Medicine and Brain Research Institute, University of Melbourne, Victoria, Australia

ANN C. MCKEE, MD
Center for the Study of Traumatic Encephalopathy and Alzheimer's Disease
Center, Boston University; Associate Professor of Neurology and Pathology, Director,
Neuropathology Core, Departments of Neurology and Pathology, Boston University
School of Medicine, Boston; Bedford Veterans Affairs Medical Center, Bedford,
Massachusetts

DAVID F. MEANEY, PhD
Professor, Department of Bioengineering, University of Pennsylvania, Philadelphia,
Pennsylvania

WILLIAM P. MEEHAN III, MD
Director, Sports Concussion Clinic, Division of Sports Medicine, Department
of Orthopedics; Division of Emergency Medicine, Department of Medicine,
Children's Hospital Boston, Boston, Massachusetts

CHRISTOPHER J. NOWINSKI, AB
Co-Director, Center for the Study of Traumatic Encephalopathy, Department
of Neurology, Boston University School of Medicine, Boston; Co-Founder, Sports Legacy
Institute, Waltham, Massachusetts

JOHN ORPHANOS, MD
Department of Neurosurgery, West Virginia University, Robert C. Byrd Health Sciences
Center, Morgantown, West Virginia

SUMMER D. OTT, PsyD
Co-Director, Methodist Hospital Neurological Institute Concussion Center; Clinical
Assistant Professor, Department of Neurology, University of Texas Medical Branch,
Houston, Texas

SANJAY P. PRABHU, MBBS, FRCR
Staff Pediatric Neuroradiologist, Division of Neuroradiology, Department of Radiology,
Children's Hospital Boston; Instructor of Radiology, Harvard Medical School, Boston,
Massachusetts

MARK PROCTOR, MD
Division of Neurosurgery, Department of Surgery, Children's Hospital Boston, Boston,
Massachusetts

MARGOT PUTUKIAN, MD, FACSM
Director of Athletic Medicine, Head Team Physician, Princeton University, Princeton;
Associate Clinical Professor, Robert Wood Johnson, UMDNJ, New Brunswick,
New Jersey

CARA L. SEDNEY, MD
Department of Neurosurgery, West Virginia University, Robert C. Byrd Health Sciences
Center, Morgantown, West Virginia

DOUGLAS H. SMITH, MD
Professor, Department of Neurosurgery, University of Pennsylvania, Philadelphia,
Pennsylvania

GARY S. SOLOMON, PhD
Associate Professor, Departments of Neurological Surgery and Psychiatry, Vanderbilt
University School of Medicine, Nashville, Tennessee

ROBERT A. STERN, PhD
Center for the Study of Traumatic Encephalopathy and Alzheimer's Disease Center, Boston University; Associate Professor of Neurology, Director, Clinical Core, Department of Neurology, Boston University School of Medicine, Boston, Massachusetts

ALEX M. TAYLOR, PsyD
Sports Concussion Clinic, Division of Sports Medicine, Department of Orthopedics; Department of Neurology, Children's Hospital Boston, Boston, Massachusetts

Contents

> Concussions and head injuries may never be completely eliminated from sports. However, with better data comes an improved understanding of the types of actions and activities that typically result in concussions. With this knowledge can come improved techniques and rule changes to minimize the rate and severity of concussions in sports. This article identifies the factors that affect concussion rate.

> The rising awareness of the long-term health problems associated with concussions re-emphasizes the need for understanding the mechanical etiology of concussions. This article reviews past studies defining the common mechanisms for mild traumatic brain injury and summarizes efforts to convert the external input to the head (force, acceleration, and velocity) into estimates of motions and deformations of the brain that occur during mild traumatic brain injury. Studies of how these mechanical conditions contribute to the cellular mechanisms of damage in mild traumatic brain injury are reviewed. Finally, future directions for improving understanding concussion biomechanics are discussed.

> Concussion or mild traumatic brain injury (mTBI) is a condition that affects hundreds of thousands of patients worldwide. Understanding the pathophysiology of this disorder can help manage its acute and chronic repercussions. Immediately following mTBI, there are several metabolic, hemodynamic, structural, and electric changes that alter normal cerebral function. These alterations can increase the brain's vulnerability to repeat injury and long-term disability. This review evaluates current studies from the bench to the bedside of mTBI. Acute and chronic effects of concussion are measured in both animal and clinical studies. Also, the effect of repeat concussions is analyzed. Concussion-induced pathophysiology with regards to glucose metabolism changes, mitochondrial dysfunction, axonal injury, and structural damage are evaluated. Translational studies such as functional magnetic resonance imaging, magnetic resonance

spectroscopy and diffusion tensor imaging prove to be effective clinical tools for both prognostic and treatment parameters. Understanding the neurobiology of concussion will lead to development and validation of physiological biomarkers of this common injury. These biomarkers (eg, laboratory tests, imaging, electrophysiology) will then allow for improved detection, better functional assessment and evidence-based return to play recommendations.

Sport-related concussion is a common injury that occurs in a variety of sports. In recent years, more attention has been focused on the importance of this injury as well as the long-term complications of unrecognized, repetitive, and/or severe injury. The acute presentation of concussion as well as the diagnosis of concussion is often straightforward and obvious, but it can also be subtle and difficult to discern. Most injuries are short lived with complete recovery within a couple of weeks, with a small minority taking several months to resolve. Unfortunately, it is difficult to predict which injuries will linger. This article discusses the on-field presentation, diagnosis, and management of sport-related concussion. It is important to have a concussion protocol for high-risk sports, including a preseason and postinjury assessment, and an individualized yet comprehensive approach that includes evaluating symptoms, and a neurologic examination that includes cognitive function and balance testing. A multifaceted approach to the evaluation and diagnosis of concussion is endorsed for the optimal management of this injury.

Most concussion symptoms resolve within the first week after injury. Athletes with persistent symptoms may manifest subtle behavioral and cognitive changes. The astute clinician uses various information to determine when these symptoms have cleared before allowing the athlete to return to athletic competition.

Assessment of concussion can be challenging for medical practitioners given the different factors associated with each individual injury. The use of neuropsychological testing provides an objective method in the evaluation and management of concussion. Over the last 20 years it has become increasingly useful in the realm of sports concussion and has been deemed a cornerstone of concussion management by the Concussion in Sport group at the International Symposia on Concussion in Sport. Neuropsychological assessment has evolved to using computer-based neurocognitive testing, which has become increasingly common over the last decade, especially in organized sports. Neuropsychological assessment has also proven to be effective in the detection of differences based on several individual factors, including age, gender, and history of prior concussion. Despite its documented value, neuropsychological assessment should be one of several tools used as part of the concussion assessment/management process.

Balance Assessment in the Management of Sport-Related Concussion

Kevin M. Guskiewicz

Although neuropsychological testing has proven to be a valuable tool in concussion management, it is most useful when administered as part of a comprehensive assessment battery that includes grading of symptoms and clinical balance tests. A thorough sideline and clinical examination by the certified athletic trainer and team physician is considered an important first step in the management of concussion. The evaluation should be conducted in a systematic manner, whether on the field or in the clinical setting. The evaluation should include obtaining a *history* for specific details about the injury (eg, mechanism, symptomatology, concussion history), followed by assessing *neurocognitive function* and *balance*, which is the focus of this article. The objective measures from balance testing can provide clinicians with an additional piece of the concussion puzzle, remove some of the guesswork in uncovering less obvious symptoms, and assist in determining readiness to return safely to participation.

The Role of Neuroimaging in Sport-Related Concussion

Sanjay P. Prabhu

This article describes some of the newer techniques that are being used in the clinical assessment of patients following mild to moderate TBI, addresses their use in the acute setting, and explores their potential role in long-term follow-up. Also addressed are the challenges faced before some of these newer techniques can be incorporated into routine clinical management. Large studies are needed with a special emphasis on the effects of repeated head trauma in the young athlete. This is especially relevant where conventional imaging does not demonstrate a macroscopic abnormality. The emphasis has to shift from identifying structural abnormalities on imaging studies to understanding the functional changes in the brain that may explain the long-term neuropsychological effects of concussion and mTBI.

Medical Therapies for Concussion

William P. Meehan III

Clinicians who manage sport-related concussions have excellent guidelines by which most injuries can be managed. Because sport-related concussions typically resolve within a short time frame, most can be managed with physical and cognitive rest alone. However, clinicians who specialize in the assessment and management of this diagnosis encounter patients with prolonged recovery courses, persistent symptoms, and significant deficits in cognitive functioning. These patients require more involved therapy, which may include additional education, academic accommodations, physical therapy, cognitive rehabilitation, and medication. This article reviews the main medical therapies for the management of concussive brain injury.

neurocognitive effects is mixed and not convincing at present in these groups of athletes. Selected studies of professional boxers and American professional football players are also reviewed, and the available data regarding long-term neurocognitive and neuropathologic effects are assessed. The evidence for long-term adverse neurocognitive effects in professional boxers is compelling. Suggestions for future research on relevant biopsychosocial variables affecting response to concussive injury are presented.

Chronic Traumatic Encephalopathy: A Potential Late Effect of Sport-Related Concussive and Subconcussive Head Trauma

Brandon E. Gavett, Robert A. Stern, and Ann C. McKee

Chronic traumatic encephalopathy (CTE) is a form of neurodegeneration believed to result from repeated head injuries. Originally termed *dementia pugilistica* because of its association with boxing, the neuropathology of CTE was first described by Corsellis in 1973 in a case series of 15 retired boxers. CTE has recently been found to occur after other causes of repeated head trauma, suggesting that any repeated blows to the head, such as those that occur in American football, hockey, soccer, professional wrestling, and physical abuse, can also lead to neurodegenerative changes. These changes often include cerebral atrophy, cavum septi pellucidi with fenestrations, shrinkage of the mammillary bodies, dense tau immunoreactive inclusions (neurofibrillary tangles, glial tangles, and neuropil neurites), and, in some cases, a TDP-43 proteinopathy. In association with these pathologic changes, disordered memory and executive functioning, behavioral and personality disturbances (eg, apathy, depression, irritability, impulsiveness, suicidality), parkinsonism, and, occasionally, motor neuron disease are seen in affected individuals. No formal clinical or pathologic diagnostic criteria for CTE currently exist, but the distinctive neuropathologic profile of the disorder lends promise for future research into its prevention, diagnosis, and treatment.

When to Consider Retiring an Athlete After Sports-Related Concussion

Cara L. Sedney, John Orphanos, and Julian E. Bailes

The pathophysiology of concussion may lead to a variety of both short- and long-term effects, which may lead to a decision to retire from contact sports. These effects follow a recognizable progression and may cause an athlete to opt out of play at any point along this progression. To elucidate the effect of concussion or mild traumatic brain injury and weigh in on a decision to retire, the treating physician needs to take into account the history, neurologic examination, brain imaging, and neuropsychological testing. In addition, myriad social factors surrounding play must be taken into consideration.

Future Advances and Areas of Future Focus in the Treatment of Sport-Related Concussion

Paul McCrory

The occurrence and management of sports concussion provokes more debate and concern than virtually all other sports injuries combined. In the past 3 decades, clinicians have gone from mostly anecdotal strategies to an international consensus–based approach and the early evolution of evidence-based practice. There is increasing engagement by mainstream neuroscientists in this field, which had previously been dominated by sports team physicians. However, the interchange has largely taken place in the media rather than through scientific journals. Legislators have proposed regulatory measures that restrict medical management of concussion in ways that apply to no other medical condition. This paper examines some of the key areas that are likely to be the focus of research in the next few years.

THE CLINICS ARE NOW AVAILABLE ONLINE!

Access your subscription at:
www.theclinics.com

Foreword

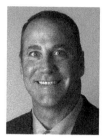

Mark D. Miller, MD
Consulting Editor

I hope this issue is a knockout! We all have seen the recent media frenzy regarding concussions in athletes and are aware of recent "consensus" statements and new evaluation tools that are available; however, much confusion persists regarding the proper management of concussions. Recent recommendations have led to a new policy for football-related concussions in the NCAA. If college football players have any concussion symptoms following an injury, they will be held out for the remainder of the game. There may be some inconsistencies in how this policy is adopted, but it certainly highlights current thinking.

This issue, edited by Drs Meehan and Micheli, is an excellent treatise on concussion. The issue begins with an analysis of the problem—how frequently do concussions occur, and what exactly happens to the brain following a concussion? The editors include recommendations on sideline management of concussion (an ever-changing field), an update on assessment tools and management of concussed athletes, as well as a look into the future. Several special populations are also considered—pediatric athletes, women athletes, and athletes with chronic concussions—as well as concussion-related sequelae.

This complete issue provides solid recommendations for the management of this difficult problem in our athletes. We must always keep in mind, however, that this is an ever-changing field! Knock yourselves out!

Mark D. Miller, MD
Department of Orthopaedic Surgery
University of Virginia
400 Ray C. Hunt Drive, Suite 330
Charlottesville, VA 22908-0159, USA

E-mail address:
mdm3p@virginia.edu

Clin Sports Med 30 (2011) xv
doi:10.1016/j.csm.2010.09.009
0278-5919/11/$ — see front matter © 2011 Elsevier Inc. All rights reserved.

Preface

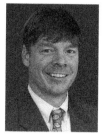 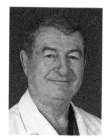

William P. Meehan III, MD   Lyle J. Micheli, MD
Guest Editors

We are privileged and honored to serve as guest editors for this edition of *Clinics in Sports Medicine*, which is entirely devoted to concussion in sports. It is estimated that 1.6-3.8 million sport-related traumatic brain injuries occur each year in the United States. The vast majority of these injuries are concussions.

The assessment and management of sport-related concussions has changed dramatically over the last 20 years. There has been renewed emphasis on this injury, which is reflected in both the amount of medical literature as well as lay media devoted to this topic. Much of this emphasis has been driven by scientific investigations and clinical studies, which have revealed several findings:

1. Concussion results in deficits in neurocognitive functioning
2. Multiple concussions can lead to long-term sequelae
3. Returning to contact or collision sports prior to complete recovery from sport-related concussion can be catastrophic
4. Some athletes will have persistent deficits in neurocognitive function, despite reporting resolution of their post-concussive symptoms.

Despite recent advances in our understanding of the epidemiology, the biomechanics, the pathophysiology, the long-term effects, the associated risks, and the natural history of concussive brain injury, no proven effective therapies or preventative measures exist. It will be the goal of many of us involved in the assessment and management of sport-related concussions to develop effective medical therapies and preventative measures in the future. To that end, this edition of *Clinics in Sports Medicine* will summarize our current understanding of sport-related concussion and review the existing data and medical literature regarding this injury.

We were fortunate to have some of the most highly respected clinicians and investigators contribute to this edition. The authors of this edition of *Clinics in Sports*

Clin Sports Med 30 (2011) xvii–xviii
doi:10.1016/j.csm.2010.09.008
0278-5919/11/$ – see front matter © 2011 Elsevier Inc. All rights reserved.

sportsmed.theclinics.com

Medicine represent both senior leaders in the field as well as some of the brightest young minds. Their names will be familiar to many readers. We are grateful they chose to lend their expertise to this project.

William P. Meehan III, MD
Sports Concussion Clinic
Division of Sports Medicine
Children's Hospital Boston
Harvard Medical School
319 Longwood Avenue
Boston, MA 02115, USA

Lyle J. Micheli, MD
Division of Sports Medicine
Children's Hospital Boston
Harvard Medical School
319 Longwood Avenue
Boston, MA 02115, USA

E-mail addresses:
William.meehan@childrens.harvard.edu (W.P. Meehan)
Lyle.micheli@childrens.harvard.edu (L.J. Micheli)

The Epidemiology of Sport-Related Concussion

Daniel H. Daneshvar, MA[a],*, Christopher J. Nowinski, AB[a,b],
Ann C. McKee, MD[c,d], Robert C. Cantu, MD[a,b,e,f,g,h]

KEYWORDS

- Concussion • Epidemiology • Equipment
- Traumatic brain injury • Sport

Each year, an estimated 44 million children and adolescents participate in organized sports in the United States.[1] In addition, 170 million adults participate in physical activities, including sports.[2] **Table 1** presents the number of high school and collegiate athletes participating in each sport from the 1982 to 1983 season through the 2007 to 2008 season.[3] Many of these activities are associated with an increased risk of traumatic brain injury (TBI).[4] In the United States, an estimated 1.7 million people sustain a TBI annually, associated with 1.365 million emergency room visits and 275,000 hospitalizations annually with associated direct and indirect costs estimated to have been $60 billion in the United States in 2000.[5,6] Additionally, the US Centers for Disease Control and Prevention (CDC) estimates that 1.6 to 3.8 million concussions

---

This work was supported by the Boston University Alzheimer's Disease Center NIA P30 AG13846, supplement 0572063345–5, the National Operating Committee on Standards for Athletic Equipment, the National Collegiate Athletic Association, the National Federation of State High School Associations, the American Football Coaches Association, and the Sports Legacy Institute.
The authors have nothing to disclose.

[a] Center for the Study of Traumatic Encephalopathy, Department of Neurology, Boston University School of Medicine, 72 East Concord Street, B7800, Boston, MA 02118, USA
[b] Sports Legacy Institute, Waltham, MA, USA
[c] Department of Neuropathology, Bedford Veterans Affairs Medical Center, 200 Springs Road, 182-B, Bedford, MA 01730, USA
[d] Departments of Neurology and Pathology, Boston University School of Medicine, Boston, MA, USA
[e] Department of Neurosurgery, Boston University School of Medicine, Boston, MA, USA
[f] Department of Neurosurgery, Emerson Hospital, John Cuming Building, Suite 820, 131 ORNAC, Concord, MA 01742, USA
[g] Department of Surgery, Emerson Hospital, John Cuming Building, Suite 820, 131 ORNAC, Concord, MA 01742, USA
[h] Neurologic Sports Injury Center, Department of Neurosurgery, Brigham and Women's Hospital, Boston, MA, USA
* Corresponding author.
E-mail address: ddanesh@bu.edu

Clin Sports Med 30 (2011) 1–17
doi:10.1016/j.csm.2010.08.006
0278-5919/11/$ – see front matter © 2011 Elsevier Inc. All rights reserved.

Table 1
Athletic participation figures by gender for 1982 to 1983 through 2007 to 2008

	High School		College	
	Men	Women	Men	Women
Baseball	10,916,754	23,517	616,947	0
Basketball	13,796,973	11,041,039	374,600	328,237
Cross country	4,546,218	3,486,467	275,202	235,937
Equestrian	621 (2004–2007)	4322 (2004–2007)	1268 (2003–2007)	6245 (2003–2007)
Field hockey	2781	1,431,676	0	145,133
American football	35,623,701	17,872	1,929,069	0
Golf	480,989 (2005–2008)	199,721 (2005–2008)	24,844 (2005–2008)	12,197 (2005–2008)
Gymnastics	98,169	637,467	15,298	38,775
Ice hockey	722,874	72,537	99,626	17,309
Lacrosse	858,712	589,973	151,309	106,153
Rowing	16,147 (2001–2007)	17,111 (2001–2007)	14,107 (2001–2007)	47,310 (2001–2007)
Skiing	154,979 (1994–2007)	131,660 (1994–2007)	16,923	15,052
Soccer	7,175,341	5,184,875	429,603	321,982
Softball	29,743	8,141,872	0	322,777
Swimming	2,242,814	2,919,225	203,271	231,394
Tennis	3,677,132	3,832,588	199,274	203,695
Track	13,266,497	10,747,774	933,764	728,059
Volleyball	536,747 (1994–2007)	5,364,475 (1994–2007)	15,391 (1994–2007)	182,530 (1994–2007)
Water polo	220,778	189,126	25,543	10,266 (1998–2006)
Wrestling	6,235,016	46,361	175,353	0
Total	100,602,986	54,067,623	5,501,432	2,953,051

Data from Mueller FO, Cantu RC. Catastrophic sport injury research 26th annual report: fall 1982–spring 2008. National Center for Catastrophic Injury Research. Chapel Hill (NC): Spring; 2008. Available at: http://www.unc.edu/depts/nccsi/AllSport.pdf. Accessed August 12, 2010.

occur in sports and recreational activities annually.[7] However, these figures vastly underestimate total TBI burden, because many individuals suffering from mild or moderate TBI do not seek medical advice.[5,7]

A concussion is a TBI induced by an impulsive force transmitted to the head resulting from a direct or indirect impact to the head, face, neck, or elsewhere.[8] These concussions may present with a wide range of clinical signs and symptoms, including physical signs (eg, loss of consciousness, amnesia), behavioral changes (eg, irritability), cognitive impairment (eg, slowed reaction times), sleep disturbances (eg, drowsiness), somatic symptoms (eg, headaches), cognitive symptoms (eg, feeling as if in a fog), or emotional symptoms (eg, emotional lability).[9] Because these impairments in neurologic function often present with a rapid onset and resolve spontaneously, many concussions are neither recognized by athletes nor observed by coaches or athletic trainers.[10–13] As a result, a large proportion of concussions are simply unreported.

This issue is further complicated by the fact that many coaches, athletic trainers, and other sports medicine professionals do not properly use current guidelines for concussion assessment and management.[14,15] To help educate these professionals on proper concussion identification and treatment, the CDC launched the *Heads Up* program, which includes educational materials aimed at youth coaches, high school coaches, parents, athletes, school administrators, and medical professionals. These resources have been shown to improve high school coaches' knowledge regarding how to evaluate and properly manage concussions.[16,17] In part because of awareness measures like these, the number of concussions reported to the National Collegiate Athletic Association (NCAA) through its Injury Surveillance System (ISS) showed an average annual increase of 7.0% from the 1988 to 1989 through the 2003 to 2004 seasons ($P<.01$).[18] **Table 2** displays the concussion rate in each sport from the 2005 to 2006 NCAA ISS database. **Table 3** displays the rate of concussion stratified into high school and collegiate play and compares concussion rate in practice versus competition. Additionally, the concussion rate observed through the ISS doubled from 0.17 per 1000 athlete exposures (A-E; with an exposure defined as one athlete playing in one game or practice) in 1988 to 1989 to 0.34 per 1000 A-Es in 2003 to 2004.[18] This increased rate of concussion may also be caused, in part, by an increase in the true rate of concussion over the past several decades. However, even with new resources, proper identification of concussion remains a problem.[16] Many of these concussions could be prevented outright with proper medical care and safety precautions, such as implementation of safer rules, proper conditioning, and standardized coaching techniques.

SPORT-SPECIFIC FINDINGS
American Football

Participation
Of all sports played in the United States, American football is the sport associated with the greatest number of traumatic brain injuries, but it also has the largest number of participants. As shown in **Table 1**, between the 1982 to 1983 season and the 2007 to 2008 season, a total of 35,641,573 high school athletes and 1,929,069 collegiate athletes competed in football.[3,19] For purposes of this article, an athlete is defined as one player playing one season. Because many high school and college players play multiple years of football, the number of unique participants is much lower. However, that data is not available. Currently, the National Federation of State High School Associations estimates that there are approximately 1,500,000 high school,

Table 2
Frequency and rates of concussion in NCAA from 1988 to 1989 through 2003 to 2004

	Percentage of All Injuries (%)	Injury Rate per 1000 Athletic Exposures	95% Confidence Interval
Men's baseball	2.5	0.07	0.06, 0.08
Men's basketball	3.2	0.16	0.14, 0.17
Women's basketball	4.7	0.22	0.20, 0.17
Women's field hockey	3.9	0.18	0.15, 0.21
Men's football	6.0	0.37	0.36, 0.38
Women's gymnastics	2.3	0.16	0.12, 0.20
Men's ice hockey	7.9	0.41	0.37, 0.44
Women's ice hockey[a]	18.3	0.91	0.71, 1.11
Men's lacrosse	5.6	0.25	0.23, 0.29
Women's lacrosse	6.3	0.25	0.22, 0.28
Men's soccer	3.9	0.28	0.25, 0.30
Women's soccer	5.3	0.41	0.38, 0.44
Women's softball	4.3	0.14	0.12, 0.16
Women's volleyball	2.0	0.09	0.07, 0.10
Men's wrestling	3.3	0.25	0.22, 0.27
Men's spring football	5.6	0.54	0.50, 0.58
Total concussions	5.0	0.28	0.27, 0.28

[a] Data collection for women's ice hockey began in 2000 to 2001.
Data from Hootman JM, Dick R, Agel J. Epidemiology of collegiate injuries for 15 sports: summary and recommendations for injury prevention initiatives. J Athl Train 2007;42(2):311–9.

junior high school, and nonfederation school football participants. The NCAA, the National Association of Intercollegiate Athletics, and the National Junior College Athletic Association estimate that there are currently 75,000 collegiate football participants, including estimates of athletes at schools not associated with any national organization. A total of 225,000 participants are estimated to compete in fully padded, organized, nonprofessional football (sandlot) and professional football. Combined, these figures indicate that approximately 1,800,000 total athletes participated in football in the United States during the 2009 football season.[19]

Injuries
Because of the aforementioned difficulties in examining concussion specifically, total incidence of catastrophic head injuries may be a better comparator for injury trends over time. Catastrophic head injury is defined as a head injury caused by direct contact during competition resulting in a fatal, nonfatal permanent, or serious nonpermanent injury. Since the 1982 to 1983 season, there have been 133 football players with incomplete neurologic recovery from catastrophic head injury. A total of 120 of these injuries occurred in high school athletes, 11 occurred in college participants, 2 occurred in sandlot players, and none occurred in professional football players. In 2009, all 9 cerebral injuries with incomplete recovery were in high school athletes.[20]

Although there have been significant reductions in these injuries following rule changes in the 1970s, the rate of head injuries has been increasing in recent years.

Table 3
Concussion rates in US high school and collegiate athletes in practice and competition, 2005 to 2006

Sport	Division	Rates more than 1000 Athlete Exposures			Overall Rate Comparison Collegiate vs High School		
		Practice	Competition	Overall	Rate Ratio	95% CI	P value
Football	High school	0.21	1.55	0.47	—	—	—
	Collegiate	0.39	3.02	0.61	1.31	1.09, 1.58	<0.01
Men's soccer	High school	0.04	0.59	0.22	—	—	—
	Collegiate	0.24	1.38	0.49	2.26	1.43, 3.57	<0.01
Women's soccer	High school	0.09	0.97	0.36	—	—	—
	Collegiate	0.25	1.80	0.63	1.76	1.21, 2.57	<0.01
Volleyball	High school	0.05	0.05	0.05	—	—	—
	Collegiate	0.21	0.13	0.18	3.63	1.39, 9.44	<0.01
Men's basketball	High school	0.06	0.11	0.07	—	—	—
	Collegiate	0.22	0.45	0.27	3.65	2.01, 6.63	<0.01
Women's basketball	High school	0.06	0.60	0.21	—	—	—
	Collegiate	0.31	0.85	0.43	1.98	1.31, 3.01	<0.01
Wrestling	High school	0.13	0.32	0.18	—	—	—
	Collegiate	0.35	1.00	0.42	2.34	1.26, 4.34	0.01
Baseball	High school	0.03	0.08	0.05	—	—	—
	Collegiate	0.03	0.23	0.09	1.88	0.79, 4.46	0.22
Softball	High school	0.09	0.04	0.07	—	—	—
	Collegiate	0.07	0.37	0.19	2.61	1.17, 5.85	0.03
Men's sport total	High school	0.13	0.61	0.25	—	—	—
	Collegiate	0.30	1.26	0.45	1.78	1.52, 2.08	<0.01
Women's sport total	High school	0.07	0.42	0.18	—	—	—
	Collegiate	0.23	0.74	0.38	2.04	1.59, 2.64	<0.01
Overall total	High school	0.11	0.53	0.23	—	—	—
	Collegiate	0.28	1.02	0.43	1.86	1.63, 2.12	<0.01

Collegiate data provided by the National Collegiate Athletic Association Injury Surveillance System.
High School data provided by the High School Sports-Related Injury Surveillance System.
Abbreviation: CI, confidence interval.
Data from Gessel LM, Fields SK, Collins CL, et al. Concussions among United States high school and collegiate athletes. J Athl Train 2007;42(4):495–503.

Over the 10-year span from 2000 to 2009, there was an average of 6.2 cerebral injuries annually with incomplete recovery in football. The prior 10 years averaged 4.5 cerebral injuries annually. The 10 cerebral injuries in 2008 and 9 in 2006 and 2009 were the highest incidences since 1984.[20]

Because concussion awareness and diagnosis has changed significantly over the past few decades, there is wide variability in the literature on the rate of concussion in football athletes. One study evaluating concussions reported to medical professionals over a 3-season span from 1995 to 1997 found that high school football players had a rate of 3.66 concussions per 100 player seasons, meaning that there were 3.66 concussions every season for every 100 athletes.[21] However, a postseason retrospective survey of 233 football players after the 1996 to 1997 season found that 110 (47.2%) reported having experienced at least 1 concussion. Multiple concussions were noted in 81 (34.9%) of the athletes.[22] Additionally, the NCAA ISS found a concussion rate of 0.37 per 1000 A-E (95% confidence interval [CI] = 0.36, 0.38) from the 1988 to 1989 season through the 2003 to 2004 season.[18] Recent studies indicate even higher rates of reported concussions in football players. In one study, examining the concussions reported by 425 athletic trainers from 100 US high schools and 180 US colleges, the rates of concussion were compared between high school and collegiate athletes. The high school athletic trainers reported 201 concussions over the 2005 to 2006 season, which yielded a concussion rate of 0.21 per 1000 A-E in practice and 1.55 concussions per 1000 A-E in competitions. Together, these rates averaged 0.47 per 1000 A-E overall. As expected, each game carries a statistically significant increased risk of concussion with an injury proportion ratio (PR) of 1.39 (95% CI = 1.01, 1.91). A total of 245 concussions were reported in the collegiate athletes, resulting in a concussion injury rate of 0.39 per 1000 A-E in practice, and a rate of 3.02 concussions per 1000 A-E in competitions (resulting in an overall rate of 0.61 per 1000 A-E).[23] These results indicate a statistically significant increase in the rate of diagnosed concussions between high school and collegiate athletes. Because college athletes tend to have greater access to and more interaction with medical professionals, the increase may be because of medical infrastructure rather than differences in the number of actual concussions sustained.

The same study evaluated the types of collisions that resulted in concussions and found that tackling and being tackled were responsible for 67.6% of the concussions observed in these football players.[23] Concussive impacts may produce different signs based on the age of the athlete. Although the high school and college groups did not differ in presentation of symptoms, such as confusion or retrograde amnesia, college athletes did experience a high rate of loss of consciousness (34%) compared with the high school athletes (11%). Despite this lower rate of loss of consciousness, studies have shown that high school athletes who have experienced a concussion show worse recovery, in the form of prolonged memory dysfunction, as compared with concussed collegiate athletes. College athletes, despite having more concussions throughout the season, typically recover and match control subjects by day 3 following the concussive blow. However, the high school athletes continue to perform significantly worse than control subjects for up to 7 days following the injury (F = 2.90; $P<.005$).[12] This age-based disparity in performance on neuropsychological testing is not correlated with self-report of postconcussion symptoms.[12]

Of note is the fact that high school athletes appear to recover more poorly as compared with collegiate athletes, despite the latter typically incurring more acutely severe injuries as a result of being bigger, faster, and stronger. There are several possible explanations for this disparity between high school and collegiate football players: the brain may not yet be fully developed, resulting in a lower injury threshold; the blood vessels may tear more easily in the less developed brain; the skull is thinner, which could provide less protection to the brain; there may be fewer medical staff members available at high school games; or poor body control and technique might make younger players more susceptible to brain injury following a poorly executed tackle.[24] In fact, one explanation may be that for various reasons, including having weaker necks, high school football players were found to sustain more absolute force to brain per hit while playing football that college athletes.[25] However, football players who have a history of previous concussions are at a greatly increased risk of experiencing future concussions as compared with athletes without a history of such impacts.[26]

Baseball/Softball

Participation

Between the fall of 1982 and the spring of 2008, 10,916,754 high school men and 23,517 high school women competed in baseball. An additional 616,947 men competed at the collegiate level.[3] Approximately 419,000 men and 900 women compete in baseball at the high school level annually.[4]

A similar number of athletes competed in softball. Between the 1982 to 1983 season and the 2007 to 2008 season, approximately 30,000 men and 8.1 million women competed in high school softball, and an additional 323,000 women competed at the collegiate level.[3] Annually, approximately 313,000 female and 1,100 male softball players compete at the high school level.[4]

Injuries

As previously addressed, early reports of concussion incidence were complicated because of underdiagnosis by trainers, coaches, and medical professionals. From 1995 to 1997, 246 certified athletic trainers reported a rate of 0.23 concussions per 100 player seasons in high school baseball players, meaning that there were 0.23 concussions every season for every 100 athletes.[21] A 15-year survey of the NCAA ISS from the 1988 to 1989 academic year through 2003 to 2004 academic year found that the rate of concussion was 0.07 per 1000 A-E (95% CI = 0.06, 0.08).[18] An analysis of both high school and collegiate athletes during the 2005 to 2006 season, which stratified rates of injury by practice and competitive play, found that high school baseball players had a rate of concussion of 0.03 per 1000 A-E in practice and 0.08 per 1000 A-E in games (0.05 overall). This study reported similar findings to the NCAA ISS, with collegiate athletes experiencing 0.03 concussions per 1000 A-E in practice and 0.23 per 1000 A-E in games (0.09 overall).[23] Concussions account for 2.9% of all injuries that occur in practice and 4.2% of all injuries occurring in games (injury PR = 3.8, $P<.01$).[27]

In softball, from the same group of athletic trainers studied from 1995 to 1997, a rate of 0.46 concussions per 100 player seasons was reported.[21] A more recent study analyzing high school softball athletes over the 2005 to 2006 season found a concussion rate of 0.09 injuries per 1000 A-E during practice and 0.04 injuries per 1000 A-E during games (overall 0.07 concussions per 1000 A-E).[23] This high school concussion rate is slightly less than that observed in college. The NCAA ISS survey reported a concussion rate of 0.14 per 1000 A-E (95% CI = 0.12, 0.16) in collegiate athletes between the 1988 to 1989 season and the 2003 to 2004 season.[18] Furthermore, over the 2005 to 2006 season, collegiate athletes experienced a rate of 0.07 concussions per 1000 A-E in practices, and 0.37 concussions per 1000 A-E in games (overall = 0.19).[23] Concussions occurring in practice accounted for 4.1% of all softball injuries; whereas, concussions in games constituted 6.4% of all softball injuries (injury PR = 2.5, $P<.01$).[27]

Although differing in form, softball and baseball are related sports with similar methods of play. As such, a recent study comparing softball athletes to baseball athletes in high school found that players in both sports experienced similar rates of concussion (0.07 concussions and 0.05 concussions per 1000 A-Es, respectively; relative risk [RR] = 1.48; 95% CI = 0.60, 3.63; P = .53). However, concussions represented a significantly greater proportion of total injuries in softball players than in baseball players (5.5% and 2.9%, respectively; injury PR = 1.91; 95% CI = 1.81, 2.01; P<.01). Additionally, the concussive injury in baseball players was more typically caused by contact with the ball than in softball players (91.4% and 59.1%, respectively; injury PR = 1.55; 95% CI = 1.50, 1.59; P<.01). Therefore, as expected, concussions in baseball players were more associated with being hit by a pitch than in softball players (50.6% and 6.9%, respectively; injury PR = 7.32; 95% CI = 6.44, 8.32; P<.01).[23]

These differences in mechanism of injury manifest in differing rates of recovery between the two sports. By 6 days after injury, symptoms were resolved in slightly more of the softball players than the baseball players (68.8% and 64.2%, respectively; injury PR = 1.07; 95% CI = 1.03, 1.11; P<.01). Despite this delayed course of symptom resolution, a greater proportion of baseball players versus softball players returned to play within 6 days (52.9% and 15.5%, respectively; injury PR = 3.42; 95% CI = 3.13, 3.73; P<.01).[23]

Basketball

Participation
One of the most popular sports across both genders, basketball was played by approximately 13.8 million high school men and 11 million high school women between the fall of 1982 and the spring of 2008.[3] An additional 375,000 men and 328,00 women competed in college.[3]

Injuries
In a survey of high school athletic trainers evaluating athletes over the 1995 to 1997 seasons, men experienced a rate of 0.75 concussions per 100 player seasons. This rate was slightly less than the rate of 1.04 concussions per 100 player seasons experienced by women.[21] In college athletes, a 15-year analysis of the NCAA ISS found that men had a rate of 0.16 concussions per 1000 A-E (95% CI = 0.14, 0.17) as compared with a rate of 0.22 concussions per 1000 A-E in women (95% CI = 0.20, 0.24).[18] An analysis over the 2005 to 2006 season in high school showed a similar relationship between male and female basketball players, with men experiencing a lower concussion rate than women (0.07 and 0.21 concussions per 1000 A-Es, respectively; RR = 2.93; 95% CI = 1.64, 5.24; P<.01). This difference was largely accounted for by concussions during competition. Men and women both had a rate of 0.06 concussions per 1000 A-E in practice; whereas, women had a rate of 0.60 concussions per 1000 A-E in games as compared with 0.11 in men. In college basketball, men experienced fewer concussions in both practices (0.22 versus 0.31 concussions per 1000 A-E) and games (0.45 versus 0.85 concussions per 1000 A-E).[23]

Concussions represented a greater proportion of the total injuries experienced by women as compared with men (11.7% and 3.8%, respectively; injury PR = 3.09; 95% CI = 2.98, 3.20; P<.01).[23] In men's high school basketball, concussions accounted for 4.1% of all the injuries sustained during practices and 5.0% of those sustained during games; this difference was not significant.[27] Women, however, experienced 3.4 times the risk of suffering a concussion during a game versus practice, with concussions accounting for 4.7% of all injuries during practice and 8.5% during games.[27] This relationship between practice and games was confirmed in another study, indicating that women have a significant increase in risk at games (injury PR = 5.82; 95% CI = 2.06, 16.49), but men had no significant difference.[28]

While playing basketball, concussions are associated with different activities in men than in women. Women receive a greater proportion of their concussions while ball handling/dribbling (19.0% versus 10.4%; injury PR = 1.83; 95% CI = 1.65, 2.02; P = .01) and while defending (22.2% versus 13.4%; injury PR = 1.66; 95% CI = 1.52, 1.81; P<.01). Men, on the other hand, experience a greater proportion of their concussions chasing loose balls (26.0% versus 10.6%; injury PR = 2.46; 95% CI = 2.28, 2.64; P<.01) and rebounding (30.5% versus 16.6%; injury PR = 1.83; 95% CI = 1.72, 1.95; P<.01). A higher proportion of men than women experienced a concussion from collision with the playing surface (34.0% and 22.0%, respectively; injury PR = 1.54; 95% CI = 1.46, 1.63; P<.01). Some women, but no men, reported a concussion caused by contact with the ball (6.0%).[23]

Male and female basketball players also have differing rates of symptom resolution and return to play. Two days after concussion, significantly more men returned to play than women (39% and 15%, respectively; injury PR = 38.21; 95% CI = 30.44, 47.96; P<.01).[23]

Cheerleading

Participation
The number of athletes participating in cheerleading is increasing as the sport becomes more popular. Annually, there are currently an estimated 3.5 million cheerleading participants who are at least 6 years of age. Based on these estimates, the number of cheerleading participants in the United States has increased 18% since 1990.[29]

Injuries
In addition to becoming increasingly popular, cheerleading has become increasingly associated with risk for catastrophic head and spine injury, especially for the flier.[3] In the past 30 years, cheerleading has transitioned from principally using toe-touch jumps, splits, and claps, to increasingly incorporating routines, such as gymnastic tumbling runs, human pyramids, lifts, catches, and tosses.[30] These moves are associated with increasing risk for injury. The Consumer Product Safety Commission (CPSC) reported that cheerleading injuries had resulted in an estimated 4954 hospital emergency room visits in 1980. This number rose to 21,906 by 1999 and reached 28,414 in 2004. In 2007, the numbers decreased slightly to 26,786, but remained 5 times higher than the number of emergency room visits 27 years earlier.[4,31,32] Many of these injuries are to the head and neck. Many result in concussions.[4]

A study looking at all injuries in North Carolina high school competitive cheerleaders from 1996 to 1999 found that 6.3% of all injuries were concussions.[33] In 2006, head injuries were associated with 1070 concussions. In 2007, head injuries were associated with 783 concussions.[4] A 1-year study of 143 cheerleading teams from 2006 to 2007 found that the majority of concussions and closed head injuries occurred in practices rather than athletic events (82% and 18%, respectively). Additionally, college cheerleaders were significantly more likely to experience a concussion or closed head injury than were cheerleaders of different levels (P = .02; odds ratio [OR] = 3.10; 95% CI = 1.20, 8.06).[34]

Gymnastics

Participation
From the fall of 1982 through spring 2008, nearly 100,000 men and 640,000 women competed in high school gymnastics. An additional 15,000 men and 40,000 women

competed collegiately.[3] Approximately 3800 men and 24,500 women participate in gymnastics annually.[4]

Injuries
A study of high school gymnasts from 1990 to 2005 found an incidence of concussion and closed head injury of 1.7%. These concussions and closed head injuries were more likely to occur while individuals were performing headstands than among individuals performing other skills (RR = 7.14; 95% CI = 3.15–16.19; $P<.002$). As the age of the athlete increased, the frequency of concussions and closed head injuries decreased.[35] From the 1988 to 1989 season through the 2003 to 2004 season, the rate of concussions reported to the ISS was 0.16 per 1000 A-E (95% CI = 0.12, 0.20).[18]

Ice/Field Hockey

Participation
Total concussions in ice hockey athletes are low because of lower participation in ice hockey at the high school and collegiate level. Approximately 723,000 men and 72,500 women competed in high school ice hockey between the fall of 1982 and the spring of 2008. Approximately 100,000 additional men and 17,000 additional women competed in college.[3] An average of approximately 27,800 men and 2800 women play ice hockey each year.[4] Field hockey is also associated with few total concussions, again because of lower athletic participation. Between the fall of 1982 and the spring of 2008, approximately 3000 men and 1.43 million women competed in high school field hockey; whereas, 145,000 additional women competed collegiately.[3]

Injuries
Both forms of hockey are associated with a high rate of concussions, considering their comparatively lower participation rate. According to the information reported to the ISS from 1988 through 2004, the rate of concussions in male collegiate athletes was 0.41 per 1000 A-E (95% CI = 0.37, 0.44), compared with 0.91 per 1000 A-E in female collegiate athletes (95% CI = 0.71, 1.11).[18] Concussions in hockey players account for 6.3% of practice injuries and 10.3% of game injuries (injury PR = 15.5; $P<.01$).[27] Although the relationship between age and concussion in hockey players remains unclear, recent evidence in youth hockey players indicates that players in Bantam (aged 13–14 years) and Pee Wee (aged 11–12 years) had a higher risk of concussion (RR = 4.04 and 3.14, respectively) when compared with players in Atom (aged 9–10 years).[36,37] There is also a question as to what extent league rules, such as body checking, are associated with concussion. A meta-analysis of 4 studies evaluating the effect of body-checking rules found that body checking in a league is associated with an increased risk of concussions (OR =1.71; 95% CI = 1.2, 2.44).[36–39]

Although there are some similarities between ice and field hockey, the proportion of concussions was higher in ice hockey players (3.9%) than in field hockey players (1.4%) (injury PR = 2.75; 95% CI = 1.17, 6.46).[40] In a survey of athletic trainers from 1995 to 1997, concussions in high school field hockey were reported at a rate of 0.46 per 100 player seasons.[21] In college, the NCAA ISS reported that female field hockey athletes had a rate of 0.18 concussions per 1000 A-E (95% CI = 0.15, 0.21) from the 1988 to 1989 season through the 2003 to 2004 season.[18] Concussions accounted for a higher proportion of all injuries in games as compared with those in practices (7.2% and 3.7%, respectively; RR 6.4).[27]

Lacrosse

Participation
From the fall of 1982 through the spring of 2008, approximately 860,000 men and 587,000 women played high school lacrosse, with an additional 151,000 men and

106,000 women competing at the college level.[3] High school lacrosse has approximately 33,000 male and 22,000 female participants each year. College participation figures reveal that there are approximately 5819 men and 4000 women lacrosse players each year.[4]

Injuries

Although lacrosse is not associated with a large number of total concussions, the rate of concussion is high when compared with other sports. The rate of concussion in collegiate athletes reported to the NCAA ISS was 0.26 per 1000 A-E in men (95% CI = 0.23, 0.39) and 0.25 per 1000 A-E in women (95% CI = 0.22, 0.28) from the 1988 to 1989 season through the 2003 to 2004 season.[18] Concussions accounted for 8.6% of all injuries in lacrosse competitions, with athletes 9 times more likely to experience a concussion in a game as compared with practice (1.08 versus 0.12 injuries per 1000 A-E; injury PR = 9.0; 95% CI = 7.1, 11.5). 78.4% of concussions resulted from a collision with another person; whereas, 10.4% resulted from collision with a stick.[41] Another study stratified concussion rate by gender and confirmed that games are associated with significantly more concussions than practice in both genders (injury PR = 13.32 in men and 6.3 in women; $P<.01$).[27] Concussions accounted for 9.8% of all female injuries, and women had approximately 5 times the rate of concussion during games as compared with practices (0.70 and 0.15 injuries per 1000 A-E, respectively; injury PR = 4.6; 95% CI = 3.5, 6.0). More than half the time, the concussions in female lacrosse players resulted from contact with a stick.[42]

Although the rate of concussions has increased dramatically in many sports, some have argued that this observation in men's lacrosse may be, in part, explained by the introduction of a new helmet. One study compared the rate of concussion in the years immediately following the helmet's introduction (1996–1997 to 2003–2004) to the preceding years (1988–1989 to 1995–1996). In practices, the rate increased by 0.14 concussions per 1000 A-E (95% CI = 0.09, 0.19; $P<.01$). In games, the rate increased by 0.84 (95% CI = 0.52, 1.16; $P<.01$).[41] However, this increase is certainly caused, in part, by improved detection and diagnosis of concussion during that time frame.

Soccer

Participation

In the United States, soccer is growing in popularity. Between 1982 and 2008, approximately 7.2 million men and 5.2 million women played soccer at the high school level. An additional 430,000 men and 322,000 women competed in college.[3]

Injuries

In a study of athletic trainers from 1995 to 1997, the rate of concussions in male soccer players was found to be 0.92 injuries per 100 player seasons.[21] According to data reported to the NCAA ISS, men in college had a rate of 0.28 concussions per 1000 A-E (95% CI = 0.25, 0.30) over the time period from the 1988 to 1989 season through the 2003 to 2004 season.[18] One study examining the 2005 to 2006 season found that high school men experienced a rate of 0.04 concussions per 1000 A-E in practice and 0.59 concussions per 1000 A-E in games (0.22 concussions per 1000 A-E overall). It was reported that college soccer players experienced 0.24 concussions per 1000 A-E in practice and 1.38 concussions per 1000 A-E in games (0.49 concussions per 1000 A-E overall).[23] Significantly more concussions occurred in games than in practice (injury PR = 6.94; 95% CI = 2.01, 23.95).[28]

Concussions in male soccer players typically occur as a result of head to head collisions in the act of heading the ball (40.5%). As expected, concussions were responsible for 64.1% of injuries that occurred while heading the ball. Another common cause of concussions in soccer players was contact with another person (85.3%). Goalies were significantly more likely to experience a concussion; 21.7% of all injuries to goalkeepers were concussions as compared with 11.1% of all injuries to other players (injury PR = 1.96; 95% CI = 1.92, 2.00; P<.01).[23]

In the aforementioned study of athletic trainers from 1995 to 1997, the rate of concussions in women was 1.14 injuries per 100 player seasons.[21] According to data from the NCAA ISS, women in college had a rate of 0.41 concussions per 1000 A-E (95% CI = 0.38, 0.44) from the 1988 to 1989 season through the 2003 to 2004 season.[18] In the previously mentioned study of the 2005 to 2006 season, high school women were shown to have a rate of 0.09 concussions per 1000 A-E in practice and 0.97 concussions per 1000 A-E in games (0.36 concussions per 1000 A-E overall). In college, female soccer players experienced 0.25 concussions per 1000 A-E in practice and 2.80 concussions per 1000 A-E in games (0.63 concussions per 1000 A-E overall).[23] Concussions accounted for 11.4% of the injuries experienced by women during games and 2.4% of all the injuries experienced during practice.[27] Like men, women were significantly more likely to experience concussions in games as opposed to practice (injury PR = 16.7; P<.01).[28]

As with men, concussions in female soccer players typically occur as a result of head-to-head collisions while heading the ball (36.7%). Women experienced fewer concussions as a result of contact with another person (58.3%; injury PR = 1.46; 95% CI = 1.45, 1.48; P<.01). On the other hand, women experienced more concussions than men as a result of contact with the ground (22.6% and 6.0%, respectively; injury PR = 3.77; 95% CI = 3.56, 4.00; P<.01) and contact with the soccer ball (18.3% and 8.2%, respectively; injury PR = 3.68; 95% CI = 3.45, 3.92; P<.01).[23]

There appear to be differences in the rate of recovery from concussion between high school and collegiate athletes. College athletes, despite experiencing a higher rate of loss of consciousness, recovered by the third day after sustaining a concussion. An athlete's self-report of postconcussion symptoms may not be associated with return to baseline performance on neuropsychologic testing, as most high school athletes reported recovery by the fifth day after sustaining a concussion, but experienced neuropsychological deficits 7 days following the injury.[12]

Skiing/Snowboarding

Participation
Between 1994 and 2007, approximately 155,000 men and 132,000 women participated in organized skiing in high school. An additional 17,000 men and 15,000 women skied in college during that time.[3] Annually, approximately 580 women participate in college skiing.[4] However, the majority of skiers and snowboarders are taking part recreationally, not as part of an organized sport.

Injuries
An estimated 15% to 20% of the approximately 600,000 annually reported skiing and snowboarding injuries are head injuries.[43] Most of these head injuries occurred early in the season and were mild TBI (69.4%) as opposed to severe TBI, based on the Glascow Coma Scale.[44] Concussions represent 9.6% of all injuries in skiers, 14.7% of all injuries in snowboarders, and 5.7% of all injuries in snowbladers.[45] A comparison of skiers and snowboarders found that both have similar rates of head injury (0.005 and 0.004 per 1000 participants, respectively), but skiers had a greater proportion of concussions (60% versus 21%); whereas, snowboarders had a much higher proportion of severe brain injuries (29% versus 15%).[46]

Additionally, there is evidence that more male than female skiers tend to be injured as a result of collisions with trees; whereas, more female than male skiers tend to be injured as a result of collisions with other skiers.[44,45] Male skiers are more likely to sustain a head injury than female skiers (OR = 2.23).[44,45]

Volleyball

Participation
Between 1994 and 2007, approximately 540,000 men and 5.4 million women played volleyball in high school, with another 15,000 men and 182,500 women playing volleyball in college.[3]

Injuries
A study of athletic trainers from 1995 to 1997 found that high school volleyball players had a concussion rate of 0.14 injuries per 100 player seasons.[21] Data reported to the NCAA ISS found that college volleyball athletes had a concussion rate of 0.09 per 1000 A-E (95% CI = 0.07, 0.10) from the 1988 to 1989 season through the 2003 to 2004 season.[18] One study reported that concussions account for 1.3% of all injuries reported in volleyball players during practices and 4.1% of those reported during games. In the same study, volleyball athletes were at a 3.8 times greater risk of sustaining a concussion during a game than a practice session.[27]

Wrestling

Participation
Like hockey, wrestling has low participation in comparison to the number of concussions sustained by wrestlers. Approximately 6.2 million men and 46,000 women wrestled in high school, and 175,000 additional men in college, from the fall of 1982 through the spring of 2008.[3] Annually, there is an average of approximately 239,000 male and 1700 female high school wrestlers, and 6700 male college wrestlers.[4]

Injuries
High school wrestlers accounted for the greatest number of direct injuries in all winter sports.[4] High school athletic trainers, from 1995 to 1997, reported a concussion rate of 1.58 injuries per 100 player seasons.[21] A study of high school athletic trainers from the 2005 to 2006 season found that concussions occurred at a rate of 0.13 concussions per 1000 A-E in practice, as compared with 0.32 per 1000 A-E concussions in games (0.18 per 1000 A-E overall).[23] The NCAA ISS determined that college wrestlers experienced 0.25 concussions per 1000 A-E (95% CI = 0.22, 0.27) from 1988 to 1989 through the 2003 to 2004.[18] In 2005 to 2006, collegiate data was further analyzed and wrestlers were found to have experienced 0.35 concussion per 1000 A-E in practice and 1.00 concussions per 1000 A-E in games (0.42 concussions per 1000 A-E, overall).[23] Concussions accounted for 6.6% of all injuries that occurred during matches and 4.5% of those injuries that were reported during practice.[27]

In wrestling, takedowns were the most common cause of concussions (42.6%) and were more likely to lead to a concussion than other wrestling maneuvers (7.6% versus 4.5%; injury PR = 1.69; 95% CI = 1.61, 1.78; $P<.01$). The majority of these concussions occurred as result of contact with another person (60.1%); whereas, the remainder occurred as a result of contact with the ground (26.9%).[23]

DISCUSSION

The rate of concussion has been increasing steadily over the past two decades. This trend is likely caused by improvement in the detection of concussion, but may also reflect an increase in the true number of concussive impacts occurring. As athletes get bigger, stronger, and faster, it is logical that the forces associated with their collisions would also increase in magnitude. It is important to realize that there is currently no effective headgear that prevents concussions; therefore, as the number of forceful collisions increase, the number of concussions would be expected to increase.

In general, athletes tend to have a higher risk of concussion in competition as compared with practice. However, given the higher frequency of practices compared with games, and the resulting total number of concussions occurring in practice, one way to quickly and drastically reduce a sport's concussion risk would be to limit unnecessary contact in practice. The majority of concussions in high school athletes resulted from participation in football, followed by women's soccer, men's soccer, and women's basketball.

Within a given sport, females tend to report higher rates of concussion than males. Within comparable sports, evidence indicates that female athletes may be at a greater risk of concussions than male athletes.[47] The evidence also indicates that, in general, concussions result in cognitive impairment in females more frequently than in males.[48] These variations may be caused by biomechanical differences, such as differences in body mass, head mass, or neck strength. They may also be explained by cultural differences, such as reluctance among males to report injury, and physiologic differences, including hormones.

In general, there are simple things that can be done to reduce the incidence of concussion in sports. Preparticipation examinations should be mandatory. If a physician or coach has questions about an athlete's readiness to compete, the athlete's safety should not be risked. At this session, or at a stand-alone meeting, concussion education should be afforded to all athletes, especially for those competing in a collision or contact sport. Proper strength and conditioning, especially focused on strengthening the muscles of the neck, is a suitable way to limit the forces experienced by the head. Properly trained coaches, athletic trainers, and medical staff are on the front line in concussion education, diagnosis, and management, and are crucial to reducing the incidence and severity of concussions. Finally, quality officiating can help to identify potentially dangerous situations and ensure the activity does not result in injury.

SUMMARY

Concussions and head injuries may never be completely eliminated from sports. However, with better data comes an improved understanding of the types of actions and activities that typically result in concussions. With this knowledge can come improved techniques and rule changes to minimize the rate and severity of concussions in sports. This article identifies the factors that affect concussion rate.

REFERENCES

1. Report on trends and participation in youth sports. Stuart (FL): National Council Of Youth Sports; 2001. Available at: http://www.ncys.org/publications/2008-sports-participation-study.php. Accessed August 12, 2010.
2. National Center for Chronic Disease Prevention & Health Promotion. Behavioral risk factor surveillance system: exercise. CDC; 2006.
3. Cantu RC, Mueller FO. The prevention of catastrophic head and spine injuries in high school and college sports. Br J Sports Med 2009;43(13):981–6.
4. Mueller FO, Cantu RC. Catastrophic sport injury research 26th annual report: fall 1982-Spring 2008. National Center for Catastrophic Injury Research. Chapel Hill

(NC): Spring; 2008. Available at: http://www.unc.edu/depts/nccsi/AllSport.pdf. Accessed August 12, 2010.

5. Faul M, Xu L, Wald MM, et al. Traumatic brain injury in the United States: emergency department visits, hospitalizations and deaths 2002–2006. Atlanta (GA): Centers for Disease Control and Prevention, National Center for Injury Prevention and Control; 2010.

6. Finkelstein E, Corso P, Miller T. The incidence and economic burden of injuries in the United States. New York: Oxford University Press; 2006.

7. Langlois JA, Rutland-Brown W, Wald MM. The epidemiology and impact of traumatic brain injury: a brief overview. J Head Trauma Rehabil 2006;21(5): 375–8.

8. Concussion (mild traumatic brain injury) and the team physician: a consensus statement. Med Sci Sports Exerc 2006;38(2):395–9.

9. McCrory P, Meeuwisse W, Johnston K, et al. Consensus statement on concussion in sport–the 3rd international conference on concussion in sport, held in Zurich, November 2008. J Clin Neurosci 2009;16(6):755–63.

10. Valovich McLeod TC, Bay RC, Heil J, et al. Identification of sport and recreational activity concussion history through the preparticipation screening and a symptom survey in young athletes. Clin J Sport Med 2008;18(3):235–40.

11. Delaney JS, Lacroix VJ, Leclerc S, et al. Concussions among university football and soccer players. Clin J Sport Med 2002;12(6):331–8.

12. Field M, Collins MW, Lovell MR, et al. Does age play a role in recovery from sports-related concussion? A comparison of high school and collegiate athletes. J Pediatr 2003;142(5):546–53.

13. Cusimano MD. Canadian minor hockey participants' knowledge about concussion. Can J Neurol Sci 2009;36(3):315–20.

14. Notebaert AJ, Guskiewicz KM. Current trends in athletic training practice for concussion assessment and management. J Athl Train 2005;40(4):320–5.

15. Covassin T, Elbin R 3rd, Stiller-Ostrowski JL. Current sport-related concussion teaching and clinical practices of sports medicine professionals. J Athl Train 2009;44(4):400–4.

16. Sarmiento K, Mitchko J, Klein C, et al. Evaluation of the centers for disease control and prevention's concussion initiative for high school coaches: "Heads Up: concussion in high school sports". J Sch Health 2010;80(3):112–8.

17. Sawyer RJ, Hamdallah M, White D, et al. High school coaches' assessments, intentions to use, and use of a concussion prevention toolkit: centers for disease control and prevention's heads up: concussion in high school sports. Health Promot Pract 2010;11(1):34–43.

18. Hootman JM, Dick R, Agel J. Epidemiology of collegiate injuries for 15 sports: summary and recommendations for injury prevention initiatives. J Athl Train 2007;42(2):311–9.

19. Mueller FO, Colgate B. Annual survey of football Injury research. Chapel Hill (NC): National Center for Catastrophic Injury Research; 2010. Available at: http://www. unc.edu/depts/nccsi/. Accessed August 12, 2010.

20. Mueller FO, Cantu RC. Catastrophic football injuries annual report. Chapel Hill (NC): National Center for Catastrophic Injury Research; 2009. Available at: http://www.unc.edu/depts/nccsi/. Accessed August 12, 2010.

21. Powell JW, Barber-Foss KD. Traumatic brain injury in high school athletes. JAMA 1999;282(10):958–63.

22. Langburt W, Cohen B, Akhthar N, et al. Incidence of concussion in high school football players of Ohio and Pennsylvania. J Child Neurol 2001;16(2):83–5.

23. Gessel LM, Fields SK, Collins CL, et al. Concussions among United States high school and collegiate athletes. J Athl Train 2007;42(4):495–503.

24. Boden BP, Tacchetti RL, Cantu RC, et al. Catastrophic head injuries in high school and college football players. Am J Sports Med 2007;35(7):1075–81.

25. Broglio SP, Sosnoff JJ, Shin S, et al. Head impacts during high school football: a biomechanical assessment. J Athl Train 2009;44(4):342–9.

26. Guskiewicz KM, McCrea M, Marshall SW, et al. Cumulative effects associated with recurrent concussion in collegiate football players: the NCAA Concussion Study. JAMA 2003;290(19):2549–55.

27. Covassin T, Swanik CB, Sachs ML. Epidemiological considerations of concussions among intercollegiate athletes. Appl Neuropsychol 2003;10(1):12–22.

28. Rechel JA, Yard EE, Comstock RD. An epidemiologic comparison of high school sports injuries sustained in practice and competition. J Athl Train 2008;43(2): 197–204.

29. Mueller FO, Cantu RC. Catastrophic sport injury research 26th annual report: fall 1982–Spring 2003: National center for catastrophic injury research. Chapel Hill (NC): Spring; 2003.

30. Giannone L, Williamson TL. A philosophy of safety awareness. In: S George GS, editor. American association of cheerleading coaches and administrators cheerleading safety manual. Memphis, TN: UCA Publications Department; 2006. p. 1–4.

31. Shields BJ, Smith GA. Cheerleading-related injuries to children 5 to 18 years of age: United States, 1990–2002. Pediatrics 2006;117(1):122–9.

32. Shields BJ, Smith GA. Cheerleading-related injuries in the United States: a prospective surveillance study. J Athl Train 2009;44(6):567–77.

33. Schulz MR, Marshall SW, Yang J, et al. A prospective cohort study of injury incidence and risk factors in North Carolina high school competitive cheerleaders. Am J Sports Med 2004;32(2):396–405.

34. Shields BJ, Fernandez SA, Smith GA. Epidemiology of cheerleading stunt-related injuries in the United States. J Athl Train 2009;44(6):586–94.

35. Singh S, Smith GA, Fields SK, et al. Gymnastics-related injuries to children treated in emergency departments in the United States, 1990–2005. Pediatrics 2008;121(4):e954–60.

36. Emery CA, Hagel B, Decloe M, et al. Risk factors for injury and severe injury in youth ice hockey: a systematic review of the literature. Inj Prev 2010;16(2):113–8.

37. Emery CA, Meeuwisse WH. Injury rates, risk factors, and mechanisms of injury in minor hockey. Am J Sports Med 2006;34(12):1960–9.

38. Macpherson A, Rothman L, Howard A. Body-checking rules and childhood injuries in ice hockey. Pediatrics 2006;117(2):e143–7.

39. Hagel BE, Marko J, Dryden D, et al. Effect of body checking on injury rates among minor ice hockey players. CMAJ 2006;175(2):155–60.

40. Yard EE, Comstock RD. Injuries sustained by pediatric ice hockey, lacrosse, and field hockey athletes presenting to United States emergency departments, 1990–2003. J Athl Train 2006;41(4):441–9.

41. Dick R, Romani WA, Agel J, et al. Descriptive epidemiology of collegiate men's lacrosse injuries: national collegiate athletic association injury surveillance system, 1988–1989 through 2003–2004. J Athl Train 2007;42(2):255–61.

42. Dick R, Lincoln AE, Agel J, et al. Descriptive epidemiology of collegiate women's lacrosse injuries: national collegiate athletic association injury surveillance system, 1988–1989 through 2003–2004. J Athl Train 2007;42(2):262–9.

43. Mueller BA, Cummings P, Rivara FP, et al. Injuries of the head, face, and neck in relation to ski helmet use. Epidemiology 2008;19(2):270–6.

44. Levy AS, Hawkes AP, Hemminger LM, et al. An analysis of head injuries among skiers and snowboarders. J Trauma 2002;53(4):695–704.
45. Bridges EJ, Rouah F, Johnston KM. Snowblading injuries in Eastern Canada. Br J Sports Med 2003;37(6):511–5.
46. Hentschel S, Hader W, Boyd M. Head injuries in skiers and snowboarders in British Columbia. Can J Neurol Sci 2001;28(1):42–6.
47. Dick RW. Is there a gender difference in concussion incidence and outcomes? Br J Sports Med 2009;43(Suppl 1):i46–50.
48. Broshek DK, Kaushik T, Freeman JR, et al. Sex differences in outcome following sports-related concussion. J Neurosurg 2005;102(5):856–63.

Biomechanics of Concussion

David F. Meaney, PhD[a],*, Douglas H. Smith, MD[b]

KEYWORDS

- Biomechanics • Tolerance • Mild traumatic Brain injury
- Concussion

INTRODUCTION AND SCOPE

The recent public awareness of mild traumatic brain injury (TBI) (concussion) and the possible long-term consequences on brain function has raised the profile of the disorder and also highlighted the lack of knowledge on how to effectively treat this disease. For decades, much of the research community concentrated on the most devastating forms of TBI, with the hopes of significantly improving outcome in this patient population. On a relative basis, the incidence of mild TBI far exceeds the number of TBI-related fatalities and moderate/severe TBIs, with some estimates suggesting its frequency is at least 10 times more common than moderate and severe TBI.[1,2] Perhaps equally important, comparing the prevalence of patients showing long-term impairment from mild TBI to other diseases is startling: approximately 225,000 new patients each year show long-term deficits from mild TBI, approximately equal to the number of patients diagnosed annually with breast cancer, multiple sclerosis, and traumatic spinal cord injury combined. The emergence of blast-induced TBI from the Iraq and Afghanistan conflicts[3–5] only heightens the need for a long-term treatment and prevention solution for mild TBI.

The purpose of this article is to provide a review of the past work directed at understanding the biomechanical etiology of concussions. The broad scale of knowledge on this topic is presented, ranging from the measurable mechanical parameters associated with concussion to the underlying mechanisms responsible for tissue damage and the molecular substrates that could form the basis of the immediate, transient impairment observed during a typical concussion episode. Possible future directions are reviewed briefly.

Funding provided by NIH NS35712, HD41699, and NS056202.

The authors declare no competing financial interests.

[a] Department of Bioengineering, University of Pennsylvania, 240 Skirkanich Hall, 210 South 33rd Street, Philadelphia, PA 19104-6392, USA

[b] Department of Neurosurgery, University of Pennsylvania, 105D Hayden Hall, 240 South 33rd Street, Philadelphia, PA 19104-6392, USA

* Corresponding author.

E-mail address: dmeaney@seas.upenn.edu

THE MECHANICAL ORIGINS OF CONCUSSION—HOW DOES THE HEAD MOVE?

There is often confusion about the mechanical etiology of concussions. One primary component of the confusion stems from the many different head motions that can occur when a head is struck with an object or when a head strikes a surface. The protected (helmeted) head has similar variety in the mechanical response. This complex variety of responses makes each injury-causing situation nearly unique. Two broad categories of forces—contact and inertial—encompass the important causal forces associated with TBIs. Both contact and inertial forces occur during impact loading, where the head is struck (or strikes) a surface. Only inertial (acceleration) loading occurs from impulsive head motions, which are defined by the absence of the head striking an object.

Primary injures caused by direct contact loading can occur both in the region of impact and in regions distant from the impact site. Focal forces are linked to skull fracture and, when focused over a small area, depressed skull fracture. These fractures can lead to subsequent injuries (eg, some linear skull fractures can cause epidural bleeding when the fracture line extends over the blood vessels within the dural membrane). Similarly, there is some evidence suggesting that these stress waves can cause fracture in sites remote from the impact where the skull shows a reduction in its structural or mechanical properties.[6] The tolerance of the brain to the forces causing these types of contusive injuries is now better characterized[7] as is the fracture tolerance of the skull to either blunt or more focused impact.[8,9] These focal brain injuries are common in moderate and severe brain injury but are largely absent in mild TBI.[10,11] For this reason, the remainder of this review focuses on the inertial forces that cause the concussive injuries common in mild TBI.

There is considerable evidence showing that the primary cause of concussive injuries is the inertial, or acceleration, loading experienced by the brain at the moment of impact. With the head/neck motions that occur during a typical impact, there are two components of acceleration that occur in nearly every instance of concussion—linear and rotational acceleration.

Early efforts to understand the biophysical basis of concussion concentrated on how *linear accelerations* measured during impact correlated to the corresponding injury thresholds in animals. Recordings of pressure throughout brain surrogates during an impact event showed a good correlation between the peak acceleration and peak pressure at a point within the brain.[12,13] Although the pressure within the brain during an impact varied, this strong correlation between an internal response (brain pressure) and external input (linear acceleration) led several investigators to study the effects of pressures within the living brain. Several studies established that the transient increase in pressure within the brain causes neurologic dysfunction, with the level of dysfunction correlating with the peak pressure achieved during the injury period.[14–16]

In parallel with these studies on animals, investigators systemically examined the tolerance of the human skull/brain structure to impact loading, with the goal of establishing a primary tolerance curve for injury in humans. Due to their nature—using postmortem samples and filling the cranial vault with gelatin—these studies did not have an ability to measure directly concussion threshold. These studies did, however, measure the relative onset of skull fracture. Some tests also measured the pressures within the brain caused during these impact conditions, providing a reference measure to pressure thresholds derived from animal studies. The tests conducted included drops onto flat surfaces, instrumented samples to measure the acceleration and pressure over time, and correlation of these measurements to the presence/absence of skull fracture. The resulting injury tolerance curve, known commonly as the Wayne State Tolerance Curve, provided the basis for a continuing series of studies to improve the ability to correlate known physical parameters (eg, linear acceleration) to head injury.[17–19] Largely stimulated by these initial data, there are now testing standards that are used for designing protective equipment and automotive safety systems that use measures of linear acceleration for determining injury risk.

Rotational acceleration is a second type of acceleration that is common during either impact or impulsive head loading. Due to the physical properties of the highly organized brain,[20–24] brain tissue deforms more readily in response to shear forces compared with other biologic tissues. Rapid head rotations generate shear forces throughout the brain, and, therefore, rotational accelerations have a high potential to cause shear-induced tissue damage. The importance of shear forces were confirmed in series of studies across different laboratories, leading to the conventional wisdom that shear deformation caused by rotational acceleration is the predominant mechanism of injury in concussion.[25–27] If the head motion is constrained to exclude any rotational motion, it is difficult to produce traumatic unconsciousness. In comparison, introducing or allowing a rotational component after impact substantially increases the likelihood of an unconscious episode.[28] This injury mechanism applies across the severity spectrum; the primary difference across the spectrum is the amount of brain tissue injured and the severity of injury at a given site within the brain.[26]

MECHANISMS OF DAMAGE—HOW DOES THE MECHANICAL ENERGY OF MOTION TRANSFER TO THE TISSUE?

A critical component of concussive injuries is how the mechanical energy from the external input (acceleration) is transferred to the brain and vascular tissue at the tissue and microscale. This energy transfer process—both how the acceleration moves and deforms the brain tissues and the effect of this physical stimulus on the living tissue and neural/glial networks—is the key step in understanding the basis for concussion. The critical common denominator in assessing the biomechanics of concussion is defining conditions that cause internal responses (eg, strain and pressure) within the brain and understanding the combination of external input conditions resulting in these conditions.

Brain is one of the softest biologic materials, shows nonlinear behavior, and changes its properties in response to the applied loading rate.[20–24] Composed largely of water, brain material is resistant to changing its shape when subjected to either slow or transient pressures. Brain tissue deforms easily, however, when shearing forces are applied. These two internal responses (pressure and shear) are the main metrics used to describe the mechanical response of the brain to an applied external loading input.

Past work shows that linear acceleration correlates well as a predictor of the peak pressures that occur within the brain.[29] A simple model of the hydrostatic gradients generated within the brain can provide a rudimentary approximation of these pressures and can also predict the effect of pressure-relieving openings (eg, foramen magnum) on the resulting pressure gradients.[30] Experimental measures of the human surrogate response to impact loading also provide key insight into how local impact from a blunt impactor causes a subsequent acceleration of the head and pressure gradient within the cranial contents. Based on these data, the ability to predict, a priori, the pressures generated within the brain under a known external loading condition has improved substantially with the advancement of computationally based finite element models in the past two decades (for recent publications, see Refs.[20,31–35]). Some versions of these computational models are becoming highly detailed, allowing investigators to examine if the ventricular system and/or blood vessel network influences measured pressure gradients within the tissue during inertial loading.[36] Similarly, the effects of these pressure gradients on the deformations that can occur within the brain are also better known. Early studies using photoelastic gelatin indicate that pressure gradients during linear acceleration-based motions can create strains at the craniocervical junction. Subsequent work studying common models of pressure-induced brain injury in animals show a similar type of ability to enhance strains in the brainstem.[37] These data also indicate, however, that the strains induced by pressure gradients within the brain are much smaller than the strains caused by rotational accelerations, primarily because the brain material deforms little in response to pressure. When considering strictly the pressures generated within the brain during typical acceleration conditions associated with concussions, this past work provides a solid foundation for prescribing the accurate pressure conditions at any point within the brain.

In contrast to pressures generated within the brain during impact or impulsive loading, the tissue deformation (strain) is influenced primarily by the applied rotational accelerations, the intracranial partitioning membranes, and the material properties of the brain tissue. For a given magnitude of rotational acceleration, the resulting patterns of strain within the brain are markedly different if the acceleration is applied in the coronal (lateral), horizontal (axial), or sagittal plane. Experimental data show the effect of rotational acceleration direction on the corresponding impairment, with lateral (coronal) plane accelerations in humans showing the most likelihood for producing damage within the deep internal structures of the brain.[26] Although neurologic impairment (loss of consciousness) is produced most readily with coronal plane motions, it is possible to generate similar impairment with rotational motions along the horizontal and sagittal planes, albeit these acceleration magnitudes are higher. The principle of directionally dependent brain damage is confirmed in a series of studies across different species[26,38] and is a critical factor in understanding the human tolerance to injuries, such as concussion. The ventricular system may have an important damping effect on the strains that appear throughout the brain during rotational motions, and the membranes that partition the cerebral hemispheres and the cerebellum from the cerebrum also influence the patterns on deformation that appear for a given head motion.[39,40]

The ability to predict the strains that appear throughout the brain during rotational motions is challenging, because the large deformations that appear during typical injury-causing situations often require advanced computational and experimental methods. Initial efforts to model the behavior of brain surrogates in simplified models of the human brain/skull showed encouraging correlation with experimental data.[20,31] Next-generation models included more accurate anatomic detail of the brain structures along specific anatomic planes and suggested the complex interface between white and gray matter, as well as the presence of fluid-filled ventricles, were important 2-D model features affecting the predicted mechanical response of the brain.[41]

Studies extending these computational models into 3-D representations of the living brain are ongoing and proceeding along two complementary directions. First, development of a more idealized 3-D geometry with the inclusion of major anatomic features is under continuous development. Published work shows that this simplified model produces approximately the same brain motions measured in human surrogate tests and that this tool can scan many possible injury scenarios quickly for a quick assessment of the situations that could produce focal or more diffuse brain injuries.[20,31] One of the initial goals of this project—developing rapid computational results on a desktop computer—makes this approach most feasible for the designers of safety and protective equipment to quickly assess the brain injury risk for any loading input. One primary benefit of this simplified computational tool is the use as a proactive design tool for testing and developing new protective equipment.

The second approach uses a more highly detailed 3-D model of the brain within the skull and can produce exceptionally detailed predictions on the local and global response of the brain to any impact or impulsive loading scenario (example studies are included in Refs.[32,34,35,42–46]). Multiscale modeling techniques with this highly detailed approach suggest it may be even possible to predict the deformations applied to networks of blood vessels and neural/glial cells, opening up a critically important window in understanding how the externally applied loading can cause local changes in vascular, neural, and glial behavior.[36] With this detailed knowledge, there is a substantial increase in the computational time needed to develop predictions. As computational power and modeling algorithms becomes more advanced, these models will eventually become available for rapid use on desktop computers. The most widely used current role for these models, however, is for researchers and not designers.

HOW IS THE BRAIN AFFECTED FROM THE MECHANICAL ENERGY TRANSFER DURING CONCUSSION?
Studying the Effect at the Microscale—What Is Known

As more was learned about the transfer of the external input (contact and inertial loading) into the brain mechanical response, it became clear that the key to understanding the basis for the immediate impairment in mild TBI was measuring the effect of these mechanical forces on the blood vessels and cellular networks within the brain. Studying these effects is technically challenging, because the forces need to be applied quickly (<50 milliseconds). In addition, the modeling of impact response showed that the deformations within the brain can be significant during injury and the systems for studying the effects at the microscale needed to apply these large deformations quickly. Finally, the deformation field occurring within the brain needed to be recreated accurately in these microinjury models.

Despite these technical challenges, several groups showed that the effect of an appropriately tuned mechanical stimulation is broad and complex. In dissociated cells, much of the early work focused on how a single, rapid deformation of cell monolayers (astrocytes, endothelial cells, and mixed cultures of neurons and glia) would cause alterations in acute biochemical signaling and affect long-term viability. Astrocytes respond to a focal mechanical stimulation by propagating intercellular waves through their network. Mechanically stimulated astrocyte networks show changes in the cytoskeleton, organelle function, and biochemical cascades over time.[47–54] Many of these initial changes point to an alteration in the homeostatic mechanisms of astrocyte regulation.

The response of neurons to microinjury is probably the most well characterized, with the most diverse approaches developed to study this response. It is possible to measure the response of cellular populations. The range of physical manipulations spans the spectrum from a mild physical insult with no obvious structural changes to an insult capable of transecting subcellular elements. Early evidence showed that these physical insults can affect the properties of important synaptic glutamate receptors that can regulate neurotransmission and plasticity in networks.[55] Moreover, inhibitory synaptic receptor functions can be altered with a physical force, showing that the balance of excitation/inhibition coupling is important to consider when assessing the effects of these physical forces.[56] Perhaps equally important is the alteration in the receptor composition and intracellular signaling that occurs after a microinjury. Several studies indicate that an initial injury to neuronal culture can lead to subsequent change in the response of neurons to an agonist stimulation, some of which are linked to the appearance of new glutamate receptor types at the synapse.[33,57,58] Moreover, there is clear evidence that physical injury can lead to activation of different neuronal death pathways, with the physical coupling of glutamate receptors potentially explaining part of this activation process.[59–61] Studies indicate the response of neural networks to repeated injuries is not simply the superposition of the response to an individual insult.[62] This is a critical observation for studying concussive brain injuries.

Rather than coupling the mechanical insult directly to intracellular signaling through mechanoactivated receptors and channels, several studies indicate an alternative mechanism of damage—an immediate, nonspecific increase in plasma membrane permeability.[63–65] The increase in membrane permeability is not long-lasting, because data suggest membrane resealing within 10 to 15 minutes.[64] The relative influence of this mechanism to the mechanoactivation of receptors and channels remains to be fully described. But there is work suggesting the deformation field applied to monolayers (eg, stretch applied in one direction versus two perpendicular directions) is a primary determinant that dictates the contributing role of each mechanism.[66] This relative threshold would help explain the diversity of responses in the literature; some studies do not show any immediate change in membrane permeability whereas others attribute the entire postinjury response to this mechanism of damage.

The technologies for studying injury at the microscale extend to the study of subcellular elements, which may be particularly important for neurons, where the subcellular organization is key for network function. Early technologies studied how the transection of a neuronal process affects signaling within the soma and defined a critical distance between the soma and the lesion site to effect changes on nuclear gene expression.[67,68] Technology to mechanically injure processes first appeared more than a decade ago, where networks of axons bridging two populations of neurons could be stretched and studied over time.[69,70] The corresponding threshold for immediate changes in biochemical (calcium-mediated) signaling was established as were approximate thresholds for structural changes and tearing of the axonal processes. Moreover, studies using this system showed that the voltage-gated sodium channels are mechanoactivated from the stretch event and undergo a rapid proteolysis that can lead to a sustained elevation of axoplasmic calcium.[71,72] This proteolysis is activated at stretch levels below the structural failure threshold and are, therefore, potentially relevant for concussive type injuries where axonal transection is rare, if present at all.

An advantage of the microscale technologies (discussed previously) is that many of these methods are scalable to more complex tissue preparations. A more advanced representation of living tissue is the organotypic brain slice culture, which contains both the neural and glial network in an architecture that more closely resembles the in vivo brain. With the ability to culture slices of the brain for long periods of time (approximately 3–4 weeks), these cultures can be mechanically stretched to mimic the deformations that occur within the brain over the entire severity spectrum of TBI.[73–75] To date, reports show the ability to study the expression of different genes in response to injury levels below the threshold to cause neuronal death, to study the effect of targeted therapeutic treatments when the level of mechanical injury exceeds the tolerance for cell death, and to define region-specific thresholds for cell death in critical brain regions (eg, hippocampus) associated with mild TBI.[76–78] Recent advances in multielectrode array recording make it possible to record changes in the network ensemble after mechanical injury on stretchable array platforms.[79–83]

The versatility of this technology has yet to be fully developed, but this shows promise in providing a number of possible output parameters (function, biochemical, and genomic) in a more realistic tissue environment compared with monolayer cultures.

The second major category of mechanical input in concussion situations is the pressure generated transiently through the brain. In cultured cells, the effects of pressure are studied much less than the effects of deformation. Slowly applied pressure can alter cell function in astrocytes and neurons, but the tested pressures are much higher than the pressure experienced during a typical concussion-type insult.[84] Applying rapid pressure changes to a fluid-filled chamber containing either brain slice or primary cell cultures can lead to biochemical changes and neural dysfunction, but thresholds for these changes are not well established.[85–89] Repeated impacts of a fluid-filled chamber into a striking plate also caused primary changes in neural cultures. It is difficult, however, to separate the effects of the deceleration during the repeated impacts from the pressures generated in the chamber for these impacts.[90]

Studying the Effects at the Microscale—What Is Not Known

At the microscale, work in the past two decades shows that the mechanical forces in the brain during TBI are capable of triggering both initial and postacute changes in function. In some studies, the forces applied are enough to cause cell death over the ensuing hours and days.[73,77] The mechanisms that regulate the response of the networks have been well studied. Less attention has been paid to the mechanical threshold for triggering these changes. Already, work is emerging to define regional thresholds for cell death in important regions of the brain (eg, hippocampus), with obvious impact on the function of networks in the affected brain region. The threshold at which a deficit appears, however, may be much lower than the level necessary to cause neuronal or glial death. This functional threshold may have an important bearing on conditions associated with concussion. For example, a recent study shows the threshold for astrocyte reactivity is well below the threshold for causing changes in astrocyte viability after stretch. This threshold is also below the level necessary to cause neuronal death.[47] These data lead to obvious questions—How does the neural network behave in the presence of these reactive astrocytes? Does this lead to a change in the synaptic plasticity of the network? The effects from the mechanical force insult may have long-lasting changes in the network that occur from interactions among two or more cell types. Defining the persistence of these changes over time will have an important bearing on understanding when forces at the microscale have a corresponding effect on function at either the micro- or macroscale.

MERGING THE MICROSCALE WITH THE MACROSCALE: ROLE OF EMERGING FIELD STUDIES

In parallel with the efforts to describe the effect of mechanical forces on neural and glial cell networks, there is a renewed emphasis on defining the field conditions associated with concussions. In many sports, the emergence of concussion as a major health issue has occurred within the past 10 years, possibly from the increased awareness of how multiple concussions early in life can affect the risk for developing neurodegenerative disease later in life.[91–93] Defining the externally applied forces and accelerations experienced by the head at the time of concussive brain injury is a critically important complement to past work and ongoing studies. Normally, work at this level is difficult to match with work at the other end of the spectrum, namely microscale injury studies. Because of the advances of computational models that bridge the gap between applied external loading and the intracranial strains, however, there is now a clear opportunity to merge knowledge across the scales to define a more comprehensive view of concussions.

In an analysis of professional football players, Pellman, and colleagues[94,95] surveyed concussions occurring in the field of play and used reconstruction techniques to establish a concussion threshold. In comparison to reconstructing single concussion cases, recent technology embedding accelerometers into helmets (head impact telemetry system [HITS]) allows researchers to constantly sample the accelerations experienced by players during game and practice situations.[96–98] The data collected between the two methods show some similarity and will provide important information for basic researchers to estimate the real world scenarios that cause concussion. Moreover, these monitoring efforts will likely inform new product designs and also offer the ability to track the effectiveness of these new helmet designs in the field of play to complement design studies conducted in the laboratory.

LOOKING TO THE FUTURE

Although the biomechanics of concussion is a research area that spans many length scales, there is now substantial work across these scales that establish a coordinated approach for better understanding of concussive brain injury and how new technologies can be developed to reduce the incidence of concussion. Methods are in place to estimate how the brain moves and deforms under common conditions associated with concussion; these computational methods are increasingly robust for predicting the mechanical response of the brain under many different situations. In parallel, field studies are defining the real world situations that cause concussions and comparing them to similar situations that do not cause concussions. These surveillance data provide critical input for the computational tools that will continue to improve the resolution and accuracy of estimating strains within specific anatomic regions. With new techniques to map these deformations to strains of cellular and vessel networks within the brain, a wealth of information from microscale studies will merge with information from large-scale studies. These combined efforts will define how different cell types are damaged during concussion and provide a method to rationally develop new technologies for reducing or preventing concussions in the field.

REFERENCES

1. Bazarian JJ, McClung J, Shah MN, et al. Mild traumatic brain injury in the United States, 1998–2000. Brain Inj 2005;19(2):85–91.
2. Langlois JA, Rutland-Brown W, Wald MM. The epidemiology and impact of traumatic brain injury: a brief overview. J Head Trauma Rehabil 2006;21(5):375–8.
3. Eibner C, Schell TL, Jaycox LH. Care of war veterans with mild traumatic brain injury. N Engl J Med 2009;361(5):537 [author reply: 537–8].
4. Preiss-Farzanegan SJ, Chapman B, Wong TM, et al. The relationship between gender and postconcussion symptoms after sport-related mild traumatic brain injury. PM R 2009;1(3):245–53.
5. Xydakis MS, Robbins AS, Grant GA. Mild traumatic brain injury in U.S. soldiers returning from Iraq. N Engl J Med 2008;358(20):2177 [author reply: 2179].
6. McElhaney JH, Hopper RH Jr, Nightingale RW, et al. Mechanisms of basilar skull fracture. J Neurotrauma 1995;12(4):669–78.
7. Shreiber DI, Smith DH, Meaney DF. Immediate in vivo response of the cortex and the blood-brain barrier following dynamic cortical deformation in the rat. Neurosci Lett 1999;259(1):5–8.

8. Raymond D, Van Ee C, Crawford G, et al. Tolerance of the skull to blunt ballistic temporo-parietal impact. J Biomech 2009;42(15):2479–85.
9. Yoganandan N, Pintar FA. Biomechanics of temporo-parietal skull fracture. Clin Biomech (Bristol, Avon) 2004;19(3):225–39.
10. Graham DI, Adams JH, Nicoll JA, et al. The nature, distribution and causes of traumatic brain injury. Brain Pathol 1995;5(4):397–406.
11. Adams JH, Doyle D, Graham DI, et al. The contusion index: a reappraisal in human and experimental non-missile head injury. Neuropathol Appl Neurobiol 1985;11(4):299–308.
12. Gurdjian ES, Lissner HR, Evans FG, et al. Intracranial pressure and acceleration accompanying head impacts in human cadavers. Surg Gynecol Obstet 1961; 113:185–90.
13. Thomas LM, Roberts VL, Gurdjian ES. Experimental intracranial pressure gradients in the human skull. J Neurol Neurosurg Psychiatr 1966;29(5):404–11.
14. Lindgren S, Rinder L. Experimental studies in head injury. II. Pressure propagation in "percussion concussion". Biophysik 1966;3(2):174–80.
15. Gurdjian ES, Lissner HR, Webster JE, et al. Studies on experimental concussion: relation of physiologic effect to time duration of intracranial pressure increase at impact. Neurology 1954;4(9):674–81.
16. Denny-Brown DE, Russell WR. Experimental concussion: (section of neurology). Proc R Soc Med 1941;34(11):691–2.
17. Gurdjian ES, Webster JE, Lissner HR. The mechanism of skull fracture. J Neurosurg 1950;7(2):106–14.
18. Gurdjian ES, Webster JE, Lissner HR. Studies on skull fracture with particular reference to engineering factors. Am J Surg 1949;78(5):736–42 [Disc 749–51].
19. Gurdjian ES, Lissner HR, Webster JE. The mechanism of production of linear skull fracture; further studies on deformation of the skull by the stresscoat technique. Surg Gynecol Obstet 1947;85(2):195–210.
20. Takhounts EG, Crandall JR, Darvish K. On the importance of nonlinearity of brain tissue under large deformations. Stapp Car Crash J 2003;47:79–92.
21. Miller K, Chinzei K. Constitutive modelling of brain tissue: experiment and theory. J Biomech 1997;30(11–12):1115–21.
22. Donnelly BR, Medige J. Shear properties of human brain tissue. J Biomech Eng 1997;119(4):423–32.
23. Arbogast KB, Thibault KL, Pinheiro BS, et al. A high-frequency shear device for testing soft biological tissues. J Biomech 1997;30(7):757–9.
24. Prange MT, Meaney DF, Margulies SS. Defining brain mechanical properties: effects of region, direction, and species. Stapp Car Crash J 2000;44:205–13.
25. Unterharnscheidt F, Higgins LS. Traumatic lesions of brain and spinal cord due to nondeforming angular acceleration of the head. Tex Rep Biol Med 1969;27(1): 127–66.
26. Gennarelli TA, Thibault LE, Adams JH, et al. Diffuse axonal injury and traumatic coma in the primate. Ann Neurol 1982;12(6):564–74.
27. Adams JH, Graham DI, Murray LS, et al. Diffuse axonal injury due to nonmissile head injury in humans: an analysis of 45 cases. Ann Neurol 1982;12(6):557–63.
28. Ommaya AK, Gennarelli TA. Cerebral concussion and traumatic unconsciousness. Correlation of experimental and clinical observations of blunt head injuries. Brain 1974;97(4):633–54.
29. Nahum AM, Smith R, Ward CC. Intracranial pressure dynamics during head impact. in 21st Annual Stapp Car Crash Conference. 1977: Society of Automotive Engineers.

30. Stalhammar D, Olsson Y. Experimental brain damage from fluid pressures due to impact acceleration. Acta Neurol Scand 1975;52:38–55.
31. Takhounts EG, Ridella SA, Hasija V, et al. Investigation of traumatic brain injuries using the next generation of simulated injury monitor (SIMon) finite element head model. Stapp Car Crash J 2008;52:1–31.
32. Ishikawa R, Kato K, Kubo M, et al. Finite element analysis and experimental study on mechanism of brain injury using brain model. Conf Proc IEEE Eng Med Biol Soc 2006;1:1327–30.
33. Bell JD, Ai J, Chen Y, et al. Mild in vitro trauma induces rapid Glur2 endocytosis, robustly augments calcium permeability and enhances susceptibility to secondary excitotoxic insult in cultured Purkinje cells. Brain 2007;130(Pt 10): 2528–42.
34. Franklyn M, Fildes B, Zhang L, et al. Analysis of finite element models for head injury investigation: reconstruction of four real-world impacts. Stapp Car Crash J 2005;49:1–32.
35. Zhang L, Yang KH, Dwarampudi R, et al. Recent advances in brain injury research: a new human head model development and validation. Stapp Car Crash J 2001;45:369–94.
36. Zhang L, Bae J, Hardy WN, et al. Computational study of the contribution of the vasculature on the dynamic response of the brain. Stapp Car Crash J 2002;46: 145–64.
37. Thibault LE, Meaney DF, Anderson BJ, et al. Biomechanical aspects of a fluid percussion model of brain injury. J Neurotrauma 1992;9(4):311–22.
38. Smith DH, Nonaka M, Miller R, et al. Immediate coma following inertial brain injury dependent on axonal damage in the brainstem. J Neurosurg 2000;93(2):315–22.
39. Ivarsson J, Viano DC, Lovsund P. Influence of the lateral ventricles and irregular skull base on brain kinematics due to sagittal plane head rotation. J Biomech Eng 2002;124(4):422–31.
40. Ivarsson J, Viano DC, Lovsund P, et al. Strain relief from the cerebral ventricles during head impact: experimental studies on natural protection of the brain. J Biomech 2000;33(2):181–9.
41. Nishimoto T, Murakami S. Relation between diffuse axonal injury and internal head structures on blunt impact. J Biomech Eng 1998;120(1):140–7.
42. Zhang L, Yang KH, King AI. A proposed injury threshold for mild traumatic brain injury. J Biomech Eng 2004;126(2):226–36.
43. Takahashi T, Kato K, Ishikawa R, et al. 3-D finite element analysis and experimental study on brain injury mechanism. Conf Proc IEEE Eng Med Biol Soc 2007;2007:3613–6.
44. Li J, Zhang J, Yoganandan N, et al. Regional brain strains and role of falx in lateral impact-induced head rotational acceleration. Biomed Sci Instrum 2007;43:24–9.
45. Zhang J, Yoganandan N, Pintar FA, et al. Role of translational and rotational accelerations on brain strain in lateral head impact. Biomed Sci Instrum 2006; 42:501–6.
46. Zhang L, Yang KH, King AI. Comparison of brain responses between frontal and lateral impacts by finite element modeling. J Neurotrauma 2001;18(1):21–30.
47. Miller WJ, Leventhal I, Scarsella D, et al. Mechanically induced reactive gliosis causes ATP-mediated alterations in astrocyte stiffness. J Neurotrauma 2009; 26(5):789–97.
48. Charles AC, Merrill JE, Dirksen ER, et al. Intercellular signaling in glial cells: calcium waves and oscillations in response to mechanical stimulation and glutamate. Neuron 1991;6(6):983–92.

49. Di X, Goforth PB, Bullock R, et al. Mechanical injury alters volume activated ion channels in cortical astrocytes. Acta Neurochir Suppl 2000;76:379–83.
50. Floyd CL, Rzigalinski BA, Weber JT, et al. Traumatic injury of cultured astrocytes alters inositol (1,4,5)-trisphosphate-mediated signaling. Glia 2001;33(1):12–23.
51. Hoffman SW, Rzigalinski BA, Willoughby KA, et al. Astrocytes generate isoprostanes in response to trauma or oxygen radicals. J Neurotrauma 2000;17(5): 415–20.
52. Ahmed SM, Rzigalinski BA, Willoughby KA, et al. Stretch-induced injury alters mitochondrial membrane potential and cellular ATP in cultured astrocytes and neurons. J Neurochem 2000;74(5):1951–60.
53. Rzigalinski BA, Willoughby KA, Hoffman SW, et al. Calcium influx factor, further evidence it is 5, 6-epoxyeicosatrienoic acid. J Biol Chem 1999;274(1):175–82.
54. Lamb RG, Harper CC, McKinney JS, et al. Alterations in phosphatidylcholine metabolism of stretch-injured cultured rat astrocytes. J Neurochem 1997;68(5): 1904–10.
55. Zhang L, Rzigalinski BA, Ellis EF, et al. Reduction of voltage-dependent Mg2+ blockade of NMDA current in mechanically injured neurons. Science 1996; 274(5294):1921–3.
56. Kao CQ, Goforth PB, Ellis EF, et al. Potentiation of GABA(A) currents after mechanical injury of cortical neurons. J Neurotrauma 2004;21(3):259–70.
57. Spaethling JM, Klein DM, Singh P, et al. Calcium-permeable AMPA receptors appear in cortical neurons after traumatic mechanical injury and contribute to neuronal fate. J Neurotrauma 2008;25(10):1207–16.
58. Bell JD, Park E, Ai J, et al. PICK1-mediated GluR2 endocytosis contributes to cellular injury after neuronal trauma. Cell Death Differ 2009;16(12):1665–80.
59. Cui H, Hayashi A, Sun HS, et al. PDZ protein interactions underlying NMDA receptor-mediated excitotoxicity and neuroprotection by PSD-95 inhibitors. J Neurosci 2007;27(37):9901–15.
60. Aarts M, Liu Y, Liu L, et al. Treatment of ischemic brain damage by perturbing NMDA receptor- PSD-95 protein interactions. Science 2002;298(5594):846–50.
61. Sattler R, Xiong Z, Lu WY, et al. Specific coupling of NMDA receptor activation to nitric oxide neurotoxicity by PSD-95 protein. Science 1999;284(5421):1845–8.
62. Weber JT, Rzigalinski BA, Willoughby KA, et al. Alterations in calcium-mediated signal transduction after traumatic injury of cortical neurons. Cell Calcium 1999; 26(6):289–99.
63. LaPlaca MC, Cullen DK, McLoughlin JJ, et al. High rate shear strain of three-dimensional neural cell cultures: a new in vitro traumatic brain injury model. J Biomech 2005;38(5):1093–105.
64. Geddes DM, Cargill RS 2nd, LaPlaca MC. Mechanical stretch to neurons results in a strain rate and magnitude-dependent increase in plasma membrane permeability. J Neurotrauma 2003;20(10):1039–49.
65. Geddes DM, LaPlaca MC, Cargill RS 2nd. Susceptibility of hippocampal neurons to mechanically induced injury. Exp Neurol 2003;184(1):420–7.
66. Geddes-Klein DM, Schiffman KB, Meaney DF. Mechanisms and consequences of neuronal stretch injury in vitro differ with the model of trauma. J Neurotrauma 2006;23(2):193–204.
67. Lucas JH. Proximal segment retraction increases the probability of nerve cell survival after dendrite transection. Brain Res 1987;425(2):384–7.
68. Lucas JH, Gross GW, Emery DG, et al. Neuronal survival or death after dendrite transection close to the perikaryon: correlation with electrophysiologic, morphologic, and ultrastructural changes. Cent Nerv Syst Trauma 1985;2(4):231–55.

69. Wolf JA, Stys PK, Lusardi T, et al. Traumatic axonal injury induces calcium influx modulated by tetrodotoxin-sensitive sodium channels. J Neurosci 2001;21(6):1923–30.
70. Smith DH, Wolf JA, Lusardi TA, et al. High tolerance and delayed elastic response of cultured axons to dynamic stretch injury. J Neurosci 1999;19(11):4263–9.
71. von Reyn CR, Spaethling JM, Mesfin MN, et al. Calpain mediates proteolysis of the voltage-gated sodium channel alpha-subunit. J Neurosci 2009;29(33):10350–6.
72. Iwata A, Stys PK, Wolf JA, et al. Traumatic axonal injury induces proteolytic cleavage of the voltage-gated sodium channels modulated by tetrodotoxin and protease inhibitors. J Neurosci 2004;24(19):4605–13.
73. Morrison B 3rd, Cater HL, Wang CC, et al. A tissue level tolerance criterion for living brain developed with an in vitro model of traumatic mechanical loading. Stapp Car Crash J 2003;47:93–105.
74. Morrison B 3rd, Meaney DF, Margulies SS, et al. Dynamic mechanical stretch of organotypic brain slice cultures induces differential genomic expression: relationship to mechanical parameters. J Biomech Eng 2000;122(3):224–30.
75. Morrison B 3rd, Eberwine JH, Meaney DF, et al. Traumatic injury induces differential expression of cell death genes in organotypic brain slice cultures determined by complementary DNA array hybridization. Neuroscience 2000;96(1):131–9.
76. Elkin BS, Morrison B 3rd. Region-specific tolerance criteria for the living brain. Stapp Car Crash J 2007;51:127–38.
77. Cater HL, Sundstrom LE, Morrison B 3rd. Temporal development of hippocampal cell death is dependent on tissue strain but not strain rate. J Biomech 2006;39(15):2810–8.
78. Morrison B 3rd, Cater HL, Benham CD, et al. An in vitro model of traumatic brain injury utilising two-dimensional stretch of organotypic hippocampal slice cultures. J Neurosci Methods 2006;150(2):192–201.
79. DeRidder MN, Simon MJ, Siman R, et al. Traumatic mechanical injury to the hippocampus in vitro causes regional caspase-3 and calpain activation that is influenced by NMDA receptor subunit composition. Neurobiol Dis 2006;22(1):165–76.
80. Yu Z, Elkin BS, Morrison B. Quantification of functional alterations after in vitro traumatic brain injury. Conf Proc IEEE Eng Med Biol Soc 2009;2009:1135–8.
81. Yu Z, Graudejus O, Lacour SP, et al. Neural sensing of electrical activity with stretchable microelectrode arrays. Conf Proc IEEE Eng Med Biol Soc 2009;2009:4210–3.
82. Yu Z, Morrison B 3rd. Experimental mild traumatic brain injury induces functional alteration of the developing hippocampus. J Neurophysiol 2010;103(1):499–510.
83. Yu Z, Graudejus O, Tsay C, et al. Monitoring hippocampus electrical activity in vitro on an elastically deformable microelectrode array. J Neurotrauma 2009;26(7):1135–45.
84. Murphy EJ, Horrocks LA. A model for compression trauma: pressure-induced injury in cell cultures. J Neurotrauma 1993;10(4):431–44.
85. Panizzon KL, Shin D, Frautschy S, et al. Neuroprotection with Bcl-2(20-34) peptide against trauma. Neuroreport 1998;9(18):4131–6.
86. Girard J, Panizzon K, Wallis RA. Azelastine protects against CA1 traumatic neuronal injury in the hippocampal slice. Eur J Pharmacol 1996;300(1–2):43–9.
87. Wallis RA, Panizzon KL, Girard JM. Traumatic neuroprotection with inhibitors of nitric oxide and ADP-ribosylation. Brain Res 1996;710(1–2):169–77.
88. Panizzon KL, Dwyer BE, Nishimura RN, et al. Neuroprotection against CA1 injury with metalloporphyrins. Neuroreport 1996;7(2):662–6.

89. Wallis RA, Panizzon KL. Felbamate neuroprotection against CA1 traumatic neuronal injury. Eur J Pharmacol 1995;294(2–3):475–82.
90. Lucas JH, Wolf A. In vitro studies of multiple impact injury to mammalian CNS neurons: prevention of perikaryal damage and death by ketamine. Brain Res 1991;543(2):181–93.
91. Kiraly M, Kiraly SJ. Traumatic brain injury and delayed sequelae: a review—traumatic brain injury and mild traumatic brain injury (concussion) are precursors to later-onset brain disorders, including early-onset dementia. ScientificWorldJournal 2007;7:1768–76.
92. Guskiewicz KM, Marshall SW, Bailes J, et al. Association between recurrent concussion and late-life cognitive impairment in retired professional football players. Neurosurgery 2005;57(4):719–26 [discussion: 719–26].
93. Stern MB. Head trauma as a risk factor for Parkinson's disease. Mov Disord 1991; 6(2):95–7.
94. Viano DC, Casson IR, Pellman EJ. Concussion in professional football: biomechanics of the struck player–part 14. Neurosurgery 2007;61(2):313–27 [discussion: 327–8].
95. Pellman EJ, Viano DC, Tucker AM, et al. Concussion in professional football: location and direction of helmet impacts-Part 2. Neurosurgery 2003;53(6):1328–40 [discussion: 1340–1].
96. Manoogian S, McNeely D, Duma S, et al. Head acceleration is less than 10 percent of helmet acceleration in football impacts. Biomed Sci Instrum 2006; 42:383–8.
97. Brolinson PG, Manoogian S, McNeely D, et al. Analysis of linear head accelerations from collegiate football impacts. Curr Sports Med Rep 2006;5(1):23–8.
98. Duma SM, Manoogian SJ, Bussone WR, et al. Analysis of real-time head accelerations in collegiate football players. Clin J Sport Med 2005;15(1):3–8.

The Molecular Pathophysiology of Concussive Brain Injury

Garni Barkhoudarian, MD[a,*], David A. Hovda, PhD[b,c,d],
Christopher C. Giza, MD[e,f,g]

KEYWORDS

- Concussion • Traumatic brain injury • Pathophysiology
- Molecular mechanisms

Concussion (or mild traumatic brain injury, mTBI) is a biomechanically induced neurological injury, resulting in an alteration of mental status, such as confusion or amnesia, which may or may not involve a loss of consciousness.[1] Concussion affects about 1.6 million to 3.8 million athletes yearly, most commonly in contact sports such as American football and boxing.[2,3] Early clinical effects of concussion include but are

This work was supported by: NS057420, NS27544, NS058489 and by the UCLA Brain Injury Research Center.

These authors have nothing to disclose.

[a] Department of Neurosurgery, David Geffen School of Medicine at UCLA, 10833 Le Conte Boulevard, Los Angeles, CA 90095, USA

[b] Department of Neurosurgery, UCLA Brain Injury Research Center, Semel Institute, David Geffen School of Medicine at UCLA, Room 18-228A, 10833 Le Conte Boulevard, Los Angeles, CA 90095, USA

[c] Department of Medical and Molecular Pharmacology, UCLA Brain Injury Research Center, Semel Institute, David Geffen School of Medicine at UCLA, Room 18-228A, 10833 Le Conte Boulevard, Los Angeles, CA 90095, USA

[d] Interdepartmental Program for Neuroscience, UCLA Brain Injury Research Center, Semel Institute, David Geffen School of Medicine at UCLA, 10833 Le Conte Boulevard, Los Angeles, CA 90095, USA

[e] Department of Neurosurgery, UCLA Brain Injury Research Center, Semel Institute, David Geffen School of Medicine at UCLA, Mattel Children's Hospital–UCLA, Room 18-218B, 10833 Le Conte Boulevard, Los Angeles, CA 90095, USA

[f] Division of Pediatric Neurology, Department of Pediatrics, UCLA Brain Injury Research Center, Semel Institute, David Geffen School of Medicine at UCLA, Mattel Children's Hospital–UCLA, Room 18-218B, 10833 Le Conte Boulevard, Los Angeles, CA 90095, USA

[g] Interdepartmental Programs for Neuroscience and Biomedical Engineering, UCLA Brain Injury Research Center, Semel Institute, David Geffen School of Medicine at UCLA, Mattel Children's Hospital–UCLA, 10833 Le Conte Boulevard, Los Angeles, CA 90095, USA

* Corresponding author.

E-mail address: gbarkhoudarian@mednet.ucla.edu

Clin Sports Med 30 (2011) 33–48

doi:10.1016/j.csm.2010.09.001

0278-5919/11/$ – see front matter. Published by Elsevier Inc.

sportsmed.theclinics.com

not limited to behavioral changes, impairments of memory and attention, headache, unsteadiness, and rarely, catastrophic severe brain injury (sometimes described as second impact syndrome). More recently, the consequences of repetitive mTBI from multiple concussions in a sports setting are becoming evident. Repeated concussions have been associated with greater severity of symptoms, with longer recovery time, and chronically with earlier onset of age-related memory disturbances and dementia. As a result and in contradistinction to the decades-earlier perception that these injuries were benign, sports medicine professionals are now increasingly being instructed to recognize and manage concussions as soon as they occur.

Over a decade ago, the American Association of Neurology developed a grading system to help diagnose and treat concussions.[4] Early symptoms (minutes to hours) include headaches, dizziness, nausea, vomiting, and lack of awareness. Later symptoms (days to weeks) include persistent headaches, sleep disturbance, diminished concentration and attention, memory dysfunction, and irritability. The ability to recognize mTBI and prevent a second, possibly more severe injury, is key in the algorithm; however, the algorithm was based more on expert consensus than on evidence-based medicine and is currently being revised and updated to reflect ever-accumulating data. Many other groups have provided guidelines or recommendations as to the identification and/or management of sports-related concussions, with the Concussion in Sport Group (CiSG) consensus statements being, perhaps, the most widely used.[5] The CiSG statements have been updated twice since 2001 (in 2005 and in 2009) and reflect both the current published literature as well as the consensus of many recognized experts in the field. The CiSG statements focus less on attempting to grade concussion severity and more on controlling the timing of an athlete's return to play based on the presence or absence of symptoms or demonstrable neuropsychological impairments.

Although clinical studies have focused predominantly on descriptive or observational investigations into qualitative symptoms or semiquantitative analysis of cognitive impairments, important elements of the underlying pathophysiology of mTBI or concussion have been delineated through experimental models. There are several different experimental models of mTBI or concussion, mostly using rodents, such as mice and rats. Some of the most frequently used techniques are closed-skull weight drop,[6,7] closed-skull controlled impact,[8,9] and lateral fluid percussion injury (FPI).[10,11] These experimental paradigms can provide clinically relevant mechanistic insights and are helpful to characterize molecular alterations, ionic and neurotransmitter disturbances, synaptic perturbations, and structural changes. More recent technology such as high-resolution magnetic resonance imaging (MRI) has allowed for real-time imaging of structural and molecular changes without killing the animal. Imaging findings in these animals can be used to delineate pathophysiologic mechanisms that may then be correlated with imaging studies in humans. The translational capability of this technology is evident and has begun to show utility in allowing for a faster bench-to-bedside research approach.[7,8,12–14] Recent human studies of traumatic brain injury (TBI) include using structural and functional MRI to further understand axonal disruption, molecular disturbances, and the time course of these changes.[15] More invasive techniques include microdialysis analysis of the injured brain as well as histopathologic evaluation while operating for TBI.[16,17] The application of advanced imaging is endless, with exciting research opportunities presenting regularly.

NEUROMETABOLIC CASCADE OF CONCUSSION

Immediately after a mechanical trauma to the brain, acceleration and deceleration forces initiate a complex cascade of neurochemical and neurometabolic events.

These events begin with a disruption of the neuronal cell membranes and axonal stretching, causing indiscriminate flux of ions through previously regulated ion channels and probably transient physical membrane defects.[18] This process then causes widespread release of a multitude of neurotransmitters, particularly excitatory amino acids (EAAs),[19,20] resulting in further ionic flux. The Na$^+$/K$^+$ ATP-dependent pump then works at maximal capacities to reestablish ionic balance, depleting energy stores (**Fig. 1**). These molecular cascades may result in subsequent cerebral hypofunction or permanent damage.[21,22] In the setting of a single mTBI or concussion, it is considered that these changes are generally self-limited and transient, although there is evidence that repeat injuries may result in a more lasting pathobiologic condition.

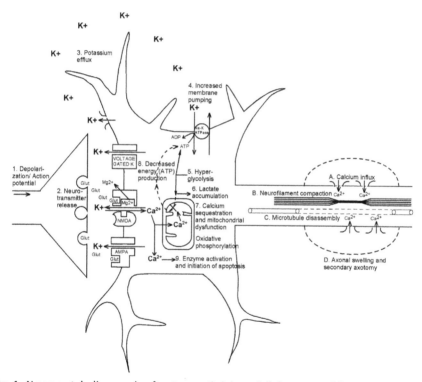

Fig. 1. Neurometabolic cascade after traumatic injury. Cellular events: (1) nonspecific depolarization and initiation of action potentials, (2) release of excitatory neurotransmitters (EAAs), (3) massive efflux of potassium, (4) increased activity of membrane ionic pumps to restore homeostasis, (5) hyperglycolysis to generate more ATP, (6) lactate accumulation, (7) calcium influx and sequestration in mitochondria, leading to impaired oxidative metabolism, (8) decreased energy (ATP) production, (9) calpain activation and initiation of apoptosis. Axonal events: (A) axolemmal disruption and calcium influx, (B) neurofilament compaction via phosphorylation or sidearm cleavage, (C) microtubule disassembly and accumulation of axonally transported organelles, (D) axonal swelling and eventual axotomy. AMPA, D-amino-3-hydroxy-5-methyl-4-isoxazolepropionic acid; Glut, glutamate; NMDA, N-methyl-D-aspartate. (*From* Giza CC, Hovda DA. The neurometabolic cascade of concussion. J Athl Train 2001;36(3):230.)

GLUTAMATE RELEASE AND IONIC FLUX

After a biomechanical injury to the brain, the neuronal membrane deforms, resulting in an excessive potassium efflux into the extracellular space. The same membrane deformity results in indiscriminate release of EAAs, particularly glutamate, that binds to the kainate, N-methyl-D-aspartate (NMDA), and D-amino-3-hydroxy-5-methyl-4-isoxazolepropionic acid (AMPA) ionic channels. NMDA receptor activation in particular causes further depolarization and influx of calcium ions. These ionic perturbations are mediated predominantly through NMDA receptors (NMDARs) because these effects are resistant to tetrodotoxin application but are attenuated by kynurenic acid (an NMDAR antagonist).[20] The resulting depolarization results in a widespread relative suppression of neurons, creating a condition resembling spreading depression.[23-25] The pathophysiology of spreading depression was originally described by Leao and has been proposed as an underlying mechanism for migraine; however, it may also be implicated in seizures and was more recently implicated with secondary neural injury after more severe TBI.[26-29]

To restore the ionic balance, ATP-dependent Na^+/K^+ pumps are activated, requiring high levels of glucose metabolism, most of which is conducted aerobically under normal conditions. After injury, however, ionic pump activation quickly reduces intracellular energy stores and causes the neurons to work overtime via rapid, but inefficient, glycolysis. This increase in glucose metabolism occurs immediately and may last from 30 minutes to 4 hours after an experimental TBI in rats.[22] Concurrently, oxidative metabolism is disrupted, likely from mitochondrial dysfunction.[30,31] Lactate production is rampant and this results in its extracellular accumulation.[32] Lactate accumulation can contribute to local acidosis, increased membrane permeability, and cerebral edema.[33] Lactate may also be used as an energy source by neurons, once mitochondrial function resumes.[34-36]

GLUCOSE METABOLISM AND MITOCHONDRIAL EFFECTS

After a concussive injury, 2 major alterations of glucose metabolism have been described, hyperglycolysis and oxidative dysfunction. Local cerebral metabolic rates for glucose are increased within the first 30 minutes after a lateral FPI, up to 30% to 46% above control levels.[21,22,37-39] After 6 hours, there is a relative glucose hypometabolism (approximately 50%, depending on the brain region) that can last up to 5 days. A similar profile of hyperglycolysis followed by glucose hypometabolism has been reported based on fluorodeoxyglucose F 18–positron emission tomography measurements after a TBI in humans. The duration of late hypometabolism may last months after a moderate to severe TBI.[40] Post-TBI hypometabolism is believed to recover more rapidly after milder injuries, although short-duration, longitudinal, within-subject positron emission tomographic studies have not yet been conducted in patients with concussions.

Activation of NMDA channels after concussive brain injury results in a significant influx of Ca^{++} which then accumulates in mitochondria, causing concomitant glucose oxidative dysfunction.[30,31,41,42] Molecular metabolic biomarkers such as ATP/ADP ratio, $NADH/NAD^+$ ratio, and N-acetylaspartate (NAA) levels were all decreased after repeat mTBI in rats.[7] This decrease was maximal for injuries with an interval of 3 days. Cytochrome oxidase expression, a marker of mitochondrial oxidative function, is downregulated after FPI. This enzyme activity, as determined by histochemistry, is decreased out to 10 days.[43]

This combination of cellular ionic disturbances, decreased cerebral blood flow (CBF), and glucose metabolic dysfunction has been hypothesized to set the stage for more severe brain injury after a repeated concussion, described clinically as the second impact syndrome.[44] However, definitive description of this clinical entity has been controversial,[5] and the role of glucose hypometabolism on brain injury has not yet been determined to be protective or exacerbating after a second insult.[45]

Alternative energy sources may be used by neuronal cells in the uninjured brain, as well as after injury. However, recent studies in rats noted a decrease in creatine (Cr), creatine phosphate (CrP), NAA, and phosphatidylcholine levels and in ATP/ADP ratio after a mTBI. The decreased NAA/Cr ratios were confirmed on magnetic resonance spectroscopy (MRS) in concussed athletes.[46] A more recent study further suggests that the Cr/CrP system is not a useful source of ATP for the injured brain.[47]

Ketone bodies have been known to be an alternative fuel source for the body during times of stress or starvation. Emerging data suggest that although glucose metabolism is perturbed after a concussive TBI, glucose may not be the best fuel for the injured brain.[48] Rats that were in ketosis or had a ketogenic diet demonstrated decreased glucose metabolism in an age-dependent fashion.[14] Subsequent studies suggest that cerebral contusion volume and behavioral outcomes improve with a ketogenic diet.[49–51] Ketosis induced by fasting may be most applicable in the first 24 hours after a moderate, but not severe, TBI.[52] The neuroprotective implications of ketosis after mTBI have yet to be investigated systematically.

CBF

The effects of severe TBI on CBF are well characterized,[53] although there is ongoing debate about the degree of post-TBI ischemia.[17,54] Based on inpatient studies of cerebral arteriovenous delivery of oxygen, cerebral metabolic oxygen consumption, and vasospasm (measured by transcranial Doppler ultrasonography), there seems to be a triphasic response to severe TBI. On postinjury day 0, there is cerebral hypoperfusion with an average CBF of 32.3 mL/100 g/min. During postinjury days 1 to 3, there is cerebral hyperemia with an average CBF of 46.8 mL/100 g/min and elevated middle cerebral artery velocities (86 cm/s). Subsequently, during postinjury days 4 to 15, there is a period of cerebral vasospasm with decreased CBF of 35.7 mL/100 g/min and elevated middle cerebral artery velocities (96.7 cm/s).[53] This triphasic response may occur in mTBI to a lesser extent; however, this has not yet been well studied.

Animal studies confirm the presence of cerebral edema in some models or severities of TBI. Perilesional edema in the ipsilateral hippocampus is viewed via MRI for 4 days after severe experimental TBI (cortical impact). The edema gradually recovered over the next 2 weeks and its recovery correlated with the neuroscore (a behavioral scale of neurologic function).[55] Restricted diffusion and reduced CBF were reported in the first few hours after a milder experimental injury (FPI),[56] but no major imaging abnormalities were observed after a weight-drop injury that induced cognitive symptoms without overt histopathologic findings.[57]

AXONAL INJURY

Diffuse axonal injury, also termed traumatic axonal injury, is a well-described phenomenon that occurs after severe blunt head injury. The mechanical stretching of the axonal cell membranes has a multitude of effects including ionic flux and diffuse depolarization, calcium influx and mitochondrial swelling,[58,59] and neurofilament compaction. Neurofilament compaction can occur in the acute phase (5 minutes–6 hours) by either phosphorylation or calpain-mediated proteolysis of sidearms.[60–63] From 6 to 24 hours postinjury, the calcium influx can also destabilize the microtubules.[64,65] These pathophysiologic processes have been shown to interfere with axonal transport, resulting in axonal blebbing and eventual disconnection.[65–67]

Although traumatic axonal injury has been best described after severe TBI, there is some evidence that it also occurs, perhaps reversibly, after mTBI. Molecular studies in mice evaluating cell body, myelin integrity, and axonal damage (via amyloid precursor protein) after mTBI suggest predominant damage at the axonal level, with minimal effect to the neuronal cell bodies or myelin sheaths.[68] This axonal damage was found to progress through various cortical and subcortical structures over 4 to 6 weeks, and this effect correlated with impaired navigation in the Morris water maze (MWM) test, a sign of spatial learning and memory deficits.

Advances in neuroimaging studies, using high-resolution (3-tesla) MRI and diffusion tensor imaging (DTI) sequences, have confirmed axonal damage in mTBI in humans. Axonal damage has been demonstrated in pediatric, adolescent, and adult patients after mTBI/concussion and, in some cases, was correlated with subtle findings of cognitive deficits.[69–71] Fractional anisotropy (FA), a measure of linear water diffusion, decreases when directionality of white matter tracts is disturbed, as might occur after axonal disconnection or damage to myelin sheaths.[72,73] Increase in FA values occurs with ongoing developmental myelination, but after injury, the increase has been hypothesized to be related to transient axonal swelling.[70]

FA value is decreased in white matter subcortical regions (inferior frontal, superior frontal, and supracallosal) but unchanged in the corpus callosum in pediatric TBI patients.[74] Motor speed, executive function, and behavioral ratings showed a correlation with these findings.

Decreases in FA values are also seen chronically after mTBI in adults, affecting regions such as the genu of the corpus callosum, the cingulum, the anterior corona radiata, and the uncinate fasciculus (Fig. 2). In this study, there was a direct correlation between decreased FA values in specific white matter structures and specific cognitive deficits.[75]

Corpus callosal findings of increased FA values were seen in the adolescent brain early (6 days) after mTBI. These findings correlated with postconcussive symptoms confirmed by cognitive, affective, and somatic scores on the Rivermead Post-Concussion Symptoms Questionnaire and the Brief Symptom Inventory.[70] The increased FA was hypothesized to be indicative of axonal swelling in the early post-concussive phase, and is in distinction to other more chronic studies showing reduced FA.

These studies suggest that DTI of axonal injury is a sensitive and effective measure of the effects from mTBI. Future research in this field is necessary to further understand the relationship between altered FA, cognition, and axonal pathophysiology.

ALTERED BRAIN ACTIVATION

Calcium regulation after TBI depends on various factors including membrane permeability, excitatory neurotransmitter release, and glutamate receptor modulation. The NMDAR is especially interesting because it requires 2 signals to be activated: membrane voltage change and glutamate binding. The voltage change releases a Mg^{++} ion within its working channel and glutamate binding then allows calcium flux into the neuron. The channel is a tetramer consisting of 2 NR1 subunits and 2 NR2 subunits. During development, there is a shift from NR2B (slower channels) predominant expression to NR2A (faster channels) predominant expression in the rat brain.[76]

After lateral FPI in pediatric (postnatal day 19) rats, the relative expression of the NR2A subunit is downregulated by postinjury days 2 to 4.[10] This downregulation

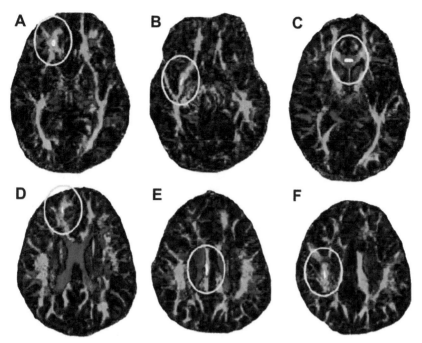

Fig. 2. Region of interest (ROI) placement for DTI. Shown are the corresponding ROIs for the right hemisphere. The solid ellipse within yellow outline indicates the location and size of the ROI. (A) uncinate fasciculus, (B) inferior longitudinal fasciculus, (C) genu of corpus callosum, (D) anterior corona radiata, (E) cingulum bundle, and (F) superior longitudinal fasciculus. (From Niogi, Mukherjee P, Ghajar J, et al. Structural dissociation of attentional control and memory in adults with and without mild traumatic brain injury. Brain 2008;131:3212.)

returns to normal by postinjury day 7. There is no apparent change in NR2B or NR1 subunit expression, suggesting a possible intrinsic neuroprotective mechanism of calcium ion regulation after TBI.

The NMDA channels have a strong association with learning, specifically long-term potentiation (LTP) and long-term depression.[77,78] Not surprisingly, after an experimental TBI, LTP induction is impaired at postinjury day 2 but seems to recover by postinjury days 7 through 15.[79,80] However, maintenance of LTP deficient up to 8 weeks postinjury.[81]

Clinically, after concussion patients can demonstrate cognitive deficits associated with abnormal activation of neural circuits. Blood oxygen level–dependent sequences obtained in functional MRI before and after cognitive tasks demonstrate a hyperactivation in the postconcussive brain at week 1 (**Fig. 3**).[82] When abnormal activation is seen after a concussive brain injury, the affected athletes seem to have a more prolonged clinical recovery.[83,84]

ACUTE RESPONSES TO REPEAT CONCUSSION

Aside from the acute effects of concussion and the subjective and objective symptoms that limit the patient, a major concern for return to activity is the second impact syndrome.[44,85,86] This syndrome is a catastrophic cerebral edema after an apparent mTBI/concussion. It results in coma and severe neurologic deficits and is often fatal.

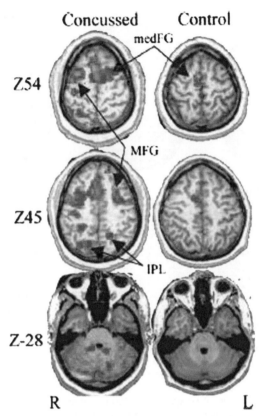

Fig. 3. Representative individual z score differences between baseline and either a postconcussion session (concussed, left) or postseason baseline sessions (control, right). Colored areas show regions of activity that significantly increased from the baseline value of the bimanual sequencing task. Although both concussed and control subjects demonstrate some increases in region of activity, those of the concussed players are considerably larger. Activity is significantly increased in the medial frontal gyrus (medFG), middle frontal gyrus (MFG), inferior parietal lobe (IPL), and bilateral cerebellum. (*From* Jantzen Anderson B, Steinberg FL, et al. A prospective functional MR imaging study of mild traumatic brain injury in college football players. AJNR Am J Neuroradiol 2004;25(5):741.)

Although the clinical consequences of individual concussions have been described in some detail, the predictive factors and the interval for return to activity are still heavily debated. Although avoiding possible second impact syndrome is the more dramatic rationale put forth for delaying return to play, the stronger argument may simply be that cerebral physiologic conditions are disturbed after concussion and this physiologic disturbance renders the brain less functional and more vulnerable. In other words, concussion-induced pathophysiologic conditions, as manifested by metabolic perturbations, altered blood flow, axonal injury, and abnormal neural activation, reduce cerebral performance and make the brain more susceptible to cellular injury. Several animal studies focusing on mTBI-induced dysfunction have been described, and current data support the concept of transient metabolic and physiologic vulnerabilities that may be exacerbated by repeated mild injuries within specific time windows of impairment.[7,8,87]

As described in the previous sections, the concussed brain acutely experiences significant alterations in ionic balance, neurotransmitter activation, axonal integrity, and energy metabolism. Logically, a patient with such a metabolically stressed state is ready neither for optimal performance nor to sustain a second injury. Vagnozzi and colleagues[6] demonstrated in a rat weight drop experiment that levels of NAA and ATP and the ATP/ADP ratio decreased significantly when measured 2 days after repeat concussion. Maximal metabolic abnormalities were seen when the occurrence of 2 mild injuries were separated by a 3-day interval; in fact, the metabolic abnormalities in these animals were similar to those occurring after a single severe experimental TBI. In a follow-up study, similar perturbations were found to persist as late as 7 days after double impact, indicating prolonged metabolic effects from repeat mTBI in this model.[7]

The metabolites analyzed are a reflection of the energy status of the brain, particularly the reductive capacity of the mitochondria. Other markers of impaired reductive capacity include the lactate/pyruvate ratio. This ratio is commonly measured and is found to be increased in patients with severe TBI.[17,88] Therefore, a significant contributor to acute TBI and its susceptibility for repeat injury is likely mitochondrial dysfunction.

Clinically, markers for this altered metabolism are observed using MRS in athletes with concussions.[46] Thirteen athletes who sustained concussions were studied with 3-tesla MRS at specific postinjury time points. The NAA/Cr ratio of injured patients versus age-matched control patients was diminished by 18.5% (1.8 vs 2.2, $P<.05$) at 3 days postinjury. This ratio improved but was still low at 15 days (1.88) and was back to control values by 30 days postinjury. Interestingly, 3 patients sustained a repeat concussion 3 to 15 days after their initial injury. These patients had a similar initial decrease in their NAA/CA ratio (1.78) but had further decrease at 15 days (1.72) rather than a partial resolution. These ratios took 45 days to resume to control levels. The patients who sustained a single concussion reported no symptoms during the 3-day study, whereas the patients who sustained double concussions stated the same at the 30-day time point. However, no standardized symptom assessments or questionnaires were administered and no symptom assessment was conducted at intermediate time points. These findings have recently been reported in a larger cohort of concussed athletes in a multicenter study.[89]

Axonal damage occurs concurrently after experimental mTBI. Interestingly, this effect is amplified with repeat mTBI.[9,90] A repeat-concussion animal model with a 3-day interval between injuries demonstrated a significant increase in cytoskeletal damage and axonal injury.[8] As mentioned earlier, white matter abnormalities have been described using DTI after mTBI in humans[69,70,91]; although these findings are not universal,[92,93] there are no specific human studies of DTI conducted early after repeated concussive injuries.

Behavioral deficits are a chronic difficulty in a subset of patients postconcussion. Acutely, animal studies have shown that repeat mTBI induces spatial memory deficits in tests such as the MWM and these impairments are related to the impact severity and the number and timing of repeated injuries.[9,12,94] In the National Collegiate Athletic Association concussion study, athletes who sustained repeat concussions (3 or more) were at a higher risk of an additional concussion. More importantly, a larger proportion of multiple-concussed athletes these had a significantly longer duration of postconcussive symptoms than those with only 1 concussion (30% vs 14.6%).[2]

POTENTIAL FOR CUMULATIVE INJURY AND CHRONIC SEQUELAE

Chronically, multiple concussions have been associated with cumulative effects on cerebral function and cognition, including early onset of memory disturbances and even dementia. Molecular markers associated with this decline in function include amyloid and tau protein deposition, presence of apolipoprotein E-4 allele (ApoE-4), and overall structural damage, particularly axonal injury.

In transgenic mice overexpressing human amyloid precursor protein, repetitive mTBI resulted in significant deposition of amyloid-β peptide (Aβ) and isoprostanes. There was an associated increased latency in the MWM test for these transgenic injured animals.[95] Others have shown increased hippocampal cell death after injury, with concomitant Aβ deposition.[96,97]

More recently, tau protein deposition has been described in chronic traumatic encephalopathy, demonstrated on brain histopathology in autopsies from boxers, football players, and other contact sport athletes. Immunohistochemistry demonstrates neurofibrillary tangles and neuritic threads consistent with a generalized tauopathy.[98–100] Multiple animal studies also show TBI-induced abnormalities in tau and other cytoskeletal proteins.[101–104]

Apolipoprotein E subtypes have been associated with different risks of posttraumatic cognitive disturbances and dementia. Specifically, the ApoE-4 allele is linked with the development of clinical signs and symptoms of chronic traumatic encephalopathy.[105] In boxers who sustain chronic TBI, there is a correlation with increased cognitive deficits, the number of boxing matches, and the ApoE-4 allele. Particularly, all patients with severe impairment as measured by the chronic brain injury scale have at least one ApoE-4 allele.[106] Animal models of Alzheimer disease used in TBI experiments reflect this link, with ApoE-4 transgenic mice developing more diffuse plaques than controls.[107] This finding has yet to be proven in repeat TBI animal models.

Similarly, chronic TBI has a lasting effect on axonal integrity. Professional boxers demonstrate evidence of increased axonal injury via DTI. FA and whole brain diffusion coefficients are significantly altered in boxers compared with nonboxers.[108] This finding has not yet been confirmed in chronic TBI animal models.

In long-term studies of professional football players, there is an increased incidence of cognitive deficits and early Alzheimer disease development. In addition, there are behavioral findings including early depression. This finding was significantly associated in players who had sustained 3 or more cumulative concussions.[109,110]

SUMMARY

Concussion, or mTBI, has both acute and chronic consequences on the brain. After concussion, there is a cascade of molecular changes in the brain that affect performance acutely and increase vulnerability for repeat injury. Repeat brain injury causes a multitude of cerebral deficits that are studied clinically, histopathologically, and by neuroimaging. These effects can be long-lasting and potentially debilitating. Prevention of single and repeat concussions should be the goal of athletes and their physicians, whether amateur or professional. Following a concussion, adequate time for physiological recovery should be allowed to minimize the risk of recurrent injury or development of cumulative impairments.

REFERENCES

1. Kelly JP, Nichols JS, Filley CM, et al. Concussion in sports. Guidelines for the prevention of catastrophic outcome. JAMA 1991;266(20):2867–9.
2. Guskiewicz KM, McCrea M, Marshall SW, et al. Cumulative effects associated with recurrent concussion in collegiate football players: the NCAA Concussion Study. JAMA 2003;290(19):2549–55.

3. Langlois JA, Rutland-Brown W, Wald MM. The epidemiology and impact of traumatic brain injury: a brief overview. J Head Trauma Rehabil 2006;21(5): 375–8.
4. Practice parameter: the management of concussion in sports (summary statement). Report of the Quality Standards Subcommittee. Neurology 1997;48(3):581–5.
5. McCrory P, Meeuwisse W, Johnston K, et al. Consensus Statement on Concussion in Sport: the 3rd International Conference on Concussion in Sport held in Zurich, November 2008. Br J Sports Med 2009;43(Suppl 1):i76–90.
6. Vagnozzi R, Signoretti S, Tavazzi B, et al. Hypothesis of the postconcussive vulnerable brain: experimental evidence of its metabolic occurrence. Neurosurgery 2005;57(1):164–71 [discussion: 164–71].
7. Vagnozzi R, Tavazzi B, Signoretti S, et al. Temporal window of metabolic brain vulnerability to concussions: mitochondrial-related impairment–part I. Neurosurgery 2007;61(2):379–88 [discussion: 88–9].
8. Longhi L, Saatman KE, Fujimoto S, et al. Temporal window of vulnerability to repetitive experimental concussive brain injury. Neurosurgery 2005;56(2): 364–74 [discussion: 364–74].
9. Prins ML, Hales A, Reger ML, et al. Repeat traumatic brain injury in the juvenile rat is associated with increased axonal injury and cognitive impairments. Dev Neurosci 2010;32(4).
10. Giza CC, Maria NS, Hovda DA. N-methyl-D-aspartate receptor subunit changes after traumatic injury to the developing brain. J Neurotrauma 2006;23(6): 950–61.
11. Gurkoff GG, Giza CC, Shin D, et al. Acute neuroprotection to pilocarpine-induced seizures is not sustained after traumatic brain injury in the developing rat. Neuroscience 2009;164(2):862–76.
12. DeFord SM, Wilson MS, Rice AC, et al. Repeated mild brain injuries result in cognitive impairment in B6C3F1 mice. J Neurotrauma 2002;19(4):427–38.
13. Henninger N, Sicard KM, Li Z, et al. Differential recovery of behavioral status and brain function assessed with functional magnetic resonance imaging after mild traumatic brain injury in the rat. Crit Care Med 2007;35(11):2607–14.
14. Prins ML, Hovda DA. The effects of age and ketogenic diet on local cerebral metabolic rates of glucose after controlled cortical impact injury in rats. J Neurotrauma 2009;26(7):1083–93.
15. Difiori JP, Giza CC. New techniques in concussion imaging. Curr Sports Med Rep 2010;9(1):35–9.
16. Hillered L, Vespa PM, Hovda DA. Translational neurochemical research in acute human brain injury: the current status and potential future for cerebral microdialysis. J Neurotrauma 2005;22(1):3–41.
17. Vespa P, Bergsneider M, Hattori N, et al. Metabolic crisis without brain ischemia is common after traumatic brain injury: a combined microdialysis and positron emission tomography study. J Cereb Blood Flow Metab 2005;25(6):763–74.
18. Farkas O, Lifshitz J, Povlishock JT. Mechanoporation induced by diffuse traumatic brain injury: an irreversible or reversible response to injury? J Neurosci 2006;26(12):3130–40.
19. Faden AI, Demediuk P, Panter SS, et al. The role of excitatory amino acids and NMDA receptors in traumatic brain injury. Science (New York, NY) 1989; 244(4906):798–800.
20. Katayama Y, Becker DP, Tamura T, et al. Massive increases in extracellular potassium and the indiscriminate release of glutamate following concussive brain injury. J Neurosurg 1990;73(6):889–900.

21. Kawamata T, Katayama Y, Hovda DA, et al. Administration of excitatory amino acid antagonists via microdialysis attenuates the increase in glucose utilization seen following concussive brain injury. J Cereb Blood Flow Metab 1992;12(1):12–24.

22. Yoshino A, Hovda DA, Kawamata T, et al. Dynamic changes in local cerebral glucose utilization following cerebral conclusion in rats: evidence of a hyper- and subsequent hypometabolic state. Brain Res 1991;561(1):106–19.

23. Giza CC, Hovda DA. The neurometabolic cascade of concussion. J Athl Train 2001;36(3):228–35.

24. Kubota M, Nakamura T, Sunami K, et al. Changes of local cerebral glucose utilization, DC potential and extracellular potassium concentration in experimental head injury of varying severity. Neurosurg Rev 1989;12(Suppl 1):393–9.

25. Somjen GG, Giacchino JL. Potassium and calcium concentrations in interstitial fluid of hippocampal formation during paroxysmal responses. J Neurophysiol 1985;53(4):1098–108.

26. Fabricius M, Fuhr S, Willumsen L, et al. Association of seizures with cortical spreading depression and peri-infarct depolarisations in the acutely injured human brain. Clin Neurophysiol 2008;119(9):1973–84.

27. Hartings JA, Strong AJ, Fabricius M, et al. Spreading depolarizations and late secondary insults after traumatic brain injury. J Neurotrauma 2009;26(11): 1857–66.

28. Strong AJ, Fabricius M, Boutelle MG, et al. Spreading and synchronous depressions of cortical activity in acutely injured human brain. Stroke 2002;33(12):2738–43.

29. Leao AA. Further observations on the spreading depression of activity in the cerebral cortex. J Neurophysiol 1947;10(6):409–14.

30. Verweij BH, Muizelaar JP, Vinas FC, et al. Mitochondrial dysfunction after experimental and human brain injury and its possible reversal with a selective N-type calcium channel antagonist (SNX-111). Neurol Res 1997;19(3):334–9.

31. Xiong Y, Gu Q, Peterson PL, et al. Mitochondrial dysfunction and calcium perturbation induced by traumatic brain injury. J Neurotrauma 1997;14(1):23–34.

32. Kawamata T, Katayama Y, Hovda DA, et al. Lactate accumulation following concussive brain injury: the role of ionic fluxes induced by excitatory amino acids. Brain Res 1995;674(2):196–204.

33. Kalimo H, Rehncrona S, Soderfeldt B. The role of lactic acidosis in the ischemic nerve cell injury. Acta Neuropathol Suppl 1981;7:20–2.

34. Magistretti PJ, Pellerin L. Cellular mechanisms of brain energy metabolism and their relevance to functional brain imaging. Philos Trans R Soc Lond B Biol Sci 1999;354(1387):1155–63.

35. Schurr A, Payne RS. Lactate, not pyruvate, is neuronal aerobic glycolysis end product: an in vitro electrophysiological study. Neuroscience 2007;147(3):613–9.

36. Tsacopoulos M, Magistretti PJ. Metabolic coupling between glia and neurons. J Neurosci 1996;16(3):877–85.

37. Andersen BJ, Marmarou A. Post-traumatic selective stimulation of glycolysis. Brain Res 1992;585(1–2):184–9.

38. Sunami K, Nakamura T, Ozawa Y, et al. Hypermetabolic state following experimental head injury. Neurosurg Rev 1989;12(Suppl 1):400–11.

39. Yoshino A, Hovda DA, Katayama Y, et al. Hippocampal CA3 lesion prevents postconcussive metabolic dysfunction in CA1. J Cereb Blood Flow Metab 1992;12(6):996–1006.

40. Bergsneider M, Hovda DA, Shalmon E, et al. Cerebral hyperglycolysis following severe traumatic brain injury in humans: a positron emission tomography study. J Neurosurg 1997;86(2):241–51.

41. Lifshitz J, Sullivan PG, Hovda DA, et al. Mitochondrial damage and dysfunction in traumatic brain injury. Mitochondrion 2004;4(5–6):705–13.

42. Robertson CL, Saraswati M, Fiskum G. Mitochondrial dysfunction early after traumatic brain injury in immature rats. J Neurochem 2007;101(5):1248–57.

43. Hovda DA, Yoshino A, Kawamata T, et al. Diffuse prolonged depression of cerebral oxidative metabolism following concussive brain injury in the rat: a cytochrome oxidase histochemistry study. Brain Res 1991;567(1):1–10.

44. Cantu RC. Second-impact syndrome. Clin Sports Med 1998;17(1):37–44.

45. McCrory PR, Berkovic SF. Second impact syndrome. Neurology 1998;50(3):677–83.

46. Vagnozzi R, Signoretti S, Tavazzi B, et al. Temporal window of metabolic brain vulnerability to concussion: a pilot 1H-magnetic resonance spectroscopic study in concussed athletes–part III. Neurosurgery 2008;62(6):1286–95 [discussion: 95–6].

47. Signoretti S, Di Pietro V, Vagnozzi R, et al. Transient alterations of creatine, creatine phosphate, N-acetylaspartate and high-energy phosphates after mild traumatic brain injury in the rat. Mol Cell Biochem 2010;333(1–2):269–77.

48. Prins ML, Giza CC. Induction of monocarboxylate transporter 2 expression and ketone transport following traumatic brain injury in juvenile and adult rats. Dev Neurosci 2006;28(4–5):447–56.

49. Appelberg KS, Hovda DA, Prins ML. The effects of a ketogenic diet on behavioral outcome after controlled cortical impact injury in the juvenile and adult rat. J Neurotrauma 2009;26(4):497–506.

50. Arun P, Ariyannur PS, Moffett JR, et al. Metabolic acetate therapy for the treatment of traumatic brain injury. J Neurotrauma 2010;27(1):293–8.

51. Prins ML, Fujima LS, Hovda DA. Age-dependent reduction of cortical contusion volume by ketones after traumatic brain injury. J Neurosci Res 2005;82(3):413–20.

52. Davis LM, Pauly JR, Readnower RD, et al. Fasting is neuroprotective following traumatic brain injury. J Neurosci Res 2008;86(8):1812–22.

53. Martin NA, Patwardhan RV, Alexander MJ, et al. Characterization of cerebral hemodynamic phases following severe head trauma: hypoperfusion, hyperemia, and vasospasm. J Neurosurg 1997;87(1):9–19.

54. Coles JP, Fryer TD, Smielewski P, et al. Incidence and mechanisms of cerebral ischemia in early clinical head injury. J Cereb Blood Flow Metab 2004;24(2):202–11.

55. Immonen R, Heikkinen T, Tahtivaara L, et al. Cerebral blood volume alterations in the perilesional areas in the rat brain after traumatic brain injury-comparison with behavioral outcome. J Cereb Blood Flow Metab 2010;30(7):1318–28.

56. Pasco A, Lemaire L, Franconi F, et al. Perfusional deficit and the dynamics of cerebral edemas in experimental traumatic brain injury using perfusion and diffusion-weighted magnetic resonance imaging. J Neurotrauma 2007;24(8):1321–30.

57. Henninger N, Dutzmann S, Sicard KM, et al. Impaired spatial learning in a novel rat model of mild cerebral concussion injury. Exp Neurol 2005;195(2):447–57.

58. Mata M, Staple J, Fink DJ. Changes in intra-axonal calcium distribution following nerve crush. J Neurobiol 1986;17(5):449–67.

59. Maxwell WL, McCreath BJ, Graham DI, et al. Cytochemical evidence for redistribution of membrane pump calcium-ATPase and ecto-Ca-ATPase activity, and calcium influx in myelinated nerve fibres of the optic nerve after stretch injury. J Neurocytol 1995;24(12):925–42.

60. Johnson GV, Greenwood JA, Costello AC, et al. The regulatory role of calmodulin in the proteolysis of individual neurofilament proteins by calpain. Neurochem Res 1991;16(8):869–73.

61. Nakamura Y, Takeda M, Angelides KJ, et al. Effect of phosphorylation on 68 KDa neurofilament subunit protein assembly by the cyclic AMP dependent protein kinase in vitro. Biochem Biophys Res Commun 1990;169(2):744–50.

62. Nixon RA. The regulation of neurofilament protein dynamics by phosphorylation: clues to neurofibrillary pathobiology. Brain Pathol 1993;3(1):29–38.

63. Sternberger NH, Sternberger LA. Neurotypy: the heterogeneity of brain proteins. Ann N Y Acad Sci 1983;420:90–9.

64. Maxwell WL, Povlishock JT, Graham DL. A mechanistic analysis of nondisruptive axonal injury: a review. J Neurotrauma 1997;14(7):419–40.

65. Pettus EH, Povlishock JT. Characterization of a distinct set of intra-axonal ultrastructural changes associated with traumatically induced alteration in axolemmal permeability. Brain Res 1996;722(1–2):1–11.

66. Povlishock JT, Pettus EH. Traumatically induced axonal damage: evidence for enduring changes in axolemmal permeability with associated cytoskeletal change. Acta Neurochir Suppl 1996;66:81–6.

67. Saatman KE, Abai B, Grosvenor A, et al. Traumatic axonal injury results in biphasic calpain activation and retrograde transport impairment in mice. J Cereb Blood Flow Metab 2003;23(1):34–42.

68. Spain A, Daumas S, Lifshitz J, et al. Mild fluid percussion injury in mice produces evolving selective axonal pathology and cognitive deficits relevant to human brain injury. J Neurotrauma 2010;27(8):1429–38.

69. Niogi SN, Mukherjee P, Ghajar J, et al. Extent of microstructural white matter injury in postconcussive syndrome correlates with impaired cognitive reaction time: a 3T diffusion tensor imaging study of mild traumatic brain injury. AJNR Am J Neuroradiol 2008;29(5):967–73.

70. Wilde EA, McCauley SR, Hunter JV, et al. Diffusion tensor imaging of acute mild traumatic brain injury in adolescents. Neurology 2008;70(12):948–55.

71. Lipton ML, Gellella E, Lo C, et al. Multifocal white matter ultrastructural abnormalities in mild traumatic brain injury with cognitive disability: a voxel-wise analysis of diffusion tensor imaging. J Neurotrauma 2008;25(11):1335–42.

72. Mac Donald CL, Dikranian K, Bayly P, et al. Diffusion tensor imaging reliably detects experimental traumatic axonal injury and indicates approximate time of injury. J Neurosci 2007;27(44):11869–76.

73. Benson RR, Meda SA, Vasudevan S, et al. Global white matter analysis of diffusion tensor images is predictive of injury severity in traumatic brain injury. J Neurotrauma 2007;24(3):446–59.

74. Wozniak JR, Krach L, Ward E, et al. Neurocognitive and neuroimaging correlates of pediatric traumatic brain injury: a diffusion tensor imaging (DTI) study. Arch Clin Neuropsychol 2007;22(5):555–68.

75. Niogi SN, Mukherjee P, Ghajar J, et al. Structural dissociation of attentional control and memory in adults with and without mild traumatic brain injury. Brain 2008;131(Pt 12):3209–21.

76. Cull-Candy S, Brickley S, Farrant M. NMDA receptor subunits: diversity, development and disease. Curr Opin Neurobiol 2001;11(3):327–35.

77. Liu L, Wong TP, Pozza MF, et al. Role of NMDA receptor subtypes in governing the direction of hippocampal synaptic plasticity. Science (New York, NY) 2004; 304(5673):1021–4.

78. Tang YP, Wang H, Feng R, et al. Differential effects of enrichment on learning and memory function in NR2B transgenic mice. Neuropharmacology 2001; 41(6):779–90.

79. Reeves TM, Lyeth BG, Povlishock JT. Long-term potentiation deficits and excitability changes following traumatic brain injury. Exp Brain Res 1995;106(2): 248–56.

80. Sick TJ, Perez-Pinzon MA, Feng ZZ. Impaired expression of long-term potentiation in hippocampal slices 4 and 48 h following mild fluid-percussion brain injury in vivo. Brain Res 1998;785(2):287–92.

81. Sanders MJ, Sick TJ, Perez-Pinzon MA, et al. Chronic failure in the maintenance of long-term potentiation following fluid percussion injury in the rat. Brain Res 2000;861(1):69–76.

82. Jantzen KJ, Anderson B, Steinberg FL, et al. A prospective functional MR imaging study of mild traumatic brain injury in college football players. AJNR Am J Neuroradiol 2004;25(5):738–45.

83. Lovell MR, Pardini JE, Welling J, et al. Functional brain abnormalities are related to clinical recovery and time to return-to-play in athletes. Neurosurgery 2007; 61(2):352–9 [discussion: 359–60].

84. McAllister TW, Sparling MB, Flashman LA, et al. Neuroimaging findings in mild traumatic brain injury. J Clin Exp Neuropsychol 2001;23(6):775–91.

85. Kissick J, Johnston KM. Return to play after concussion: principles and practice. Clin J Sport Med 2005;15(6):426–31.

86. Putukian M. Repeat mild traumatic brain injury: how to adjust return to play guidelines. Curr Sports Med Rep 2006;5(1):15–22.

87. Tavazzi B, Vagnozzi R, Signoretti S, et al. Temporal window of metabolic brain vulnerability to concussions: oxidative and nitrosative stresses–part II. Neurosurgery 2007;61(2):390–5 [discussion: 395–6].

88. Vespa P, Boonyaputthikul R, McArthur DL, et al. Intensive insulin therapy reduces microdialysis glucose values without altering glucose utilization or improving the lactate/pyruvate ratio after traumatic brain injury. Crit Care Med 2006;34(3):850–6.

89. Vagnozzi R, Signoretti S, Cristofori L, et al. Assessment of metabolic brain damage and recovery following mild traumatic brain injury: a multicentre, proton magnetic resonance spectroscopic study in concussed patients. Brain 2010. [Epub ahead of print].

90. Laurer HL, Bareyre FM, Lee VM, et al. Mild head injury increasing the brain's vulnerability to a second concussive impact. J Neurosurg 2001;95(5):859–70.

91. Huang MX, Theilmann RJ, Robb A, et al. Integrated imaging approach with MEG and DTI to detect mild traumatic brain injury in military and civilian patients. J Neurotrauma 2009;26(8):1213–26.

92. Levin HS, Wilde E, Troyanskaya M, et al. Diffusion tensor imaging of mild to moderate blast-related traumatic brain injury and its sequelae. J Neurotrauma 2010;27(4):683–94.

93. Schrader H, Mickeviciene D, Gleizniene R, et al. Magnetic resonance imaging after most common form of concussion. BMC Med Imaging 2009;9:11.

94. DeRoss AL, Adams JE, Vane DW, et al. Multiple head injuries in rats: effects on behavior. J Trauma 2002;52(4):708–14.

95. Uryu K, Laurer H, McIntosh T, et al. Repetitive mild brain trauma accelerates Abeta deposition, lipid peroxidation, and cognitive impairment in a transgenic mouse model of Alzheimer amyloidosis. J Neurosci 2002;22(2):446–54.

96. Rabadi MH, Jordan BD. The cumulative effect of repetitive concussion in sports. Clin J Sport Med 2001;11(3):194–8.
97. Smith DH, Nakamura M, McIntosh TK, et al. Brain trauma induces massive hippocampal neuron death linked to a surge in beta-amyloid levels in mice overexpressing mutant amyloid precursor protein. Am J Pathol 1998;153(3):1005–10.
98. McKee AC, Cantu RC, Nowinski CJ, et al. Chronic traumatic encephalopathy in athletes: progressive tauopathy after repetitive head injury. J Neuropathol Exp Neurol 2009;68(7):709–35.
99. Omalu BI, Hamilton RL, Kamboh MI, et al. Chronic traumatic encephalopathy (CTE) in a National Football League Player: case report and emerging medicolegal practice questions. J Forensic Nurs 2010;6(1):40–6.
100. Smith C, Graham DI, Murray LS, et al. Tau immunohistochemistry in acute brain injury. Neuropathol Appl Neurobiol 2003;29(5):496–502.
101. Genis L, Chen Y, Shohami E, et al. Tau hyperphosphorylation in apolipoprotein E-deficient and control mice after closed head injury. J Neurosci Res 2000; 60(4):559–64.
102. Hoshino S, Tamaoka A, Takahashi M, et al. Emergence of immunoreactivities for phosphorylated tau and amyloid-beta protein in chronic stage of fluid percussion injury in rat brain. Neuroreport 1998;9(8):1879–83.
103. Kanayama G, Takeda M, Niigawa H, et al. The effects of repetitive mild brain injury on cytoskeletal protein and behavior. Methods Find Exp Clin Pharmacol 1996;18(2):105–15.
104. Smith DH, Chen XH, Nonaka M, et al. Accumulation of amyloid beta and tau and the formation of neurofilament inclusions following diffuse brain injury in the pig. J Neuropathol Exp Neurol 1999;58(9):982–92.
105. Jordan BD. Chronic traumatic brain injury associated with boxing. Semin Neurol 2000;20(2):179–85.
106. Jordan BD, Relkin NR, Ravdin LD, et al. Apolipoprotein E epsilon4 associated with chronic traumatic brain injury in boxing. JAMA 1997;278(2):136–40.
107. Hartman RE, Laurer H, Longhi L, et al. Apolipoprotein E4 influences amyloid deposition but not cell loss after traumatic brain injury in a mouse model of Alzheimer's disease. J Neurosci 2002;22(23):10083–7.
108. Zhang L, Heier LA, Zimmerman RD, et al. Diffusion anisotropy changes in the brains of professional boxers. AJNR Am J Neuroradiol 2006;27(9):2000–4.
109. Guskiewicz KM, Marshall SW, Bailes J, et al. Association between recurrent concussion and late-life cognitive impairment in retired professional football players. Neurosurgery 2005;57(4):719–26 [discussion: 719–26].
110. Guskiewicz KM, Marshall SW, Bailes J, et al. Recurrent concussion and risk of depression in retired professional football players. Med Sci Sports Exerc 2007;39(6):903–9.

The Acute Symptoms of Sport-Related Concussion: Diagnosis and On-field Management

Margot Putukian, MD[a,b,*]

KEYWORDS

- Sport-related concussion • Sideline management
- Concussion protocol • Symptoms • Diagnosis
- Mild traumatic brain injury • Head injury • Sports

Concussion is diagnosed when an athlete presents with typical symptoms, signs, behaviors, and difficulties with cognition and/or balance after direct or indirect trauma.[1] Standard imaging modalities, such as computerized tomography (CT) and magnetic resonance imaging (MRI) scans, are typically normal, demonstrating that the injury is a functional problem more than a structural one. More sophisticated studies evaluating for structural injury, such as functional MRI, diffusion tensor imaging (DTI), along with neurochemical biomarkers and genetic markers may someday modify the methods by which the diagnosis of concussion is made. These tools remain research investigations, are not the emphasis of this article, and are reviewed elsewhere.[2–7]

Most (80%–90%) sport-related concussions resolve within 7 to 10 days, although for some athletes, the time for complete recovery takes much longer.[8–10] Why some athletes seem to recover quickly and others do not remains unclear. There do seem to be modifiers that may alter how concussion is managed and determine which athletes may have prolonged recovery patterns.[10] Given these sometimes complex and unpredictable injuries, it is useful to consider a team approach to concussion management, with a variety of tools for evaluation and diagnosis, and consultants for treatment and management.

Financial disclosures and/or conflicts of interest: the author has nothing to disclose.

[a] Princeton University, University Health Services, Washington Road, Princeton, NJ 08544, USA
[b] Robert Wood Johnson, University of Medicine and Dentistry of New Jersey, 125 Paterson Street, New Brunswick, NJ 08901, USA
* Corresponding author. Robert Wood Johnson, University of Medicine and Dentistry of New Jersey, 125 Paterson Street, New Brunswick, NJ 08901.
E-mail address: putukian@princeton.edu

Clin Sports Med 30 (2011) 49–61
doi:10.1016/j.csm.2010.09.005
0278-5919/11/$ – see front matter

WHAT IS REPORTED?

Athletes often minimize and/or do not report their symptoms because they want to play and believe that their symptoms are mild enough to safely play through them. Younger athletes seek to emulate older athletes and show that they are tough enough to play despite their injuries and not to let their teammates down. It is common that athletes, at all levels, assume that "having their bell rung" is part of the game, and do not realize the significant consequences of playing with concussion. Many athletes do not realize that their symptoms indicate concussion. Most athletes do not want to be taken out of play, and will go to great lengths to minimize or trivialize their symptoms.

In a study of high-school football players,[11] only 47.3% of players with a concussion reported their injury. Of those who did not report, 66.4% did think their injuries were serious enough to report, 41% did not want to be held out of play, and 36.1% did not realize their symptoms were consistent with concussion. In this study, when injuries were reported, they were most often reported to an athletic trainer. Given the serious nature of concussive injuries if untreated and/or repeated,[12–14] it is important that the culture of sport change such that athletes, parents, coaches, and health care providers understand the significance of unreported, repetitive concussive injury. This is most important at the youth level where sports-trained medical providers, such as athletic trainers and team physicians, are often lacking.

GRADING SYSTEMS

The idea of grading a concussion at the time of injury with the intent of then determining when it will be safe to return to play led to a variety of different grading and classification systems.[15–17] Although appealing, these grading scales have been abandoned, because they are not research based and assumed that loss of consciousness (LOC) denoted more severe injury. There is significant variability in injury and therefore a cookbook approach to managing concussion is ineffective.

The Zurich Guidelines[10] represent the most recent, internationally agreed consensus statement on the management of sport-related concussion. They recommend: (1) athletes with symptoms should be removed from play; (2) no athlete with symptoms, at rest or with exertion, should continue to play; (3) young athletes need to be treated more conservatively; (4) there is no role for CT or MRI in concussion; and (5) a multidisciplinary approach to management is useful.

PREDICTORS OF SEVERITY

Based on the research on sport-related concussion that has occurred in the past decade, there are some recognized symptoms and/or signs that may predict more severe outcome as measured by the length of time that symptoms, neurocognitive deficits, or balance dysfunction occurs. Although brief LOC does not correlate with severity, the presence of prolonged LOC (>1 minute) has been shown to be associated with more severe injury.[18] In addition, other studies have shown that amnesia, prolonged confusion, and persistent symptoms are associated with more severe injury.[19,20] A recent study in Australian football players found that headache longer than 60 hours, self-reported fatigue/fogginess, and those with more than 4 symptoms were more likely to have delayed recovery based on cognitive testing.[21] These symptoms should be evaluated during the sideline assessment of the concussed athlete. The severity of injury is likely best determined by the nature, burden, and duration of symptoms, as well as the time that cognitive and balance disturbances persist, and none of these can be determined at the time of injury.

SIDELINE MANAGEMENT OF CONCUSSION

For the athletic trainer and team physician taking care of athletes, the first step in sideline management is to have an emergency action plan (EAP) in place.[22,23] Providers should be familiar with the EAP and for high-risk sports it should include a concussion protocol.[24–26] The EAP is essential for all individuals involved in sport, including administrators, coaches, athletes, the team medical staff, and other health care providers. The concussion program may differ based on the resources available as well as the athletes being served, but should maintain basic principles of management including recognition of injury, assessment, disposition, follow-up, return to play (RTP), and education. Several sport and athletic organizations have developed programming and best practices that are useful in this regard.[26–28] Education is an important aspect of the concussion protocol and should include athletes as well as coaches and parents as applicable.

RECOGNITION

The first step in evaluating and managing concussion is recognition of injury. Although a big hit gathers the attention of medical staff and others present, it is important to realize that the mechanism of injury may be more subtle and not as obvious. In a study evaluating the relationship between the force of impact in college football and clinical outcome, magnitude of impact did not correlate with clinical injury.[29] This study used accelerometers embedded into the football helmet and evaluated athletes with a clinical program involving preinjury baseline testing (symptoms, neuropsychological testing, postural balance testing) and repeat postinjury testing. The postinjury measures were compared with the baseline measures. The impact magnitude of the hits in concussed athletes ranged from 60.51 to 168.71 g, yet no significant relationships between these impacts (linear or rotational, location) and the change scores for symptom severity, postural stability or neurocognitive function were found. Additional research is needed to evaluate what other biomechanical issues play a role in the causation of injury.

Many symptoms of concussion are not specific to concussion. This creates a difficult dilemma in making the diagnosis. Headache, the most common symptom in concussion, has many causes, and is the most common symptom for individuals presenting to an emergency room facility.[8,21] To diagnose a concussion, it is important that there is a history of trauma, either a blow to the head or a blow to the body that transmits an impulsive force to the head. The injury may have occurred several hours previously and can sometimes be difficult to discern. Teammates and/or coaches also often notice that an athlete is not acting normally, having difficulty remembering plays or assignments, or showing other signs of concussion. Education of coaches, athletes, parents, and health care providers regarding common signs and symptoms of concussion, as well as the importance of recognition and early management of these injuries is essential.

An athlete with signs or symptoms of concussion should be removed from play and evaluated by a health care provider.[26–28,30] The athlete should not be allowed to RTP until an evaluation occurs. Coaches and administrators, as well as teammates and parents, should be familiar with how to engage the emergency medical services available to them and arrange for evaluation.

The symptoms of concussion are one component of diagnosis with the other components including a neurologic examination, cognitive assessment, and balance evaluation. The physical examination is important to exclude other critical diagnoses, as well as determine whether additional emergent evaluation is necessary. For example, if any evidence of skull fracture or cervical spine injury is present, the athlete should be stabilized and emergently transferred to an emergency facility. Diagnoses such as skull fracture, cervical spine fracture, and/or intracranial injuries must be considered. The balance examination can indicate injury when other aspects of the examination are normal.

The first steps in evaluating the athlete on the sideline with possible concussive injury are to ensure that the athlete is stable from a cardiovascular standpoint, and exclude cervical spine injury. Emergency management principles should be followed and an EAP should be in place for all practices and competition. Part of this initial assessment includes evaluating the mental status of the athlete, including if necessary, the Glasgow Coma Scale. If the athlete is conscious, the athlete should be asked whether or not they have any neck pain. Signs and symptoms of cervical spine injury can include neck pain or neck tenderness, pain with neck movement, weakness, and/or numbness or tingling in the extremities. If the athlete is unconscious, then the assumption should be that a cervical spine injury is present; spine board immobilization and immediate transfer to an emergency facility should be arranged.

The following discussion pertains to the athlete who has been evaluated, acute cervical spine and/or neurologic emergency excluded, the athlete is stable, and concussion is the probable diagnosis.

BASELINE INFORMATION

An important feature of the concussion plan is to have a baseline evaluation for athletes participating in high-risk sports including a history of prior injuries as well as other modifiers, a baseline evaluation that includes symptoms, neurologic examination, cognitive evaluation, and balance testing. This can be incorporated into the preparticipation examination that athletes have before they participate in school sports. There are several symptom scales, cognitive evaluations, and balance-testing options that can be used. More important than which of these is used is the concept that a baseline evaluation is performed and is then repeated after injury to assess for changes reflective of concussive injury. This approach of combining a variety of tools for baseline and subsequent postinjury assessment has been found through a meta-analysis to be effective in managing sport-related concussion.[31] A multifaceted approach is especially helpful in evaluating concussion as the symptoms vary, the presentations vary, and significant individual differences between athletes exist.[8,32] There is significant benefit to having as many tools as possible to form the baseline and postinjury evaluation. This information provides the clinician with more data to consider.

Given the individualized nature of decision making in the management and RTP of concussed athletes, obtaining a history of modifiers[10] is very important in those athletes at high risk for injury, and these are provided in **Table 1**. The concussion history should include prior history of injury, the symptoms that occurred, the duration of symptoms, and the length of time out of activity. It should also include any special testing obtained as well as the temporal relationship of injuries. Additional modifiers that should be included in the baseline evaluation are a history of learning disability (eg, attention deficit hyperactivity disorder), mental health issues (eg, depression, anxiety), migraine history, and/or sleep disorders.

THE SYMPTOM CHECKLIST: WHAT SYMPTOMS ARE IMPORTANT?

The symptoms of concussion listed earlier are not specific to concussion, which can contribute to the difficulty in making a diagnosis. If an athlete is confused or having

Table 1 Concussion modifier	
Factors	**Modifier**
Symptoms	Number
	Duration (>10 days)
	Severity
Signs	Prolonged loss of consciousness (>1 min), amnesia
Sequelae	Concussive convulsions
Temporal	Frequency: repeated concussions over time
	Timing: injuries close together in time
	Recency: recent concussion or traumatic brain injury
Threshold	Repeated concussions occurring with progressively less impact force or slower recovery after each successive concussion
Age	Child and adolescent (<18 years old)
Co- and premorbidities	Migraine, depression, or other mental health disorders, attention deficit hyperactivity disorder, learning disabilities, sleep disorders
Medication	Psychoactive drugs, anticoagulants
Behavior	Dangerous style of play
Sport	High-risk activity, contact and collision sport, high sporting level

Data from McCrory P, Meeuwisse W, Johnston K, et al. Consensus statement on Concussion in Sport 3rd International Conference on Concussion in Sport. Zurich, Switzerland, November 2008. Br J Sports Med 2009;43:i76–84.

difficulties with memory, it may be easier to discern that a concussion is the diagnosis. However, if the athlete is simply dizzy or has a headache, the diagnosis can be more difficult. These symptoms are common yet can also occur in a variety of other sport-related issues such as dehydration, heat-related illness, or anemia. This underscores the importance of having a baseline score for each individual athlete and performing a complete evaluation. Headache is one of the most difficult symptoms given that there are athletes who have headache unrelated to trauma as well as defined headache disorders that are related to trauma, such as trauma-induced migraine, further complicating diagnostic decisions. In these situations, it is important to be conservative in management remembering the adage "when in doubt, sit them out."

It is beneficial in both the preseason evaluation and the postinjury evaluation to use a symptom checklist. This is most important during the postinjury evaluation, when a standardized symptom checklist is preferable to open-ended questions such as "how are you," or "are you ok," which are likely to under diagnose injury. Using a symptom checklist provides a systematic approach to the evaluation and management whereby the same scale can be used for every interaction that the athlete has with various health care providers during the time course of their injury. Many different symptom scales exist in the literature and most of these have been put together as lists without evaluating for their psychometric components. A recent systematic review of the literature on symptom scores in sport-related concussion[33] identified 6 core scales and several derivative scales, but limited information about their psychometric properties as well as limited scientific data to support their use. Common symptom checklists include the Pittsburgh Steelers Post-concussion Scale[34] and its derivatives (eg, Post-concussion Scale Revised,[35] Head Injury Scale,[36] McGill ACE Post-concussion Symptoms Scale[37]), Concussion Resolution Index,[38] Sports Concussion Assessment Tool (SCAT), Post Concussion Symptom Scale,[39] and the Concussion Symptom Inventory.[40] In addition, derivative scales were also identified but with very limited scientific data to support their use. The most recent symptom checklist published as part of the 3rd International Consensus Conference on Concussion[10] is called SCAT 2.[41] Although more research is necessary to determine the ideal symptom checklist/scale, using a scale as part of a standardized evaluation, with a baseline set of symptoms for the individual athlete, is of benefit.

The symptom scale used in the SCAT was evaluated in a group of varsity university athletes. In addition to providing individual baseline information for each athlete, they also determined normative data for this group of athletes in terms of symptoms reported.[42] They found that overall, 41.2% of participants reported a symptom score of 0, the mean baseline score for all participants was 4.29, 3.52 for men and 6.39 for women. In addition, when they differentiated athletes with a prior history of concussion versus those without a history of concussion, they found that the symptom score was higher in those with a prior history of concussion (5.25 vs 3.75). In this study, the most common baseline symptoms reported included fatigue/low energy (37%), drowsiness (23%), and neck pain (20%). A significant number of athletes also reported baseline symptoms of difficulty concentrating (18%) and difficulty remembering (18%). In addition to the gender differences seen between total baseline symptom scores, there were also gender differences for particular symptoms such as headache and emotional lability. The difference in baseline symptoms between genders as well as between athletes with or without a prior history of concussion has been noted in other studies.[43,44]

COGNITIVE TESTING

When an athlete exhibits signs and/or symptoms of concussion, it is important to perform a cognitive evaluation that determines how well the athlete's brain is working; how they respond to questions, how well their short-term memory works, how they process information or perform simple tasks. For the team physician or athletic trainer who knows the athlete well, it may be very obvious during this cognitive evaluation that the athlete is struggling and may have a concussion. How accurately they answer simple questions as well as how quickly they respond and are able to process the information can be confirmative of a concussed athlete, once other possibilities are excluded.

The cognitive evaluations that are used as part of sideline management should also be standardized such that they are also used as part of the baseline evaluation. The evaluation should emphasize mental status and questions regarding orientation as well as simple tests of memory, recall, and new learning. Although a mental status examination is important in terms of orientation ("where are we?," "what day is it?," "what is the date?," "what is the month?," "what is the year," "what is the approximate time"), it is also important to recognize that these questions might be answered incorrectly without any injury. More useful are the questions by Maddocks and colleague,[45] which ask "what venue are we at?," "what half is it?," "who scored last in this match?," "what team did we play last week/game?," "did your team win the last game?," "what was the score?" These questions are part of the SCAT2 sideline tool discussed previously.

Asking an athlete to remember 5 words, remember digit span backward (present the numbers in a series forward, and ask the athlete to say them back in reverse; ie, "if I say 5-3, you say 3-5" continuing with a longer series until the athlete fails twice) and asking them to quickly give the months in reverse order are examples of cognitive tests that are easy to perform on the sideline. These tests are part of the SCAT2, an abbreviated sideline test that includes a few cognitive tests.

Neuropsychological (NP) tests provide a reliable assessment and quantification of brain functioning by examining brain-behavior relationships.[46] These include reaction time, attention, concentration, short-term and delayed memory, new learning, and problem solving. NP test batteries, either traditional paper/pencil tests, shorter abbreviated computerized batteries (eg, Headminder, CogSport, ImPACT) and/or a hybrid model have all been used in sport-related concussion.[46–50] These tests are not appropriate for the sideline, but are useful in the postinjury setting when a more comprehensive evaluation can be considered. These tests are typically performed at least 24 to 48 hours after injury, when the athlete is symptom free, and when compared with preseason baseline tests, provide useful information to the team physician. There is typically no benefit to performing NP testing when the athlete is symptomatic, as the athlete should not RTP before being asymptomatic. However, for the very young athlete, or the athlete with prolonged symptomatology, NP testing before the resolution of symptoms may be considered. There is certainly value added by using NP testing.[51] Often symptoms resolve completely before the resolution of cognitive deficits as measured by NP testing.[8,20,51,52] However, it is essential that health care providers understand the limitations of the use of NP testing.[53–55]

In 1 study evaluating the test-retest reliability of the available computerized NP batteries, individuals were found to test in the impaired range 20% to 40% of the time when the tests were performed and compared with their baseline test, even though they were not concussed.[53] There are many test limitations and factors that affect NP testing, such as fatigue. In addition, there are subtleties that may be difficult to discern, underscoring the use of these tests as 1 component of the complete evaluation. Ideally, NP tests should be interpreted by a neuropsychologist.[10,26,56] It is also important to remember that NP testing is just one tool in the toolbox; a multipronged approach to evaluation that includes symptoms, physical and cognitive examination, and balance testing is ideal.

POSTURAL STABILITY TESTING

Postural balance testing is a component of the physical examination that is important to include at baseline and during postinjury evaluations. Balance testing is sensitive to concussion[2,57–59] and useful as 1 component of the evaluation. A variety of balance-testing options are available including the Sensory Organization Test on the NeuroCom Smart Balance Master System as well as the Balance Error Scoring System (BESS).[57] More recently, the modified BESS was included as part of a sideline tool for concussion.[41] Musculoskeletal instability issues affect the results of postural balance testing. These tests demonstrate learning/practice effects,[60] again emphasizing the importance of baseline testing as well as using a variety of tools to measure injury.

SIDELINE TOOLS

Sideline tools that are useful for the athletic trainer and team physician for evaluating sports-related concussion include the Standardized Assessment of Concussion (SAC),[61] the SCAT,[39] and the SCAT 2.[41] These tools remain an abbreviated sideline battery and are not designed to take the place of more comprehensive evaluation or NP testing. When using an abbreviated test, it is possible that an athlete with concussion will be able to perform well enough to be considered normal, despite having significant deficits on more rigorous testing. This has been demonstrated with the SAC. Although useful in differentiating concussed compared with nonconcussed athletes at the time of injury, the SAC no longer was able to differentiate these 2 groups when repeated a day later. In addition, concussed athletes scored 29% better on the SAC at the time of their injury compared with their baseline evaluation.[62] This demonstrates that though the SAC and other tools may be useful in making the diagnosis of concussion, there is a practice effect (athletes can be expected to perform better on a test if they have taken it before) and a low ceiling (the score at which one is considered normal is easy to reach) for some of these tests that should be considered. The sensitivity and specificity of these tests may be limited. The SCAT was developed during the 2nd International Consensus Conference on Concussion[39] and combined several other symptom scores, measures, and assessments, including the SAC, into 1 tool. The SCAT was further refined during the 3rd International Consensus Conference on Concussion in Sport[10] and called the SCAT2.[41] Neither the SCAT nor the SCAT 2 have been validated, yet remain, for many, a sophisticated sideline tool.

DISPOSITION

Once an athlete has been diagnosed with concussion, they should be removed from play and evaluated by the appropriate health care provider. If an appropriate health care provider is not available immediately, the athlete should not be returned to play. Appropriate referral to a health care provider should be made. The immediacy of this referral depends on the situation and should be individualized. If an appropriate health care provider is available, then the appropriate disposition should be made. If the diagnosis is concussion, then the decision rests on whether the athlete is stable and can be observed, or whether the athlete needs emergency evacuation and evaluation. Situations in which an athlete should be sent for emergency evaluation include deteriorating mental status or worsening symptoms. Particular symptoms that raise concern include worsening headache, nausea or vomiting, or increased lethargy. In addition, for the athlete presenting with significant focal deficits or any deficits on physical examination, emergent transportation to a facility that can handle neurosurgical emergencies is essential.

TAKE-HOME INFORMATION

Most sport-related concussion injuries are mild injuries that do not necessitate emergency evacuation or treatment. It is important that all athletes are removed from play and evaluated in a complete and thorough manner. Athletes should be observed for the first few hours after their injury and should not be left alone in this timeframe. They should be monitored to ensure that no deterioration occurs. It is imperative that athletes are given take-home instructions regarding concussion; the symptoms and signs that should prompt referral to an emergency room, the importance of reporting symptoms as well as avoiding both physical and cognitive work in the immediate postinjury hours. They should be told to avoid alcohol and aspirin and other medications or drugs that may affect their brain, and to avoid video games, schoolwork, as well as the computer as these may aggravate their symptoms. Athletes need to understand the significance of concussive injury both in the short- and long-term as well as the importance of being honest regarding symptoms. A plan for follow-up evaluation should be made with the athlete.

FOLLOW-UP

When the athlete is seen in follow-up, it is important to review their symptoms (using a symptom checklist) and what other difficulties, if any, they have had. This is an opportunity to again review the important features of concussion as well as the importance of both physical and cognitive rest. For athletes who are in school, special accommodations may be necessary such as extended time for tests, avoiding the computer, having someone take notes for them, and/or time away from school. Necessary accommodations are individualized and often difficult to predict.

RTP

The RTP decision is one of the most challenging decisions facing the team physician and is made more difficult given the individual nature of this injury. It is essential that the team physician takes into account the previous history of injury as well as the other modifiers for that individual in making the RTP decision. It is also important to take into account the other variables that play a role in making the RTP decision. In the past several years there has been a dramatic change in how clinicians approach the RTP decision. There has been a more conservative approach to RTP. In December 2009, the National Football League provided revised RTP guidelines that mandated that athletes diagnosed with concussion remain out of play for the remainder of the day.[27] These modified RTP guidelines set an example that other sport organizations should consider. Whether independently arrived at or not, the National Collegiate Athletics Association (NCAA)[26] and the National Federation of State High School Associations[28] have subsequently put into practice modifications that will change RTP decisions for athletes with concussion. These include being removed from play once any signs or symptoms of concussion are present, as well as the need for immediate evaluation by a health care provider trained in concussion management. Both the NCAA and NHFS state that athletes diagnosed with concussion cannot RTP the same day, and require evaluation by a physician or their designee before return to play. These more stringent RTP policies are designed to protect the health and safety of participants in sport.

It is essential that the athlete is asymptomatic both at rest and with exertion, before initiating an RTP progression. The first step in an RTP progression is to initiate cardiovascular demand without the risk for contact. This is often a trial of cardiovascular activity, lasting 15 to 20 minutes, during which the athlete increases their heart rate and work load without increasing the risk for contact. The athlete should break a sweat and an increase in their heart rate should be recognized. If the athlete is able to tolerate this load, then the intent would be to gradually increase the load as well as the risk for contact gradually. This RTP process (**Table 2**) was outlined in the 1st International Agreement Statement and is endorsed by several other more recent publications.[10,24,25,39,63,64]

The RTP process is a complex one that requires an individual approach. An injury in an athlete without any significant modifiers may take only a few days to start the RTP progression, whereas for the same injury in an athlete with several modifiers the team physician might decide that a longer symptom-free interval is necessary. In addition, for the athlete who recently sustained a concussion, it may be important to take a slower approach to progressing activity, whereby instead of a day for each stage, a longer period of time is taken for each stage. This decision is an individualized one that should factor in the specific modifiers that each athlete has.

The sideline evaluation of the concussed athlete represents one of the most difficult evaluations facing the team physician. Having an EAP that includes a concussion protocol for high-risk sports is useful in practicing the approach to this injury, although realizing that several individual factors/modifiers will need to be considered. Using a standardized sideline tool for evaluation of injury and the preseason evaluation against which to compare is useful for the clinician on the sideline. This should include a symptom checklist, a directed physical examination, a cognitive evaluation, and balance testing. The decision to remove an athlete from play when suspected signs or

	Table 2	
Graduated return to play protocol		
Rehabilitation Stage	**Functional Exercise at Each Stage of Rehabilitation**	**Objective of Each Stage**
1. No activity	Complete physical and cognitive rest	Recovery
2. Light aerobic exercise	Walking, swimming, or stationary cycling keeping intensity <70% maximum predicted heart rate No resistance training	Increase heat rate
3. Sport-specific exercise	Skating drills in ice hockey, running drills in soccer. No head impact activities	Add movement
4. Noncontact training drills	Progression to more complex training drills, eg passing drills in football and ice hockey May start progressive resistance training	Exercise, coordination, and cognitive load
5. Full contact practice	After medical clearance, participate in normal trailing activities	Restore confidence and assess functional skills by coaching staff
6. Return to play	Normal game play	

From McCrory P, Meeuwisse W, Johnston K, et al. Consensus statement on Concussion in Sport 3rd International Conference on Concussion in Sport. Zurich, Switzerland, November 2008. Br J Sports Med 2009;43:i76–84; with permission.

symptoms of concussion are present is important. Given the long-term consequences of unreported and/or recurrent injury, it is imperative that a conservative approach is used. It is important to evaluate for and exclude more emergent medical issues such as intracranial bleed, skull fracture, and/or cervical spine injury. It is important that appropriate disposition and follow-up is discussed with the athlete including specific take-home instructions. Further management may include more comprehensive neuro-psychological and balance testing, and basic principles regarding an RTP progression should be considered. It is the optimistic view of this author that if these basic principles are followed, participating in sport, no matter the activity or risk for concussive injury, remains a safe activity. Although the risk for concussion exists in sport, the assertion is that if treated promptly and appropriately, significant long-term risks are avoided and the overall the benefits of participation far outweigh the risks of participation.

REFERENCES

1. Aubry M, Cantu R, Dvorak J, et al. Summary and agreement statement of the First International Conference on Concussion in Sport, Vienna 2001. Recommendations for the improvement of safety and health of athletes who may suffer concussive injuries. Br J Sports Med 2002;36(1):6–10.
2. Davis GA, Iverson GL, Guskiewicz KM, et al. Contributions of neuroimaging, balance testing, electrophysiology and blood markers to the assessment of sport-related concussion. Br J Sports Med 2009;43:i36–45.

3. Ptito A, Chen JK, Johnston K. Contribution of functional magnetic resonance imaging (fMRI) to sport concussion evaluation. NeuroRehabilitation 2007;22:217–27.
4. Terrell TR, Bostick R, Abramson R, et al. APOE, APOE promoter, and Tau genotypes and risk for concussion in college athletes. Clin J Sport Med 2008;18:10–7.
5. Niogi SN, Mukherjee P, Ghajar J, et al. Structural dissociation of attentional control and memory in adults with and without mild traumatic brain injury. Brain 2008; 131:3209–21.
6. Chen JK, Johnston KM, Petrides M, et al. Recovery from mild head injury in sports: evidence from serial functional magnetic resonance imaging studies in male athletes. Clin J Sport Med 2008;18:241–8.
7. Chen JK, Johnston KM, Frey, et al. Functional abnormalities in symptomatic concussed athletes: an fMRI study. Neuroimage 2004;22:68–82.
8. Echemendia R, Putukian M, Mackin RS, et al. Neuropsychological test performance prior to and following sports-related mild traumatic brain injury. Clin J Sport Med 2001;11:23–31.
9. McCrea M, Guskiewicz KM, Marshall SW. Acute effects and recovery time following concussion in collegiate football players. the NCAA concussion study. JAMA 2003;290:2556–63.
10. McCrory P, Meeuwisse W, Johnston K, et al. Consensus statement on Concussion in Sport 3rd International Conference on Concussion in Sport. Zurich, Switzerland, November 2008. Br J Sports Med 2009;43:i76–84.
11. McCrea M, Hammeke T, Olsen G, et al. Unreported concussion in high school football players: implications for prevention. Clin J Sport Med 2004; 14(1):13–7.
12. Cantu RC, Voy R. Second impact syndrome; a risk in any contact sport. Phys Sportsmed 1995;23:27–34.
13. Barth JT, Diamond R, Errico A. Mild head injury and post concussion syndrome; does anyone really suffer? Clin Electroencephalogr 1996;27:183–6.
14. Cantu RC. Chronic traumatic encephalopathy in the National Football League. Neurosurgery 2007;61(2):223–5.
15. Cantu RC. Return to play guidelines after a head injury. Clin Sports Med 1998; 17(1):45–60.
16. Colorado Medical Society School and Sports Medicine Committee. Guidelines for the management of concussion in sports. Colo Med 1990;87:4.
17. Quality Standards Subcommittee. American Academy of Neurology, Practice Parameter; The management of concussion in sports. Neurology 1997;48: 581–5 (summary statement).
18. Jennett B, Bond M. Assessment of outcome after severe brain damage: a practical scale. Lancet 1975;i:480–4.
19. Erlanger D, Kausik T, Cantu R, et al. Symptom-based assessment of the severity of concussion. J Neurosurg 2003;98:34–9.
20. Collins MW, Iverson GL, Lovell MR, et al. On field predictors of neuropsychological and symptom deficit following sports-related concussion. Clin J Sport Med 2003;13:222–9.
21. Makdissi M, Darby D, Maruff P, et al. Natural history of concussion in sport; markers of severity and implications for management. Am J Sports Med 2010; 38(3):464–71.
22. Rubin AL. Safety, security, and preparing for disaster at sporting events. Curr Sports Med Rep 2004;3(3):141–5.
23. Herring SA, Bergfeld J, Boyd J, et al. Sideline preparedness for the team physician: a consensus statement. Med Sci Sports Exerc 2001;33(5):846–9.

24. Putukian M, Aubry M, McCrory P. Return to play after sports concussion in elite and non-elite athletes. Br J Sports Med 2009;43(Suppl 1):i28–31.
25. Herring SA, Bergfeld J, Indelicato P, et al. Concussion (mild traumatic brain injury) and the team physician: a consensus statement. Med Sci Sports Exerc 2005;37(11):2012–6.
26. NCAA Health and Safety Web site. NCAA required concussion management plan. Available at: http://www.ncaa.org/wps/myportal/ncaahome?WCM_GLOBAL_ CONTEXT=/ncaa/ncaa/academics+and+athletes/personal+welfare/health+and+ safety/concussion. Accessed June 15, 2010.
27. NFL Press Release. NFL outlines for players steps taken to address concussions. Available at: http://www.nfl.com/news/story/09000d5d8017cc67/article/nfl-outlines-for-players-steps-taken-to-address-concussions. Accessed May 12, 2010.
28. National Federation of High School Sports. 2009 NFHS concussion brochure. Available at: http://www.nfhs.org/sportsmed.aspx. Accessed May 1, 2010.
29. Guskiewicz KM, Mihalik JP, Shankar V, et al. Measurement of head impacts in college football players: relationship between head impact biomechanics and acute clinical outcome after concussion. Neurosurgery 2007;61(6):1244–52 [discussion: 1252–3].
30. Zack Lystedt Law. Available at: http://apps.leg.wa.gov/billinfo/summary.aspx? bill=1824. Accessed May 15, 2010.
31. Broglio SP, Puetz TW. The effect of sport concussion on neurocognitive function, self-report symptoms and postural control. A meta-analysis. Sports Med 2008; 38(1):53–67.
32. Meehan WP, Bachur RG. Sport-related concussion. Pediatrics 2009;123:114–23.
33. Alla S, Sullivan SJ, Hale L, et al. Self-report scales/checklists for the measurement of concussion symptoms: a systematic review. Br J Sports Med 2009;43:i3–12.
34. Maroon JC, Lovell MR, Norwig J, et al. Cerebral concussion in athletes: evaluation and neuropsychological testing. Neurosurgery 2000;47:659–69 [discussion: 69–72].
35. Lovell MR, Collins MW. Neuropsychological assessment of the college football player. J Head Trauma Rehabil 1998;13:9–26.
36. Piland SG, Motl RW, Ferrara MS, et al. Evidence for the factorial and construct validity of a self-report concussion symptoms scale. J Athl Train 2003;38:104–12.
37. Leclerc S. Assessment of concussion in athletes. Canada: McGill University; 2004.
38. Erlanger D, Feldman D, Kutner K, et al. Development and validation of a web-based neuropsychological test protocol for sports-related return to play decision making. Arch Clin Neuropsychol 2003;18:293–316.
39. McCrory P, Johnston K, Meeuwisse W, et al. Summary and agreement statement of the 2nd International Conference on Concussion in Sport, Prague 2004. Br J Sports Med 2005;39:196–204.
40. Randolph C, Barr WB, McCrea M, et al. Concussion symptom inventory (CSI): an empirically-derived scale for monitoring resolution of symptoms following sport-related concussion. Available at: http://www.smf.org/. Accessed February 22, 2010.
41. SCAT2. Sport concussion assessment tool 2. Br J Sports Med 2009;43:i85–8.
42. Shehata N, Wiley JP, Richea S, et al. Sport concussion assessment tool: baseline values for varsity collision sport athletes. Br J Sports Med 2009;43:730–4.
43. Covassin T, Swanik CB, Sachs M, et al. Sex differences in baseline neuropsychological function and concussion symptoms of collegiate athletes. Br J Sports Med 2006;40:923–7.

44. Bruce JM, Echemendia RJ. Concussion history predicts self-reported symptoms before and following a concussive event. Neurology 2004;63:1516–8.
45. Maddocks DL, Dicker GD, Saling MM. The assessment of orientation following concussion in athletes. Clin J Sport Med 1995;5(1):32–5.
46. Echemendia RJ. Sports neuropsychology: assessment and management of traumatic brain injury. New York: Guilford Press; 2006.
47. Erlanger DM, Kaushik T, Broshek D, et al. Development and validation of a web-based screening tool for monitoring cognitive status. J Head Trauma Rehabil 2002;17:458–76.
48. Collie A, Maruff P, Makdissi M, et al. CogSport: reliability and correlation with conventional cognitive tests used in post concussion medical evaluations. Clin J Sport Med 2003;13:28–32.
49. Lovell MR, Collins MW, Podell K, et al. Immediate post-concussion assessment and cognitive testing (version 2.0). Pittsburgh (PA): Neurohealth Systems, LLC; 2007.
50. Barth JT, Alves W, Ryan T, et al. Mild head injury in sports: neuropsychological sequelae and recovery of function. In: Levin H, Eisenberg J, Benton A, editors. Mild head injury. New York: Oxford University Press; 1989. p. 257–75.
51. Van Kampen DA, Lovell MR, Pardini JE, et al. The "value added" of neurocognitive testing after sports-related concussion. Am J Sports Med 2006;10(10):1–6.
52. Makdissi M, Darby D, Maruff P, et al. Natural history of concussion in sport: markers of severity and implications for management. Am J Sports Med 2010;38:464.
53. Broglio SP, Ferrara MS, Macciocchi SN, et al. Test-retest reliability of computerized concussion assessment programs. J Athl Train 2007;42(4):509–14.
54. Barr WB. Methodologic issues in neuropsychological testing. J Athl Train 2001; 36:297–302.
55. Randolph C, McCrea M, Barr WB. Is neuropsychological testing useful in the medical management of sport-related concussion? J Athl Train 2005;40(3): 136–51.
56. Echemendia RJ, Herring S, Bailes J. Who should conduct and interpret the neuropsychological assessment in sports-related concussion? Br J Sports Med 2009; 43:i32–5.
57. Guskiewicz KM, Ross SE, Marshall SW. Postural stability and neuropsychological deficits after concussion in collegiate athletes. J Athl Train 2001;36(3): 263–73.
58. Cavanaugh JT, Guskiewicz KM, Guiliani C, et al. Detecting altered postural control after cerebral concussion in athletes with normal postural stability. Br J Sports Med 2005;39(11):805–11.
59. Riemann BL, Guskiewicz KM. Effects of mild head injury on postural stability as measured through clinical balance testing. J Athl Train 2000;35(1):19–25.
60. Valvolich-McLeod TC, Barr WB, McCrea M, et al. Psychometric and measurement properties of concussion assessment tools in youth sports. J Athl Train 2006; 41(4):399–408.
61. McCrea M. Standardized mental status assessment of sports concussion. Clin J Sport Med 2001;11(3):176–81.
62. Hecht S, Puffer J, Clinton C, et al. Concussion assessment in football and soccer players. Clin J Sport Med 2004;14(5):310.
63. Putukian M. Repeat mild traumatic brain injury: how to adjust return to play, 64 guidelines. Curr Sports Med Rep 2006;5:15–22.
64. Guskiewicz KM, Bruce SL, Cantu RC, et al. National Athletic Trainers' Association position statement: management of sport-related concussion. J Athl Train 2004; 39(3):280–97.

Subacute Symptoms of Sports-Related Concussion: Outpatient Management and Return to Play

Pierre d'Hemecourt, MD

KEYWORDS

- Concussion • Symptom score • Neuropsychological testing
- Balance testing • Return to play criteria

Participation in contact and collision sports is on the rise worldwide. Consequently, the incidence of sports- and recreation-related concussions has been estimated at 1.6 to 3.8 million cases per year in the United States.[1] For many clinicians, the care from the time of acute injury through the management phases to the decision-making involved in returning the athlete to play is challenging. Although most athletes with concussions become symptom-free within 10 days, some symptoms—subtle and not so subtle—and neurocognitive deficits may persist.[2,3] Recently, one study reported that 35% of concussed athletes experienced neurocognitive deficits that persisted for several days after the symptoms had resolved.[4] Previous articles have focused on the acute care of the athlete in the first few days of injury. This article concentrates on athletes with persistent symptoms after the first few days and those with modifying factors that must be considered when returning the athlete to play.

The recent Zurich consensus statement defined concussion as "a complex patho-physiologic process affecting the brain, induced by traumatic biomechanical forces."[5] This functional disturbance is most often short-lived but may occasionally have prolonged symptoms. The panel recognized the similarity of mild traumatic brain injury with sports-related concussion. However, because the injury constructs were different, the terms should not be used interchangeably. Although the sports-related concussion may be an entity early on the spectrum of traumatic brain injury, it is not

The author has nothing to disclose.

Division of Sports Medicine, Children's Hospital, 300 Longwood Avenue, Boston, MA 02115, USA

E-mail address: pierre.dhemecourt@childrens.harvard.edu

always clear when the injury crosses from mild to moderate traumatic brain injury. Much of the recent experience in dealing with mild traumatic brain injury comes from the military experience. In Afghanistan and Iraq, the signature injury has been mild traumatic brain injury. This condition was previously recognized as "shell shock," the signature injury of World War I.[6] The military criteria for return to duty criteria have many similarities to the sports criteria for return to play.

CONCERNS FOR RETURN TO PLAY DECISIONS

One well-accepted criterion for return to contact/collision sports is the resolution of all concussive symptoms both at rest and with exercise.[7] Often the subtleness of symptoms lead to confusion and uncertainty in decision making. Ultimately, clinicians have three major categories of concern: second impact syndrome (SIS), a prolonged recovery from sequential concussions, and chronic traumatic encephalopathy.

Although rare, SIS is a devastating injury with a mortality rate of at least 50% and a nearly 100% morbidity rate.[8] The injury occurs in adolescent and young athletes who sustain a second concussive event while still symptomatic from a prior event. SIS may occur with either mild or significant trauma as the first or second event. Except for in boxing, it has not been reported in athletes older than 20 years.[9] The timing between events can occur as early as the same game or several weeks later. SIS is believed to be caused by a rapid loss of vascular autoregulation with massive intracerebral swelling.[10] Some controversy exists regarding the existence of SIS, because some would call it "diffuse cerebral swelling" that can occur in the younger individual with an initial minor traumatic brain injury.[11] However, most authorities concur that an initial incident precedes the catastrophic second event and is marked by incomplete recovery of symptoms. Often the vagueness of the symptoms combined with an intense desire to return to play leads to unfortunate decisions.

The second concern regarding return to contact or collision sports after a concussion is the possibility of a prolonged recovery from a second concussion. Studies have shown that high school and collegiate-level American football players with a history of concussion have a three- to sixfold increased risk of sustaining a second concussion.[12] Repeat concussions are most likely to occur in the first 10 days after the initial concussion.[13] Collins and colleagues[14] showed that athletes with a history of concussions were more likely to experience significant on-field symptoms of amnesia and confusion during repeat concussions. These symptoms may be related to a more prolonged rate of recovery. A longer recovery from second concussions was also shown in terms of balance recovery. One study stratified collegiate athletes based on single versus multiple concussions. The athletes who experienced more than a single event took longer to recover visual–kinetic integration than those who experienced a single event.[15]

Finally, concern exists over the cumulative effects of repeated traumatic brain injury, including the potential for dementia pugilistica or chronic traumatic encephalopathy (CTE). This entity has been recognized since the early 1900s.[16] Initially recognized in boxers, it has been shown in retired National Football League (NFL) players and several other collision sports.[17] The neuropathology of CTE has similar findings to those of Alzheimer disease, including cell drop-out and neurofibrillatory tangles. In CTE, however, the major areas of involvement are the septum pellucidum, the substantia nigra, and the cerebellum, and the condition is often associated with diffuse axonal loss. This involvement results in loss of intellect, memory, and balance and symptoms similar to those of Parkinson disease.[18,19]

No finite number of head injuries is equated with the development of CTE. These neuropathologic changes are often not recognized for several years after the injuries.

Hence, who is going to develop these problems is difficult to predict. However, Collins and colleagues[14] showed that athletes with multiple concussions often manifest deficits on neurocognitive testing. These subtle neurocognitive deficits may help identify which athletes with multiple concussions should consider retirement. Further investigation is necessary before this can be determined.

EVALUATION OF THE ATHLETE WITH PERSISTENT POSTCONCUSSIVE SYMPTOMS

Athletes with a concussion should undergo a full evaluation, including a history of the injury and all initial findings. Careful consideration should be given to injuries outside the spectrum of concussion. Persistent or progressive symptoms should prompt consideration of neuroimaging to exclude other potential causes of the patient's symptoms. At 1-week postinjury, MRI is the most sensitive imaging tool and lacks exposure to ionizing radiation.

The cervical spine should also be thoroughly evaluated for signs of injury. Cervical spine tenderness should initiate at least plain radiographs, with flexion and extension lateral radiographs. In the adult, further evaluation may require CT scanning. In the child athlete, upper cervical spine injuries may be evaluated with an MRI.

The sports-related concussion complex involves careful evaluation of symptoms, physical findings, cognitive impairment, and behavioral changes. The subtlety of concussion may be determined in any of these realms. The initial symptoms at injury that are somewhat predictive of a longer postconcussive course are the total symptom load and possibly amnesia and confusion.[20,21]

Symptom Assessment

Persistent symptoms may be clumped into three categories: somatic, emotional, and cognitive. Somatic symptoms include headaches, balance issues, and sleep disturbance. Emotional symptoms are often depression and anxiety. Cognitive symptoms include concentration and memory problems. A symptom checklist, such as the sideline concussion assessment tool 2 (SCAT 2), is critical in maintaining a complete evaluation log (**Fig. 1**). The checklist is used both to quantify symptoms as they resolve and to flag some symptoms that require direct treatment, such as sleep disturbance. A baseline symptom checklist is useful, because many symptoms, such as lack of concentration, may predate the injury.

Various postconcussive symptoms are possible, including headaches, photophobia, dizziness, and problems with memory and concentration. Headaches are the most common symptom but do not always correlate with concussion severity.[22,23] Fogginess, or the sense of being out of touch, correlates highly with problems in memory performance and reaction time, and is predictive of increased time to recovery.[24] Diminished sleep has also been correlated with poor recovery of cognitive function.[25] Specifically, attention deficits are increased in patients with postconcussive sleep dysfunction.[26]

Physical Findings

A thorough neurologic examination is important to assess for a focal brain deficit masking as a concussion. However, the concussion examination may elicit several findings, including vestibular and balance problems, caused by the lack of integration of the vestibular and visual systems. One sensitive tool for postural balance is the Balance Error Scoring System (BESS).[27] This test is easy to administer in the office and may stay abnormal up to several days after injury. It consists of posture in three

SCAT 2 Symptom Score
How do you feel?

You should score yourself on the following symptoms, based on how you feel now.

	None	Mild		Moderate		Severe	
Headache	0	1	2	3	4	5	6
"Pressure in head"	0	1	2	3	4	5	6
Neck Pain	0	1	2	3	4	5	6
Nausea or vomiting	0	1	2	3	4	5	6
Dizziness	0	1	2	3	4	5	6
Blurred vision	0	1	2	3	4	5	6
Balance problems	0	1	2	3	4	5	6
Sensitivity to light	0	1	2	3	4	5	6
Sensitivity to noise	0	1	2	3	4	5	6
Feeling slowed down	0	1	2	3	4	5	6
Feeling like "in a fog"	0	1	2	3	4	5	6
"Don't feel right"	0	1	2	3	4	5	6
Difficulty concentrating	0	1	2	3	4	5	6
Difficulty remembering	0	1	2	3	4	5	6
Fatigue or low energy	0	1	2	3	4	5	6
Confusion	0	1	2	3	4	5	6
Drowsiness	0	1	2	3	4	5	6
Trouble falling asleep	0	1	2	3	4	5	6
More emotional	0	1	2	3	4	5	6
Irritability	0	1	2	3	4	5	6
Sadness	0	1	2	3	4	5	6
Nervous or Anxious	0	1	2	3	4	5	6

Total number of symptoms (Maximum possible 22)

Symptom severity score

(Add all scores in table, maximum possible: 22 x 6 = 132)
Do the symptoms get worse with physical activity? Y N
Do the symptoms get worse with mental activity? Y N
Overall rating
If you know the athlete well prior to the injury, how different is the athlete acting compared to his / her usual self? Please circle one response.
no different very different unsure

Fig. 1. SCAT 2 symptom score.

stances: double leg, single leg, and tandem stance on a firm and a foam surface. Having a baseline score of the BESS is very helpful.

Cognitive (Neuropsychological) Assessment

It is well established that resolution of symptoms and neurocognitive function do not always coincide. This finding has been shown in American football players at both the high school and college levels.[20,28] The simple sideline tests, such as the Maddocks questionnaire or the Standardized Assessment of Concussion (SAC), provide good initial information with respect to confusion and amnesia. However, they do not give information on performance in the more subtle cognitive domains. Initial interest in advanced neuropsychological testing for sports-related concussion started in the 1980s at the University of Virginia.[29] The traditional "paper and pencil" testing led to the more efficient computer-based testing, which allows for more accurate assessment of some cognitive functions, such as reaction time, which is inherently better suited to computerized assessment.[30] The other measured cognitive domains include visual memory, verbal memory, and processing speed. The currently available commercial products for computer-based testing include ImPACT (Immediate Post-Concussion Assessment and Cognitive Testing), Headminder, CogState, and ANAM (Automated Neuropsychological Assessment Metric).

Neuropsychological testing is valuable in the assessment of the concussed athlete, but it is not a stand-alone tool and may not always be available. It is only one part of the multifactorial assessment of the athlete. Symptoms, physical findings (balance testing), previous concussions, and comorbid neurologic issues must all be considered in returning the athlete to competition. It is best used if a baseline was established before injury. Baseline tests should always be evaluated for validity of performance.[31] It is important for clinicians to question the athletes about difficulties with any segment of the test.

The test is often administered when the athlete becomes symptom-free. It may be used earlier in athletes with prolonged symptoms and in younger athletes, because it could help determine whether academic accommodations and cognitive rehabilitation are needed. When used in the younger athlete, testing must be sensitive to the maturation of cognitive function throughout adolescence. Neural maturation will necessitate repeated baselines every 6 months.[32,33] A neuropsychologist may be very helpful in interpreting testing in this population, especially if learning disabilities exist.

For most sports-related concussions, the return of neuropsychological function is usually within the first 2 weeks, and often in the first 7 to 10 days.[34] Furthermore, in the general population with mild traumatic brain injury, neuropsychological function will recover by 90 days postinjury in most people.[35,36] In the sports population, Makdissi and colleagues[4] showed that initial presentation of symptoms is somewhat predictive of duration of cognitive defects. Athletes that presented with more than four symptoms, a headache lasting longer than 60 hours, and the report of fogginess or fatigue took longer to recover. Furthermore, computer-based neuropsychological testing recovery lagged behind symptom recovery and was more sensitive than paper and pencil neuropsychological testing.

MANAGEMENT OF CONCUSSIVE SYMPTOMS

Management of the postconcussive state follows some general guidelines. Athletes are kept at cognitive and physical rest until the symptoms resolve and then follow a graded pathway of increasing exercise activity until they are able to return to play. However, persistent symptoms may hinder this process. Clinicians must monitor the symptoms, because they may require intervention.

Physical Rest, Cognitive Rest, and Education

Rest from all physically strenuous activity is recommended, not just from those activities that confer an increased risk of trauma to the head. A more difficult area for the athlete, parents, and teachers to understand is the importance of cognitive rest. These activities include many that are not as well understood, such as computer games and text messaging.

Academic accommodations will help the scholar athlete achieve cognitive rest. It is crucial for these athletes to understand that their visual and verbal memory processing is slowed and that academic performance will be affected. Early in the recovery period, the athlete may be kept out of school completely. As symptoms resolve, a gradual academic return is initiated, perhaps beginning with half days and no tests or reading assignments, followed by progression to limited reading and untimed tests. Much of this is dependent on the severity of the symptom score.

Rest from exercise is paramount in the early stages of recovery. Most symptoms will have cleared after the first 7 to 10 days. In cases of prolonged symptoms lasting more than 6 weeks, Leddy and colleagues[37] showed that subsymptom threshold levels of exercise are safe with close monitoring for recurrence of symptoms. Prolonged concussions often are associated with depression and anxiety.[38] Subthreshold exercise may diminish this effect.

Education for the athlete, parents, coaches, and teachers plays a major role in the recovery of sports-related concussion. Education should center on the description of cognitive deficiencies and the natural history of concussion syndrome.[39] Involving a psychologist at this point to provide cognitive behavior therapy is very helpful. Education is the cognitive component, and the behavioral component involves working with maladaptive behavior and moods that interfere with recovery.

Medications

Several principles of medication use in the setting of sports-related concussion should be understood. First, few well-designed studies have examined the use of medications specifically for sports-related concussion.[40] Second, no evidence shows that medications speed the recovery of sports-related concussions. They can be useful in mitigating the symptoms but not the overall recovery time. Finally, the general principle is to have the athlete discontinue the interventional medications before returning to sports. However, this is not always possible when dealing with underlying emotional issues, and the clinician will need to exhibit caution in these circumstances. The medications used to treat the symptoms of sport-related concussion are discussed in greater detail elsewhere in this issue.

RETURN TO PLAY CRITERIA

Before returning to play, the athlete must prove to be symptom-free at rest and with exertion. Once the symptoms have resolved, a well-accepted progression should occur before returning to contact sports:

Symptom-free state → light aerobic activity → sport-specific activities → noncontact training drills → medical clearance and full contact practice → game play.

This progression follows several principles. If any symptoms recur, the athlete is to go back one step and wait at least 1 day after symptoms resolve before progressing again. The timing between steps may be increased based on certain modifying factors, as discussed below.

Modifying Factors in Concussion Management

Age

The young athlete is managed based on similar principles as the older athlete. Given the immaturity of the brain, however, the young athlete may require more time to recover than the adult patient.[41] Therefore, the time between the steps for return to play that are listed earlier is increased for young athletes. In addition, the long-term neuropsychological effects of repetitive concussions are not well understood. Computer-based neurocognitive testing can be performed, but should be compared with age-matched controls, and requires frequently repeated baseline examinations. Interpretation may require a trained neuropsychologist, especially if learning disabilities are involved. Preinjury learning disabilities have been associated with increased cognitive disability after concussion. This symptom is possibly related to diminished cognitive reserve.[42] Cognitive rest is crucial in the young athlete and neuropsychological testing can help modify academic involvement.

Concussion Recurrence

Although a specific number of concussions has not been established to mandate seasonal or permanent retirement, experts understand that repetitive concussions are associated with more significant neurocognitive deficits.[34] The factors that prompt the consideration of conservative management include less time between concussions, progressively less force resulting in injury, and increasing duration of concussion recovery. In the future, neuropsychological testing may be helpful in these settings to determine fine changes as harbingers of permanent injury.

Symptom Description

Some symptoms may predict longer recovery. Interest has been shown in amnesia as one type of marker. But total symptom load is a more likely predictive of a prolonged recovery.[4] Fogginess and mental slowness most likely represent impaired cognitive function. Loss of consciousness for less than 1 minute has not been found to a useful predictor of prolonged recovery.[43]

Comorbidity of Learning Disabilities and Migraines

Learning disabilities in the premorbid state predict more significant cognitive injury, which makes neuropsychological testing more difficult to interpret. Involvement of a trained neuropsychologist should be considered to help interpret difficult cases. Because these athletes will exhibit more significant cognitive deficits, precautions should be taken when they return to play.

Occasionally, headaches triggered by concussive injury can complicate recovery. Athletes with preinjury migraines might be considered recovered when their migraine symptoms return to preinjury levels. However, for athletes without a history, migraines may be initiated by a sports-related concussion, often confusing the decision to return the athlete to play.[44] Clinicians must determine whether the patient has postconcussive headaches, which indicate incomplete recovery, or whether a primary migraine was triggered by the injury. In these difficult situations, it is useful to document a good description of the headache. If the headache is not exacerbated by exercise, the patient has a positive family history of migraines, all other concussion symptoms have resolved, and neuropsychological testing has returned to baseline, the clinician might consider a primary diagnosis of migraines, and therefore consider returning the athlete to play.

The subacute symptoms of sports-related concussion can be difficult to treat. Fortunately, they are usually short-lived and self-resolving. The cause of the symptoms may occasionally be confusing. A multidisciplinary approach to recovery and return to play decisions is ideal. Recent consensus statements offer useful guidelines to assist clinicians in the management of concussed athletes.

REFERENCES

1. Langlois JA, Rutland-Brown W, Wald MM. The epidemiology and impact of traumatic brain injury: a brief overview. J Head Trauma Rehabil 2006;21:375–8.
2. McCrea M, Guskiewicz KM, Marshall SW, et al. Acute effects and recovery time following concussion in collegiate football players: the NCAA concussion study. JAMA 2003;290:2556–63.
3. Macciocchi SN, Barth JT, Alves W, et al. Neuropsychological functioning and recovery after mild head injury in collegiate athletes. Neurosurgery 1996;39:510–4.
4. Makdissi M, Darby D, Maruff P, et al. Natural history of concussion in sport: markers of severity and implications for management. Am J Sports Med 2010; 38:464.
5. McCrory P, Meeuwisse W, Johnston K, et al. Consensus statement on concussion in sport: the 3rd international conference on concussion in sport held in Zurich, November 2008. Br J Sports Med 2009;43(Suppl 1):176–90.
6. Jones E, Fear N, Wessely S. Shell shock and mild traumatic brain injury: a historical review. Am J Psychiatry 2007;164:1641–5.
7. LeBlanc C, Coombs J, Davis R. The management of minor closed head injury in children. Pediatrics 2000;106(6):1524–5.
8. Cantu R. Second-impact syndrome. Clin Sports Med 2009;7:37–44.
9. Herring S, Bergfeld J, Boland A, et al. Concussion (mild traumatic brain injury) and the team physician: a consensus statement. Med Sci Sports Exerc 2005; 37(11):2012–6.
10. Kirkwood M, Yeates K, Wilson P. Pediatric sport-related concussion: A review of the clinical management of an oft-neglected population. Pediatrics 2006;117(4): 1359–71.
11. McCrory P. Does second impact syndrome exist? Clin J Sport Med 2001;11(3): 144–9.
12. Guskiewicz KM, Weaver NL, Padua DA, et al. Epidemiology of concussion in collegiate and high school football players. Am J Sports Med 2000;28:643–50.
13. McCrea M, Guskiecz K, Randolph. Effects of a symptom-free waiting period on clinical outcome and risk of reinjury after sports-related concussion. Neurosurgery 2009;65:876–83.
14. Collins M, Lovell M, Iverson G, et al. Cumulative effects of concussion in high school athletes. Neurosurgery 2002;51:1175–81.
15. Siobounov S, Siobounov E, Sebastianelli W, et al. Differential rate of recovery in athletes after first and second concussion episodes. Neurosurgery 2007;61(2): 338–44.
16. McCrory P, Meeuwisse W, Johnston K, et al. Consensus statement on concussion in sport: the 3rd international conference on concussion in sport held in Zurich 2008. Br J Sports Med 2009;43:176–84.
17. Corsellis JA, Bruton CJ, Freeman-Browne D. The aftermath of boxing. Psychol Med 1973;3:270–303.
18. Omalu BI, DeKosky ST, Hamilton RL, et al. Chronic traumatic encephalopathy in a national football league player part II. Neurosurgery 2006;59:1086–92.
19. Cantu R. Chronic traumatic encephalopathy in the National Football League. Neurosurgery 2007;61:223–5.
20. Lovell MR, Collins MW, Iverson GL, et al. Recovery from mild concussion in high school athletes. J Neurosurg 2003;98:296–301.
21. McCrory PR, Ariens T, Berkovic SF. The nature and duration of acute concussive symptoms in Australian football. Clin J Sport Med 2000;10:235–8.

22. Packard RC. Epidemiology and pathogenesis of posttraumatic headache. J Head Trauma Rehabil 1999;14:9–21.
23. Couch JR, Bearss C. Chronic daily headache in the posttrauma syndrome: relation to extent of head injury. Headache 2001;41:559–64.
24. Iverson G, Gaetz M, Lovell M, et al. Relation between subjective fogginess and neuropsychological testing following concussion. J Int Neuropsychol Soc 2004; 10:904–6.
25. Fichtenberg NL, Zafonte RD, Putnam S, et al. Insomnia in a post-acute brain injury sample. Brain Inj 2002;16:197–206.
26. Imogen L, Bloomfield M, Colin A, et al. Do sleep difficulties exacerbate deficits in sustained attention following traumatic brain injury? J Int Neuropsychol Soc 2009; 16:17–25.
27. Guskiewicz KM, Ross SE, Marshall SW. Postural stability and neuropsychological deficits after concussion in collegiate athletes. J Athl Train 2001;36: 263–73.
28. Lovell MR, Collins MW. Neuropsychological assessment of the college football player. J Head Trauma Rehabil 1998;13:9–26.
29. Barth JT, Alves WM, Ryan TV, et al. Mild head injury in sports. In: Levin HS, Eisenberg H, Benton A, editors. Mild head injury. Oxford (UK): Oxford University Press; 1989. p. 257–75.
30. Lovell M, Collins M, Bradley J. Return to play following sports-related concussion. Clin Sports Med 2004;23:421–41.
31. Lovell MR, Iverson GL, Collins MW, et al. Measurement of symptoms following sports-related concussion: reliability and normative data for the post-concussion symptom scale. Appl Neuropsychol 2006;13(3):166–75.
32. McCrory P, Collie A, Anderson V, et al. Can we manage sport related concussion in children the same as in adults? Br J Sports Med 2004;38(5):516–9.
33. Gioia G, Janusz J, Gilstein K, et al. Neuropsychological management of concussion in children and adolescents: effects of age and gender on impact [abstract]. Br J Sports Med 2004;38:657.
34. Belanger HG, Vanderploeg RD. The neuropsychological impact of sport-related concussion: a meta-analysis. J Int Neuropsychol Soc 2005;11(4): 345–57.
35. Belanger HG, Curtiss G, Demery JA, et al. Factors moderating neuropsychological outcomes following mild traumatic brain injury: a meta-analysis. J Int Neuropsychol Soc 2005;11(3):215–27.
36. McCrea M, Iverson G, McAllister T, et al. An integrated review of recovery after mild traumatic brain injury (MTBI): implications for clinical management. Clin Neuropsychol 2009;23:1368–90.
37. Leddy J, Kozlowski K, Donnelly J, et al. A preliminary study of subsymptomatic threshold exercise training for refractory post-concussion syndrome. Clin J Sport Med 2010;20:21–7.
38. McAllister TW. Neuropsychiatric sequelae of head injuries. Psychiatr Clin North Am 1992;15:395–413.
39. Ponsford J, Willmott C, Rothwell A, et al. Impact of early intervention on outcome after mild traumatic brain injury in children. Pediatrics 2001;108: 1297–303.
40. Tenovuo O. Pharmacological enhancement of cognitive and behavioral deficits after traumatic brain injury. Curr Opin Neurol 2006;19:528–33.
41. Catroppa C, Anderson VA, Morse SA, et al. Children's attentional skills 5 years post-TBI. J Pediatr Psychol 2007;32:354–69.

42. Dicker BG. Profile of those at risk for minor head injury. J Head Trauma Rehabil 1992;7:83–91.
43. Collins MW, Iverson GL, Lovell MR, et al. On-field predictors of neuropsychological and symptom deficit following sports-related concussion. Clin J Sport Med 2003;13:222–9.
44. Lenaerts ME, Couch JR. Posttraumatic headache. Curr Treat Options Neurol 2004;6:507–17.

Neuropsychological Assessment of Sport-Related Concussion

Eric W. Johnson, PsyD[a],*, Nathan E. Kegel, MSEd[a],
Michael W. Collins, PhD[b]

KEYWORDS

- Neuropsychology • Concussion • mTBI • Sports
- Assessment • Management

Evaluation and management of sports-related concussion has received unprecedented attention in both the scientific community and lay media in recent years. Assessment of concussion can be a challenging endeavor for medical practitioners given the different factors associated with each individual injury. Traditionally, clinicians have had to rely on subjective reports of athletes to determine status regarding recovery. The use of neuropsychological testing provides an objective method in the evaluation and management of concussion, and has led to its increased popularity over the past decade. The purpose of this article is to review the utility of neuropsychological testing in the management of sports concussion. The discussion begins with a brief review of the history of neurocognitive testing in sports, followed by an examination of data supporting the reliability, validity, sensitivity, and prognostic value of using neurocognitive testing during the subacute period of recovery following sports concussion. A case study demonstrating the practical use of neurocognitive testing in sports-related concussion is also presented.

HISTORY OF NEUROPSYCHOLOGICAL TESTING

Before the 1980s most brain injury research focused on severe traumatic brain injury; neurologic and neurocognitive changes following mild traumatic brain injury (mTBI) were considered inconsequential. Barth and colleagues[1] conducted the first large scale research study of neuropsychological assessment of concussion in sports that laid the foundation for current management practices. This landmark study

Disclosure: Michael Collins is the co-developer and chief clinical officer of ImPACT applications.
[a] Department of Orthopaedic Surgery, Sports Concussion Program, University of Pittsburgh Medical Center, 3200 South Water Street, Pittsburgh, PA 15203, USA
[b] Department of Orthopaedic Surgery and Neurological Surgery, University of Pittsburgh Medical Center, 3200 South Water Street, Pittsburgh, PA 15203, USA
* Corresponding author.
E-mail address: johnsonew@upmc.edu

examined recovery from concussion in collegiate athletes using a neuropsychological test battery of paper/pencil tasks. Overall, it was found that athletes experienced a significant decline in neurocognitive functioning after injury when compared with preinjury baseline testing. Data returned to normal within 10 days after injury. A few years later, neuropsychological assessment of concussion was first used in professional sports with the Pittsburgh Steelers. This eventually led to league-wide concussion programs in the National Football League (NFL; 1993),[2] the National Hockey League (1996),[3] and Major League Baseball (2004). Since then, neuropsychological testing has continued to accurately identify deficits in athletes who were otherwise asymptomatic.[4–7] As a result, neuropsychological assessment has expanded understanding of concussion and currently plays an important role in the evaluation and management of sport-related concussion.[8] However, use of traditional paper/pencil testing is neither practical nor economical for widespread use among the millions of athletes that experience concussion each year.[9]

To more greatly benefit concussed athletes at all levels and ages, computer-based neurocognitive testing has become increasingly common over the last decade, especially in organized sports. When compared with traditional neuropsychological testing, computer-based assessment has several advantages. For baseline testing, computerized assessment is efficient and economical because large numbers of athletes are able to be tested within a short period of time. Practice effects are minimal because computer-based testing allows for randomization of stimuli and multiple test versions improve reliability across multiple administrations. In addition, computer-based testing allows for more accurate measurement of reaction time to within one one-hundredth of a second, and increased validity of identifying subtle changes or deficits in cognitive speed. Computer-based testing also reduces administrator error and inter-rater reliability issues.[10] Following each administration, data is easily stored and accessed in a computer database.[11] Despite the immediate availability of test scores, however, only qualified professionals trained in both neuropsychological assessment and traumatic brain injury should interpret the results. In fact, current legislation is being instituted in multiple states that would require athletes to be removed from play until they are evaluated by a physician or psychologist.

The main disadvantage with computer-based assessment is that the examiner typically cannot directly observe the athlete taking the test. Also, computer-based tests sample from selective neuropsychological domains rather than a global assessment of cognitive function. The measured domains, such as attention, working memory, visual motor speed, reaction time, and so forth, have been shown to be selectively affected by mild traumatic brain injury and are the focus of computer-based assessment. In cases of postconcussion syndrome or protracted recovery from sports concussion, more thorough neuropsychological assessment may be indicated. For the many previously stated reasons, however, computerized assessment for concussion is not only being used at the professional level but is currently used by approximately 350 universities and 2500 high schools. There are currently multiple computer-based neuropsychological batteries that have been developed to assess athletes following concussion. Examples of available programs include ImPACT, Cog-Sport, and Headminder. Varying levels of psychometric data are available for these instruments, although all have been researched and used specifically for the management of sports concussion.[12–15]

Recent studies using functional MRI with adolescent athletes have confirmed that there is significant hyperactivation and disruption of brain physiology in even mild injuries that do not involve loss of consciousness.[16] In general, standard structural brain imaging techniques, such as CT and MRI scans of the brain, are usually unremarkable following concussion because it is a functional rather than structural injury.[17]

In conjunction with objective neuropsychological assessment, subjective reporting symptom reporting remains an important element in the evaluation of concussion. Headache is the most common physical symptom following concussion.[18] Athletes who experience headaches accompanied by typical migraine type symptoms of nausea, vomiting, vision changes, and photophobia or phonophobia may experience a greater severity of symptoms and prolonged recovery. Mihalik and colleagues[19] assessed the presentation of posttraumatic migraine via neurocognitive testing with 3 groups: a nonheadache control group, a headache group, and a group exhibiting posttraumatic migraine characteristics. Findings indicated that the posttraumatic migraine group demonstrated significantly lower neurocognitive functioning on all 4 composites areas (verbal memory, visual memory, visual motor speed, and reaction time) and reported significantly more symptoms than both the control group and headache group.[19]

In an effort to better understand symptom presentation following concussion, factor analysis was conducted on the Post-Concussion Symptom Scale,[2,7] a 22-item Likert scale completed by the athlete following a concussion. Statistical analysis revealed 4 symptom clusters: physical/somatic, cognitive, emotional, and sleep-related difficulties.[20] Please refer to **Fig. 1**. These factors should be viewed both independently and reciprocally, and represent important domains for individually tailored interventions.

THE ROLE OF NEUROPSYCHOLOGICAL ASSESSMENT

Neuropsychological assessment has long been used following traumatic brain injury because it provides specific information regarding neurocognitive and neurobehavioral status of the examinee. Over the last 20 years it has become increasingly useful in the realm of sports concussion and has been deemed a cornerstone of concussion

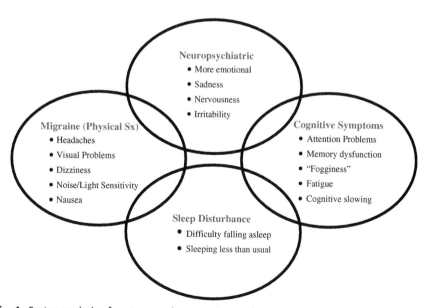

Fig. 1. Factor analysis of postconcussion symptom scale.

management by the Concussion in Sport (CIS) group at the International Symposia on Concussion in Sport.[17,21,22] Furthermore, the recommendations of the CIS group's consensus statement call for the use of baseline neuropsychological testing whenever possible.[23] Recommendations for the use of objective neuropsychological assessment in the management of sports-related concussion can also be found in the position statement of the National Athletic Trainers Association.[22] The recognition of objective neuropsychological assessment by groups comprised of varied medical professionals is an indication of its importance as an effective tool in the evaluation and management of sports-related concussion.

Clinical Utility of Neuropsychological Assessment

Neuropsychological assessment has become the preferred assessment tool for evaluating neurocognitive functioning following traumatic brain injury,[24] in part, because of its ability to detect even subtle cognitive deficits in concussed athletes.[4,11] Several studies have used neuropsychological assessment, both traditional paper and pencil and computerized, to determine duration of recovery from concussion. The results of these studies, most of which have been conducted over the past decade, are summarized in **Table 1**.

An examination of data from **Table 1** reveals several clearly observable trends. First, a comparison between days until cognitive resolution and symptom resolution indicates an apparent discrepancy and tremendous variability across studies. Computerized neuropsychological assessment appears to be more sensitive to the subtleties of recovery, indicating that symptoms resolve before return to baseline neurocognitive functioning. Overall, it appears reasonable to suggest that objective

Table 1
Cognitive and physical symptom resolution following sports-related concussion

Authors	Sample Size	Population	Tests Used	Total Days Cognitive Resolution	Total Days Symptom Resolution
Pellman et al 2005[59]	95	Pro (NFL)	Paper and pencil NP	1 d	1 d
McCrea et al 2003[60]	94	College	SAC	>1 d	7 d
McCrea et al 2003[60]	94	College	Paper and pencil NP	5–7 d	7 d
Echemendia 2001[5]	29	College	Paper and pencil NP	3 d	3 d
Guskiewicz et al 2003[37]	94	College	Balance BESS	3–5 d	7 d
Bleiberg et al 2005[61]	64	College	Computer	3–7 d	Did not evaluate
Iverson et al 2006[41]	30	High school	Computer	10 d	7 d
McClincy et al 2006[62]	104	High school	Computer	14 d	7–10 d
Lovell, et al 2007[63]	208	High school	Computer	26 d	17 d

Abbreviations: BESS, balance error scoring system; NP, neuropsychological testing; SAC, the standardized assessment of concussion.

neuropsychological testing is more sensitive to recovery than subjective symptom reporting. Every athlete, however, should have both full cognitive recovery and symptom resolution before returning to play. In addition, there is evidence indicating prolonged recovery times for younger athletes. This effect of age highlights the importance of considering individualized factors when evaluating and managing sports-related concussion.

Individualized Management

Neuropsychological assessment provides not only an objective measure of neurocognitive functioning following head injury and allows for an individualized approach to concussion management. Individual athletes vary significantly in neurocognitive ability before or after injury, so one must measure their individual differences.[25] Neuropsychological assessment has detected differences in neurocognitive performances based on several individual factors, including age, gender, and history of prior concussion.

Age

Several studies have used neurocognitive testing to demonstrate differences in child and adolescent athletes compared with adults. Field and colleagues[26] compared baseline and postconcussion neurocognitive functioning for high school and college athletes during recovery from concussion. Despite the higher rate of prior concussions for the college sample, high school athletes demonstrated longer overall recovery from in-study concussions. These finding suggest a more protracted recovery from concussion in high school athletes. Similar results have been found in comparisons between high school and professional football players.[27] Furthermore, evidence suggests that high school athletes who experienced a mild concussion, (ie, less than 15 minutes of on-field symptoms), required at least 7 days before full neurocognitive and symptom recovery was achieved.[28] Prolonged recovery in younger athletes is thought to be directly related to immature brain development, and possibly increased susceptibility to the neurometabolic changes associated with mTBI.[29–33]

Gender

The increased participation of women and girls in organized athletics has raised the question of whether gender influences concussion incidence and severity. Recently, new evidence has suggested that a potential difference exists between the way men and women experience and recover from concussion. Colvin and colleagues[34] compared a large sample of male and female soccer players, adjusting for body mass index, and found that women had significantly more postconcussive symptoms as well as poorer performance on computer-based neuropsychological testing. Several other studies have found similarly poor postconcussion neurocognitive performance in women when compared with men.[35,36] Although there appear to be gender differences in the severity of symptoms and neurocognitive functioning following concussion, the potential reasons for these differences remain unclear. There may be gender-specific differences in brain physiology or even neck strength that may contribute to these findings. Moreover, incidence of migraine is higher in women compared with men, and could potentially play a mediating role. Continued research in this area is needed to further clarify the complex factors involved in these apparent gender differences.

Prior concussion history

Identification of an athlete's concussion history is an important factor in determining whether the athlete can safely return to play. There is a growing body of evidence suggesting detrimental physical and cognitive effects of multiple concussions. Although there is a paucity of prospective evidence, a recent retrospective study surveyed a sample of retired NFL athletes and found that those who had experienced 3 or more concussions were more likely to report symptoms of cognitive impairment and depression.[37] In a study examining multiple concussions in college football players, Collins and colleagues[4] demonstrated long-term mild deficits in executive functioning and speed of information processing in athletes who sustained 2 or more concussions. In a more recent study, Colvin and colleagues[34] reported male and female high school soccer players with a history of at least 1 previous concussion performed significantly worse on computerized neuropsychological testing than those athletes who had no prior concussion history. Neurocognitive deficits in processing speed were also identified in male rugby players with a history of 3 or more concussions.[38] Other studies, however, have indicated no detrimental effects of concussion history on neurocognitive performance.[39–41] As a result, there continues to be a lack of consensus regarding the effects of multiple concussions on neurocognitive performance, which is a topic of continued empirical investigation. It is hoped that studies such as these will help to clarify the significance of individualized factors, such as age, gender, and history of multiple concussion, and ultimately help to inform effective management strategies.

Psychometric Properties and Utility of Neuropsychological Testing

The primary purpose of neuropsychological testing following concussion is to assess for possible change in cognitive functioning. Typically, clinicians attempt to estimate decline in cognitive functioning attributable to head injury. This section will examine the psychometric properties and clinical utility of neuropsychological testing in sports-related concussion.

Reliability

Adequate reliability is critically important to neuropsychological tests, but perhaps even more so for those meant specifically to assess concussion. Assessments of neurocognitive functioning following sports-related concussion often occur in brief retest intervals because of the nature of return-to-play decision-making. Several studies have attempted to demonstrate reliability of computer-based neuropsychological measures of concussion, with test-retest reliabilities generally falling in the moderate range.[42–44] Some methodological concerns have occurred in these prior studies, including the administration of multiple test batteries in the testing session, which increases the risk of interference effects and inclusion of invalid data in these analyses. In a well-controlled study examining ImPACT, Iverson and colleagues[45] looked at the psychometric properties by assessing a sample of 56 nonconcussed adolescents on 2 occasions. Results of the initial analysis were then compared with results from a group of 41 amateur athletes assessed within 72 hours of injury. Test-retest reliability coefficients for the 5 composite scores ranged from 0.65 to 0.86, which are comparable or higher than many traditional neuropsychological tests. Furthermore, the comparison of concussed and nonconcussed athletes demonstrated the sensitivity of ImPACT and allowed for the calculation of Reliable Change Indices (RCIs).[45] RCIs provide the clinician with increased confidence when determining whether or not follow-up assessments are discrepant from baseline. (The RCIs for ImPACT can be found in **Table 2**).

Overall, athletes with concussions are far more likely to have 2 or more declines exceeding reliable change across the 5 composites compared with healthy controls (63.4% versus 3.6%).[45]

Table 2		
Reliable change indices for ImPACT: 80% confidence interval		
Composite	**Declined**	**Improved**
Verbal memory	9 points	9 points
Visual memory	14 points	14 points
Processing speed	3 points	7 points
Reaction time	0.06 s	0.06 s
Postconcussion scale	10 points	10 points

Data from Iverson GL, Lovell MR, Collins MW. Interpreting change on ImPACT following sports concussion. Clin Neuropsychol 2003;17:464.

Long-term test-retest reliability for ImPACT has also been established. Schatz[46] examined a sample of collegiate athletes by administering participants' baseline assessments 2 years apart. Intraclass correlation coefficients revealed adequate stability for the visual memory, processing speed, and reaction time composites, with slightly more variability on the verbal memory composite and symptom score (**Table 3**). However, using RCIs and regression-based methods, only a small percentage of participants' scores showed reliable or significant change on the composite scores (0%–6%) or symptom scale (5%–10%).

Validity

Studies of validity of neuropsychological measures of concussion have attempted to determine a given test's ability to measure their purported cognitive constructs. Schatz and Putz[47] examined concurrent validity of several computerized neurocognitive assessment tools (eg, ImPACT, HeadMiner, CogSport) using cross-validation. First, computerized measures were shown to demonstrate significant but moderate correlations with established neuropsychological measures (eg, Trail Making Tests, Digit Span Test). In addition, computerized assessments generally demonstrated moderate correlations with one another on processing speed and reaction time domains, but not on memory indices. These results indicate that the tests share some common variance on cognitive constructs, such as processing speed and reaction time.

Neuropsychological testing is both sensitive and specific in identifying concussion. Schatz and colleagues[48] examined performance on computerized neurocognitive testing, as well as on a subjective symptom scales, and found that 82% of subjects

Table 3			
Two-year test-retest reliability for impact in collegiate athletes			
	Mean		
Composite	**Time 1 (in seconds)**	**Time 2 (in seconds)**	**ICC**
Verbal memory	87.6	87.8	.459
Visual memory	75.6	78.1	.653
Processing speed	41.2	42.0	.742
Reaction time	0.54	0.53	.676
Symptom scale	9.3	9.8	.431

Abbreviation: ICC, intraclass correlation coefficient.

Data from Schatz P. Long-term test-retest reliability of baseline cognitive assessments using ImPACT. Am J Sports Med 2010;38:47–53.

in the concussion group and 89% of subjects in the control group were correctly classified according to discriminate function analysis. Furthermore, Iverson and Brooks[49] compared healthy adolescent males to high school football players who sustained a recent concussion using an algorithm that classifies neurocognitive performance based on composite percentile ranks. Findings indicated that the majority of normal subjects (73%) and the minority of concussed athletes (21%) were classified as "broadly normal." In contrast, 56% of concussed athletes and only 8.5% of the normal subjects fell in the unusually low or extremely low classification ranges. Similar studies have demonstrated sensitivity exceeding 90% when computerized assessment measures were combined with a self-reporting measure and a brief traditional neuropsychological test battery.[50]

Added Value

Several recent studies have also demonstrated the added value of computerized neurocognitive testing relative to the use of subjective symptoms in isolation. Traditionally, clinicians have relied heavily on the subjective self-reporting of symptoms when evaluating postconcussion functioning. However, the asymptomatic athletes performed significantly lower than uninjured controls on measures of neurocognitive functioning.[6] Van Kampen and colleagues[51] found 93% of a sample of concussed athletes had either abnormal neurocognitive test results or elevated symptoms when compared with baseline, and adding neurocognitive testing resulted in a net increase in sensitivity of 19%.[51] When specific neurocognitive abilities (reaction time and memory) were examined 4 days following concussion in high school and college athletes, 11% of the concussed athletes had abnormal reaction time and 32% had abnormal memory compared with their baseline data.[52] These studies show the added value of using neurocognitive testing in conjunction with symptom evaluation when determining recovery from concussion. The addition of neuropsychological testing provides a sensitive, objective assessment tool that helps clinicians make more accurate diagnostic and return-to-play decisions.

Prognostic Utility

Neuropsychological assessment may also assist with prognosis following concussion. Prognosis is important because it alerts the clinician to the severity of the injury. As a result, specific treatment recommendations can be made or implemented. For example, depending on the severity of deficits on neurocognitive testing, specific academic accommodations can be implemented (eg, untimed tests) before experiencing significant academic difficulty stemming from the injury.

To determine whether acute examination could predict recovery occurring within 10 days, Iverson[53] administered computerized neurocognitive testing to concussed high school athletes within 72 hours of injury. This prospective study indicated that more than half the sample (56%) required more than 10 days to completely recover. A closer examination of the composite scores indicated that concussions that required more than 10 days to recover from were more likely to result in multiple scores below the tenth percentile compared with normative data. In fact, high school athletes performed worse on 3 of 4 cognitive composite scores (visual memory, processing speed, and reaction time), and approximately 95% of these athletes required greater than 10 days to recover.[53] Additional research has further identified prognostic indicators of concussion based on symptoms and neuropsychological test patterns. Lau and colleagues[54] examined 177 concussed high school football players and discovered both subjective and objective prognostic indicators when evaluating athletes within an average of 2.23 days following concussion. Self-reported migraine symptoms, perceived neurocognitive decline (eg, bradyphrenia), and decreased reaction time composite scores were most significant in predicting longer recovery times following concussion. Continued research addressing prognostic indicators may determine more accurate recovery times for acutely injured athletes.

CLINICAL EVALUATION

Existing evaluation and management techniques have been strongly influenced by the CIS group's consensus statements, which have suggested each athlete progress through standardized return-to-play guidelines.[17,21] Specifically, McCrory and colleagues[21] described 3 main components to be used with all athletes for concussion management: neuropsychological assessment, evaluation of subjective symptoms, and balance testing. These components are critical when making return-to-play decisions and should be considered in conjunction with internationally accepted return-to-play criteria outlined in the following list:

1. Athlete must be asymptomatic at rest.
2. Athlete must be asymptomatic with full physical and cognitive exertion.
3. Balance testing must be returned to baseline.
4. Neurocognitive testing must be returned to baseline.

Baseline Neurocognitive Testing

Ideally, the clinical evaluation begins with baseline testing before a concussive injury. Measuring an athlete's neurocognitive abilities before injury allows for more informed return-to-play decisions. Baseline testing is not required to successfully determine that an athlete has fully recovered because neuropsychological tests are constructed to compare injured athletes scores to healthy normal individuals of their same normative group (eg, age, gender). Despite this, baseline testing is preferred for a more accurate understanding of an athlete's premorbid neurocognitive status. It should be noted that baseline testing can be invalid for a multitude of reasons, including a distracting environment, not taking the test seriously, lack of full effort, confusion with instructions, learning disabilities, and attention-deficit/hyperactivity disorder. Thus, a thorough evaluation should address the presence of these issues.

Clinical Model

Following diagnosis (or suspicion) of a concussion, a clinician trained in neuropsychological testing evaluates the athlete. Subacute clinical evaluation of the concussed athlete should include a detailed clinical interview related to premorbid functioning; current injury; relevant patient history, including medical, social, psychiatric, school, developmental, cultural variables (eg, family environment); and behavioral observations.[27]

Athletes should return to play based on a graduated progression through several steps. Overall, any athlete with remaining symptoms or abnormal neurocognitive test results should not be returned to play. Lovell[55] provided a framework from which to base decisions. Ideally, an athlete should undergo a neuropsychological evaluation within 72 hours of the concussion. If any neurocognitive deficits are present, follow-up neuropsychological testing is best completed 5 to 7 days later,[55] and subsequently at weekly or biweekly intervals to monitor and track recovery.

Testing a symptomatic athlete allows for prognostic estimates, as previously described, and provides data-based recommendations regarding academic considerations and potential return to physical conditioning. The brief (20–25 minute) neurocognitive test may or may not temporarily exacerbate some symptoms. But the subjective information along with the objective test data helps formulate specific recommendations to expedite recovery (eg, removal from school or classroom accommodations for student athletes). However, if the athlete is severely symptomatic, it may not be necessary to test neurocognitive abilities because testing can significantly exacerbate symptoms. In these cases, cognitive and physical exertion should be eliminated or extremely limited and the athlete evaluated with computer testing after several days of recovery. In most instances, repeat testing every week or two is generally recommended and allows one to track the athlete's recovery process.

Once an athlete is asymptomatic at rest, a graded return to exertion is necessary to monitor any return of symptoms with increased heart rate and avoid severe exacerbation of symptoms. If symptoms return with exertion, modifications may be made to the athlete's cognitive or physical exertion. The athlete does not progress to the next level, but rather stays at an exertional level (both cognitive and physical exertion) that does not provoke symptoms. Thus, it is necessary to increase exertional levels from mild, then to moderate, then finally to heavy (or game pace exertion) over several days before any contact. In all cases, once the athlete is asymptomatic with heavy, noncontact exertion, a final neurocognitive test should be used to ensure that the athlete's abilities are at baseline levels before contact. If the athlete is asymptomatic, but neurocognitive testing has not returned to baseline levels, then the athlete should not be returned to play. Rather, if the athlete displays deficits on testing, an additional examination with repeat testing is recommended within 5 to 7 days. For athletes who continue to exhibit significant symptoms or test deficits despite rest, consideration should occur for more extensive medical intervention or more extensive neuropsychological testing.

Despite its documented value, neuropsychological assessment should not be used exclusively as the lone source of clinical information when treating sports concussions. Along with subjective symptoms and neurocognitive testing, a physical/vestibular examination should be included. Problems with balance occurs in up to 40% of concussed athletes.[56] Balance dysfunction can occur secondary to brain trauma or actual injury to the vestibular system. In either instance, a screening of postural sway with the athlete standing with feet together and eyes open and then eyes closed can identify grossly abnormal balance. Most athletes' dizziness or gait dysfunction resolves within a few weeks. However, recent research found vestibular rehabilitation significantly reduced dizziness, gait, and balance dysfunction in athletes.[57]

When an athlete is unable to meet the return-to-play criteria previously described, the topic of retirement becomes an issue of concern, especially because multiple concussions may result in long-term neurocognitive deficits also previously described.[4,56] Unfortunately, no specific cutoff has been established for retiring a player, and again, decisions should be made on an individual basis. However, 2 potential red flags for potential retirement include (1) lingering symptoms many weeks or months following the injury despite proper management and (2) if minimal biomechanical force is causing a reoccurrence of concussion-related symptoms.

CASE EXAMPLE

Patrick is a 15-year-old high school quarterback who sustained multiple concussions during the 2009 football season. The first injury occurred in mid September when he sustained a posterior helmet-to-turf impact after being tackled. In retrospect, he reported experiencing several acute symptoms, including vision changes, fatigue, vasovagal dizziness, headache, and general lethargy. Patrick denied these symptoms at the time of the injury and continued to play. He continued to experience headaches 3 out of 7 days per week, vasovagal dizziness, fatigue, and cognitive difficulties through October 2009 when he unfortunately sustained another head injury while playing football. This second injury again involved the posterior aspect of his helmet striking the turf following a tackle, resulting in a significant exacerbation of previous symptoms.

Patrick completed the 2009 football season without reporting the symptoms of either head injury. He reported the injuries and symptoms following the 2009 season and was seen in clinic in mid November 2009. At the time of his initial clinic visit, Patrick was experiencing daily headaches, particularly at school, that he rated as a 7 out of 10 on a pain scale. He also continued to experience vasovagal dizziness, fatigue, photosensitivity, phonophobia, and moderate to severe cognitive difficulties that were resulting in decreased academic performance. A clinical interview revealed no prior history of concussion. There was a strong family history of migraine headaches on the maternal side, as well as a proclivity for carsickness. The physical evaluation revealed deficits during vestibular-ocular screening, particularly provocation of dizziness during gaze stability testing. Neurocognitive testing was accomplished using ImPACT, and revealed statistically significant deficits in memory (verbal and visual), processing speed, and reaction time when compared with baseline (see ImPACT data).

Overall, results of the initial evaluation indicated moderate levels of post concussion syndrome resulting from multiple head injuries sustained during the 2009 football season. Patrick's symptom presentation called for several treatments. First, removal from physical exertion and reduction of cognitive exertion via academic accommodations was indicated. Patrick was placed on half days of school and provided with 50% reduction of work, extra time on tests, elimination of tests when possible, and extensions on long-term assignments. Second, Patrick was referred for pharmacologic intervention with recommendation of prescription of amantadine, a neurostimulant empirically shown to be effective in improving cognitive functioning following head injury.[58] Finally, given his difficulty during vestibular ocular screening, Patrick was referred for a formal vestibular evaluation and subsequent vestibular physical therapy.

After approximately 1 month of compliance with treatment recommendations, Patrick returned to the clinic in mid December 2009, and demonstrated improvements in both physical symptoms and neurocognitive functioning, although neither returned to baseline. He was prescribed 200 mg of amantadine (100 mg in the morning and 100 mg at lunch) and completed 1 month of vestibular therapy. Headache frequency decreased to one time per week and severity decreased to a 1 out of 10 on a pain scale. Dramatic improvements in neurocognitive functioning were observed during ImPACT testing. Verbal and visual memory scores improved considerably, but remained slightly below baseline, and processing speed and reaction time composite scores were commensurate with baseline (see ImPACT data). At this point in recovery, it was recommended that Patrick remain on prescribed medication while returning to school full time and engaging in increased amounts of noncontact physical exertion during formal physical therapy to monitor heart rate.

Patrick returned to the clinic in mid January 2010 and reported a complete resolution of physical symptoms associated with concussion. He continued his prescribed dosage of 200 mg amantadine and Patrick was no longer experiencing headache, dizziness, or fatigue despite having returned to school full time (with academic accommodations) and engaging in moderate levels of noncontact physical exertion (running and weightlifting). ImPACT data at the time of this appointment indicated 3 out of 4 composite scores within reliable change of Patrick's baseline. The lone exception was continued mild deficits in verbal memory. Because of his improved symptom presentation and near baseline neurocognitive functioning, it was recommended that Patrick be weaned off amantadine while continuing exertional physical therapy and remaining in school full-time with academic accommodations.

When he returned to clinic in February 2010, Patrick reported being completely asymptomatic from both a physical and cognitive standpoint. He had been weaned off amantadine for approximately 1 month, and continued to engage in high levels of physical exertion with no return of symptoms. In addition, academic performance returned to preinjury levels and there were no symptoms with cognitive exertion while at school. Furthermore, Patrick's neurocognitive performance on ImPACT returned to baseline. Because Patrick was completely asymptomatic with full physical exertion and demonstrated baseline neurocognitive functioning, it was determined that he met international return-to-play criteria and he was cleared for return to football. Patrick and his parents agreed to follow-up approximately 3 weeks into the next football season to be certain subtle symptoms or neurocognitive deficits did not return with contact.

This case illustrates several important issues to consider in the management of concussion. First and foremost, accurate identification of signs and symptoms on the sideline is a critical initial step in effective management. As was the case here, athletes are not always forthcoming when reporting symptoms of concussion. As a result, medical staff, athletic trainers, and coaches must be aware of subtle concussion signs and changes in mental status. Players exhibiting any sign or symptom of concussion should be removed from play and referred for medical follow-up. Athletes should never be permitted to return to the contest during which the injury took place. Second, this case highlights the potential for protracted recovery time in cases where a subsequent head injury is sustained before the first injury was completely resolved. In this case, Patrick's second head injury clearly exacerbated the unresolved first injury, and almost certainly resulted in prolonged recovery time. Finally, the use of neurocognitive assessment is a critical component in the identification and management of concussion. Computerized neurocognitive assessment tools, such as ImPACT, provide the clinician with important information for the planning of treatment recommendations and allow for progress monitoring during recovery. This information also offers the clinician increased certainty that neurocognitive deficits, which are often subtle, are completely resolved before returning an athlete to play.

ImPACT™ Clinical Report   High School Football QB

Exam Type	Baseline	Post-injury	Post-injury	Post-injury	Post-injury	Post-injury
Date Tested	08/13/2008	11/16/2009	11/30/2009	12/18/2009	01/11/2010	02/22/2010
Last Concussion	11/23/2008	09/11/2009	09/11/2009	09/11/2009	09/11/2009	09/11/2009
Exam Language	English	English	English	English	English	English
Test Version	4.5.805	4.5.805	4.5.805	4.5.805	4.5.805	4.5.805
Normative Comparison Group	M 14-15	M 14-15	M 14-15	M 14-15	M 14-15	M 14-15

Composite Scores *												
Memory composite (verbal)	91	68%	83	38%	77	18%	89	60%	83	38%	93	80%
Memory composite (visual)†	89	80%	73	36%	55	5%	83	69%	89	80%	89	80%
Visual motor speed composite	46.58	95%	29.05	19%	29.05	19%	47.33	96%	52.68	99%	53.25	99%
Reaction time composite	0.49	90%	0.78	1%	0.76	1%	0.44	97%	0.42	96%	0.45	96%
Impulse control composite	4		45		9		2		1		5	
Total Symptom Score	0		17		18		7		3		1	

SUMMARY

Neuropsychological assessment has long been used following traumatic brain injury because it provides specific information regarding neurocognitive and neurobehavioral status of the examinee. It has been deemed reliable, valid, and can be prognostic when used in the acute stages following concussion. Over the last 20 years it has become increasingly useful in the realm of sports concussion and has been deemed a cornerstone of concussion management by the CIS group at the International Symposia on Concussion in Sport.[17,21,22] As a result, evaluation and management of sports-related concussion has received unprecedented attention at the professional and collegiate levels, as well as in high school and middle school. To more greatly benefit concussed athletes at all levels and ages, computer-based neurocognitive testing has become increasingly common as well as baseline testing before injury. Despite its proven value, neuropsychological assessment should be used as one tool in a full, individualized assessment of concussion.

REFERENCES

1. Barth JT, Alves WM, Ryan TV, et al. Mild head injury in sports: neuropsychological sequelae and recovery of function. In: Levin HS, Eisenberg HM, Benton AL, editors. Mild head injury. New York: Oxford University Press; 1989. p. 257–75.
2. Lovell MR. Evaluation of the professional athlete. In: Bailes JE, Lovell MR, Maroon JC, editors. Sports-related concussion. St Louis (MO): Quality Medical Publishing; 1999. p. 200–14.
3. Lovell MR, Burke CJ. Concussion management in professional hockey. In: Cantu RE, editor. Neurologic athletic head and spine injury. Philadelphia: WB Saunders Inc; 2000. p. 109–16.
4. Collins MW, Grindel SH, Lovell MR, et al. Relationship between concussion and neuropsychological performance in college football players. JAMA 1999;282: 964–70.
5. Echemendia RJ, Putukian M, Mackin RS, et al. Neuropsychological test performance prior to and following sport-related mild traumatic brain injury. Clin J Sport Med 2001;11:23–31.
6. Fazio VC, Lovell MR, Pardini JE, et al. The relation between post concussion symptoms and neurocognitive performance in concussed athletes. NeuroRehabilitation 2007;22:207–16.
7. Lovell MR, Collins MW. Neuropsychological assessment of the college football player. J Head Trauma Rehabil 1998;13:9–26.
8. Zillmer EA, Schneider J, Tinker J, et-al. A history of sports-related concussions: a neuropsychological perpective. In: Echemendia RJ, editor. Sports neuropsychology: assessment and management of traumatic brain injury. New York: Guilford; 2006. p. 17–35.
9. Lovell MR. The management of sports-related concussion: current status and future trends. Clin Sports Med 2009;28:95–112.
10. Lovell MR, Collins MW, Fu FH, et al. Neuropsychologic testing in sports: past, present, and future. Br J Sports Med 2001;35:367–72.
11. Schatz P, Zillmer E. Computer-based assessment of sports-related concussion. Appl Neuropsychol 2003;10:42–7.
12. Collie A. Computerised cognitive assessment of athletes with sports related head injury. Br J Sports Med 2001;35:7–302.
13. Collie A, Maruff P. Computerized neuropsychological testing. Br J Sports Med 2003;37:2–3.

14. Erlanger DM, Feldman DJ, Kutner K. Concussion resolution index. NewYork: Headminder, Inc; 1999.

15. Lovell MR, Collins MW, Podell K, et al. Immediate post-concussion assessment and cognitive testing (ImPACT). Pittsburgh (PA): NeuroHealth Systems, LLC; 2000.

16. Lovell MR, Pardini JE, Welling J, et al. Functional brain abnormalities in sports-related concussion predict time to return to play. Neurosurgery 2007;6:352–9.

17. Aubry M, Cantu R, Dvorak J, et al. Summary and agreement statement of the 1st international symposium on concussion in sport, Vienna 2001. Clin J Sport Med 2002;12:6–11.

18. Guskiewicz KM, Weaver NL, Padua DA, et al. Epidemiology of concussion in collegiate and high school football players. Am J Sports Med 2000;28: 643–50.

19. Mihalik J, Stump J, Collins MW, et al. Posttraumatic migraine characteristics in athletes following sports-related concussion. J Neurosurg 2005;102:850–5.

20. Pardini D, Stump JE, Lovell MR, et al. The post-concussion symptom scale (PCSS): a factor analysis. Presented at the Second International Symposium on Concussion in Sport. Prague (Czech Republic), November 2004.

21. McCrory P, Meeuwisse W, Johnston K, et al. Consensus statement on concussion in sport: the 3rd international conference on concussion in sport held in Zurich, November 2008. Br J Sports Med 2009;43(Suppl 1):i76–90.

22. McCrory P, Johnston K, Meeuwisse W, et al. Summary and agreement statement of the 2nd international conference on concussion in sport, prague 2004. Clin J Sport Med 2005;15:48–55.

23. Guskiewicz KM, Bruce SL, Cantu RC, et al. National Athletic Trainer's Association position statement: Management of sport-related concussion. J Athl Train 2004; 39:280–97.

24. Barth JT, Broshek DK, Freeman JR. A new frontier for neuropsychology. In: Echemendia R, editor. Sports neuropsychology: assessment and management of traumatic brain injury. Guilford: New York; 2006.

25. Schatz P, Covassin T. Neuropsychological testing programs for college athletes. In: Echemendia R, editor. Sports neuropsychology: assessment and management of traumatic brain injury; 2006. p. 160–175.

26. Field M, Collins MW, Lovell MR, et al. Does age play a role in recovery from sports-related concussion? a comparison of high school and collegiate athletics. J Pediatr 2003;142:546–53.

27. Pellman EJ, Lovell MR, Viano D, et al. Concussion in professional football: recovery of NFL and high school athletes by computerized neuropsychological testing-part 12. Neurosurgery 2006;58:263–74.

28. Lovell MR, Collins MW, Iverson GL, et al. Recovery from mild concussion in high school athletes. J Neurosurg 2003;98:296–301.

29. Biagas KV, Gundl PD, Kochanek PM, et al. Posttraumatic hyperemia in immature, mature, and aged rats: autoradiographic determination of cerebral blood flow. J Neurotrauma 1996;13:189–200.

30. Bruce DA, Alavi A, Bilaniuk L, et al. Diffuse cerebral swelling following head injuries in children: the syndrome of "malignant brain edema". J Neurosurg 1981;54:170–8.

31. Grundl PD, Biagas KV, Kochanek PM, et al. Early cerebrovascular response to head injury in immature and mature rats. J Neurotrauma 1994;11:135–48.

32. McDonald JW, Johnston MV. Physiological pathophysiological roles of excitatory amino acids during central nervous system development. Brain Res Brain Res Rev 1990;15:41–70.

33. McDonald JW, Silverstein FS, Johnston MV. Neurotoxicity of N-methyl-D-aspartate is markedly enhanced in developing rat central nervous system. Brain Res 1988;459:200–3.
34. Colvin AE, Mullen J, Lovell MR, et al. The role of concussion history and gender in recovery from soccer-related concussion. Am J Sports Med 2009;37(9): 1699–704.
35. Broshek DK, Kaushik T, Freeman JR, et al. Sex differences in outcome following sports-related concussion. J Neurosurg 2005;102:856–63.
36. Covassin T, Schatz P, Swanik C. Sex differences in neuropsychological function and post-concussion symptoms of collegiate athletes. Neurosurgery 2007;61: 345–51.
37. Guskiewicz KM, McCrea M, Marshall SW, et al. Cumulative effects associated with recurrent concussion in collegiate football players: the NCAA concussion study. JAMA 2003;290:2549–55.
38. Gardner A, Shores EA, Batchelor J. Reduced processing speed in rugby union players reporting three or more previous concussions. Arch Clin Neuropsychol 2010;25:174–81.
39. Broglio SP, Ferrara MS, Piland SG, et al. Concussion history is not a predictor of computerised neurocognitive performance. Br J Sports Med 2006;40: 802–5.
40. Bruce JM, Echemendia RJ. History of multiple self-reported concussions is not associated with reduced cognitive abilities. Neurosurgery 2009;64:100–6.
41. Iverson GL, Brooks BL, Lovell MR, et al. No cumulative effects of one or two previous concussions. Br J Sports Med 2006;40:72–5.
42. Broglio SP, Ferrara MS, Macciocchi SN, et al. Test-retest reliability of computerized concussion assessment programs. J Athl Train 2007;42:509–14.
43. Segalowitz SJ, Mahaney P, Santesso DL, et al. Retest reliability in adolescents of a computerized neuropsychological battery used to assess recovery from concussion. NeuroRehabilitation 2007;22:243–51.
44. Valovich-McLeod TC, Barr WB, McCrea M, et al. Psychometric and measurement properties of concussion assessment tools in youth sports. J Athl Train 2006;41: 399–408.
45. Iverson GL, Lovell MR, Collins MW. Interpreting change on ImpACT following sports concussion. Clin Neuropsychol 2003;17:460–7.
46. Schatz P. Long-term test-retest reliability of baseline cognitive assessments using ImPACT. Am J Sports Med 2010;38:47–53.
47. Schatz P, Putz BO. Cross-validation of measures used for computer-based assessment of concussion. Appl Neuropsychol 2006;13:151–9.
48. Schatz P, Pardini JE, Lovell MR, et al. Sensitivity and specificity of the ImPACT test battery for concussion in athletes. Arch Clin Neuropsychol 2006;21:91–9.
49. Iverson GL, Brooks BL. Development of preliminary evidence-based criteria for cognitive impairment associated with sport-related concussion. Br J Sports Med 2009;43(Suppl 1):i100.
50. Broglio SP, Macciocchi SN, Ferrara MS. Sensitivity of concussion assessment battery. Neurosurgery 2007;60:1050–8.
51. Van Kampen DA, Lovell MR, Pardini JE, et al. The "value added" of neurocognitive testing after sports-related concussion. Am J Sports Med 2006;34(10): 1630–5.
52. Lovell MR, Collins MW, Van Kampen DA. Concussion evaluation using ImPACT neuropsychological testing. Presented at 2010 Big Sky Athletic Training Sports Medicine Conference. Big Sky (MT), February, 2010.

53. Iverson GL. Predicting slow recovery from sport-related concussion: the new simple-complex distinction. Clin J Sport Med 2007;17:31–7.

54. Lau B, Lovell MR, Collins MW, et al. Neurocognitive and symptom predictors of recovery in high school athletes. Clin J Sport Med 2009;19:216–21.

55. Lovell MR. Neuropsychological assessment of the professional athlete. In: Echemendia R, editor. Sports neuropsychology: assessment and management of traumatic brain injury; 2006. p. 176–189.

56. Collins MW, Lovell MR, Iverson GL, et al. Cumulative effects of concussion in high shool athletes. Neurosurgery 2002;51:1175–81.

57. Alsalaheen BA, Mucha A, Morris LO, et al. Vestibular rehabilitation for dizziness and balance disorders after concussion. J Neurol Phys Ther 2010;34:87–93.

58. Kraus MF, Smith GS, Butters M, et al. Effects of the dopaminergic agent and NMDA antagonist amantadine on cognitive function, cerebral glucose metabolism and D2 receptor availability in chronic traumatic brain injury: a study using positron emission tomography (PET). Brain Inj 2005;19:471–9.

59. Pellman EJ, Lovell MR, Viano DC, et al. Concussion in professional football: neuropsychological testing–part 6. Neurosurgery 2004;55:1290–305.

60. McCrea, Guskiewicz KM, Marshall SW, et al. Acute effects and recovery time following concussion in collegiate football players: the NCAA concussion study. JAMA 2003;290(19):2556–63.

61. Bleiberg J, Warden, D. Duration of cognitive impairment after sports concussion. Neurosurgery 2005;56:E1166.

62. McClincy MP, Lovell MR, Pardini J, et al. Recovery from sports concussion. Brain Injury 2006;20:33–9.

63. Lovell MR, Pardini J, Welling J, et al. Functional brain abnormalities are related to clinical recovery and time to return-to-play in athletes. Neurosurgery 2007;61(2): 352–60.

Balance Assessment in the Management of Sport-Related Concussion

Kevin M. Guskiewicz, PhD, ATC

KEYWORDS

- Postural stability • Equilibrium • Clinical assessment
- Traumatic brain injury

Over the past decade, there is probably no sports injury more discussed in the lay media than concussion or traumatic brain injury (TBI). There has also been a flood of publications into the peer-reviewed medical literature on the topic in recent years, and the medical community has a better understanding of concussive injury today than it did just 10 years ago. Clinicians, especially those responsible for the medical care of elite athletes, have been placed under the microscope and are being scrutinized for their management of these potentially catastrophic injuries. Concussion often presents with varying symptomatology and most experts think it should be evaluated using a multifactorial approach.[1–4] Yet many clinicians neglect the use of a comprehensive concussion assessment plan,[5] despite the complexity of this injury. Given that athletes may under-report concussions by nearly 50%,[6] significant attention has been given to the validation of objective measures for managing concussion. Although neuropsychological testing has proven to be a valuable tool in concussion management, it is most useful when administered as part of a comprehensive assessment battery that includes grading of symptoms and clinical balance tests.[2,4,7,8]

A thorough sideline and clinical examination by the certified athletic trainer and team physician is considered an important first step in the management of concussion. It is best if the clinician performing the examination knows the athlete well enough to detect changes in their disposition. The evaluation, whether on the field or in the clinical setting, should be conducted in a systematic manner. The evaluation should include obtaining a *history* for specific details about the injury (eg, mechanism, symptomatology, concussion history), followed by assessing *neurocognitive function* and *balance*, which is the focus of this article. The objective measures from balance testing

The author has nothing to disclose.
Matthew Alan Gfeller Sport-Related Traumatic Brain Injury Research Center, Department of Exercise and Sport Science, University of North Carolina at Chapel Hill, 209 Fetzer Hall, CB#8700, Chapel Hill, NC 27599-8700, USA
E-mail address: gus@email.unc.edu

Clin Sports Med 30 (2011) 89–102
doi:10.1016/j.csm.2010.09.004
0278-5919/11/$ – see front matter © 2011 Elsevier Inc. All rights reserved.

can provide clinicians with an additional piece of the concussion puzzle, remove some of the guesswork in uncovering less obvious symptoms, and assist in determining readiness to return safely to participation.

For many years, neurologic examination in the athletic setting has included Romberg's tests of balance/postural stability. However, the standard Romberg test lacks objectivity and sensitivity for evaluating concussion, especially in elite athletes who tend to normally excel with activities of coordination and agility. Recent technological developments have provided the sports medicine community with more quantitative and objective assessment tools for evaluating head injuries. A review of the balance literature indicates there are characteristic deficits following traumatic brain injury, even those classified as mild traumatic brain injury (mTBI) or cerebral concussion.

ROLE OF THE CENTRAL NERVOUS SYSTEM IN MAINTAINING POSTURAL EQUILIBRIUM

Understanding the central nervous system's (CNS) feedback mechanism for maintaining postural equilibrium is the first step in building a case for *objective balance testing* in the management of sport concussion. Maintaining equilibrium requires the CNS to process and integrate afferent information from the visual, somatosensory (proprioceptive), and vestibular systems to execute appropriate and coordinated musculoskeletal responses. Feedback, obtained from sensors housed within the 3 systems, sends commands to the muscles of the extremities, which then generate an appropriate contraction to maintain postural stability.[9–13]

The primary purposes of the human vestibular system are to (1) maintain the eyes fixed on a stationary target in the presence of head and body movement and (2) maintain balance in conjunction with additional information from visual and somatosensory inputs. To accomplish the first, the semicircular canals of the vestibular labyrinth sense angular acceleration of the head, converting it to velocity information, and sending it through the vestibuloocular reflex pathways to the ocular muscles. Secondly, balance is maintained by central integration of vestibular, visual, and somatosensory orientation information. The vestibular system provides angular information from the semicircular canals and linear acceleration information (including gravity) from the utricles and saccules of the inner ear and transmits it via the vestibulospinal spinal tract to the spinal and lower extremity muscles. Under normal conditions, visual and somatosensory information is adequate for maintenance of balance. However, in populations with known vestibular deficits, the inner ear senses of balance are essential when visual and somatosensory inputs are disrupted or provide conflicting information.[13,14]

Balance Control

Balance plays a vital role in the maintenance of fluid, dynamic movement common in sport, and is defined as the process of maintaining the center of gravity (COG) within the body's base of support. Many factors enter into the task of controlling balance within this designated area. The system involves a complex network of neural connections and centers that are related by peripheral and central feedback mechanisms. A hierarchy integrating the cerebral cortex, cerebellum, basal ganglia, brainstem, and spinal cord is primarily responsible for controlling voluntary movements.[14,15]

The highest level of the hierarchy involves areas of the brain responsible for attention, concentration, memory and emotion, as well as the association cortex for receiving and correlating input from other brain structures. The middle level involves the sensorimotor cortex, cerebellum, parts of the basal ganglia, and some brainstem nuclei. The cerebellum is likely the most important structure for coordinating and controlling balance, as it receives information from the muscles, joints, skin, eyes, ears, and even the viscera.[14,15] The afferent pathways of the reflex arcs come from 3 sources: the eyes, the vestibular apparatus, and the proprioceptors. Their collective actions are referred to as postural reflexes. The efferent pathways are the alpha motor neurons to the skeletal muscles, and the integrating centers are neuron networks in the brainstem and spinal cord.[11,14] The lowest level of the hierarchy involves the brainstem and the spinal cord from which the motor neurons exit. These structures receive information from the middle level via the descending pathways. Its function is to specify the tension of particular muscles and the angle of joints necessary to carry out the programs transmitted from the middle level.

Isolation of Sensory Input

From our knowledge of the central nervous system's involvement in maintaining upright posture, we can divide the processes into 2 components. The term *sensory organization* involves those processes that determine timing, direction, and amplitude of corrective postural actions based upon information obtained from the vestibular, visual, and somatosensory inputs. This concept is important for understanding some of the concussion assessment techniques described later, such as the Sensory Organization Test (SOT; NeuroCom International, Inc, Clackamas, OR, USA). Despite the availability of multiple sensory inputs, the central nervous system generally relies on only one sense at a time for orientation information. For healthy adults, the preferred sense for balance control comes from somatosensory information (ie, feet in contact with the support surface).[13]

The second component, muscle coordination, describes processes that determine the temporal sequencing and distribution of contractile activity among the muscles of the legs and trunk that generate supportive reactions for maintaining balance. Balance deficiencies in people with neurologic problems can result from inappropriate interaction among the 3 sensory inputs that provide orientation information to the postural control system. Patients may be inappropriately dependent on one sense for situations presenting intersensory conflict.[11,13,16]

Several studies have attempted to isolate and clarify which sensory inputs are most involved with regulating posture and how the interaction among these inputs affects postural control.[16–22] A technique described by Shumway-Cook and Horak[11] and Ingersoll and Armstrong[23] called the Clinical Test of Sensory Interaction and Balance (CTSIB) was originally used to systematically remove or conflict sensory input from 1 or more of the 3 senses. The technique used combinations of 3 visual and 2 support-surface conditions during assessment of postural sway to identify any reliance on 1 or more of the 3 senses for postural control, which was thought to be present for certain pathologic conditions, including TBI.[23]

BALANCE DEFICITS FOLLOWING TBI

Disruption of static and dynamic balance in nonathletic populations has been identified and described following pathologic conditions, such as moderate-severe traumatic brain injury,[23–31] hemiplegia and craniocerebral injury,[32] cerebellar atrophy and ataxia,[33] and whiplash.[25,34] It is thought that communication between the 3 sensory systems is lost in many of these individuals, causing moderate to severe postural instability in either the anterior-posterior direction, medial-lateral direction, or both. In most cases symptoms with visual, vestibular, or somatosensory orientation, such as dizziness, vertigo, tinnitus, lightheadedness, blurred vision, or photophobia, are reported.[23–34] These deficits may be either temporary or permanent, depending on the structures involved and the severity of the injury.

The Genesis?

Occasionally, we witness the woozily looking football player or hockey player who has just been hit trying to find his way back to the huddle, sideline, or bench. More likely, however, we hear of the subtle and less obvious balance problems a concussed athlete might complain of during the follow-up clinic evaluation. The author's 2000 study of 1003 sport-related concussions, found that balance problems are present 30% of the time following concussive injury, trailing only headache, dizziness, confusion, disorientation, and blurred vision in frequency of occurrence among a list of 18 symptoms (**Fig. 1**).[35] So what might explain this disruption in balance following TBI, be it mild, moderate, or severe? In the case of cerebral concussion and mTBI, we know that the injury produces functional rather than structural neurophysiologic changes in the cortex and brainstem's reticular formation.[36] The latter disturbance in particular is presumed to account for the autonomic, motor, and postural impairments that occur in many individuals following TBI.[23,36] Subtle vestibular deficits caused by sensory integration disruption identified in the nonathlete mTBI population[25] also occurs in sport-related concussion (see later discussion).

The transient nature of most cerebral concussion symptoms and impairments suggests that like a headache, blurred vision, or memory problems, balance deficits (when they exists) should resolve quickly. Several longitudinal studies involving high school and college athletes have demonstrated a typical pattern of recovery using both high-technology (computerized dynamic posturography) and low-technology (clinical balance) methods. In the sports medicine setting, similar balance deficits have been identified, but fortunately have been shown to resolve within 3 to 10 days after injury.[4,7,37–43] High-technology and low-technology balance assessment tools have been validated for assessing the initial deficits and tracking recovery following concussive injury.

HIGH-TECHNOLOGY BALANCE ASSESSMENT FOLLOWING SPORT-RELATED CONCUSSION

Studies of postural stability and balance following concussion have used a variety of methodologies and metrics. For example, in one of the earliest studies assessing balance deficits in concussed athletes, the author used a modified CTSIB on a force plate to systematically remove or conflict sensory inputs.[37] The author recorded

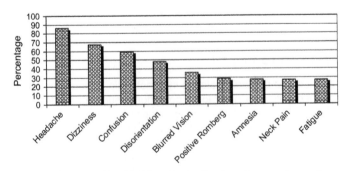

Fig. 1. Percentage of total injured athletes experiencing signs and symptoms associated with concussion. Positive Romberg test represents balance problems. (*Reprinted from* Guskiewicz KM, Weaver NL, Padua DA, et al. Epidemiology of concussion in collegiate and high school football players. Am J Sports Med 2000;28(5):643–50; with permission.)

2 indices of center of pressure displacement about a fixed, central reference point to quantify impairments in postural stability in college and high school athletes with cerebral concussion. Concussed subjects, matched to healthy comparison controls, demonstrated decreased postural stability compared with their own baseline scores and to their matched controls during the initial 3 days after injury. The degree of balance impairment in the concussed subjects increased with increasing task demands, such as altering the visual, vestibular, or somatosensory feedback during the trial. The author attributed the overall balance deficits to a sensory interaction problem (ie, difficulty using various combinations of somatosensory, visual, and vestibular information) for controlling upright posture during the first few days following concussion.

More recently, the SOT has been used to assess balance following concussion.[7,38–44] The SOT technical force plate system is designed to systematically disrupt the sensory selection process by altering the orientation information available to the somatosensory or visual inputs while at the same time measuring the patients' ability to maintain a quiet stance. Sway referencing is used throughout the test because the movement of the platform beneath the patients' feet and the environmental surround move in response to the athlete's anterior-posterior (A-P) sway. The SOT uses 6 different conditions; each condition is performed 3 times to assess balance (**Fig. 2**). The test protocol consists of 3 20-second trials under 3 different visual conditions (eyes open, eyes closed, sway referenced) and 2 different surface conditions (fixed, sway referenced) (see **Fig. 2**). Patients are asked to stand as motionless as possible for each of the 20-second trials in a normal stance with the feet shoulder width apart. The term *sway referencing* involves the tilting of the support surface or visual surround

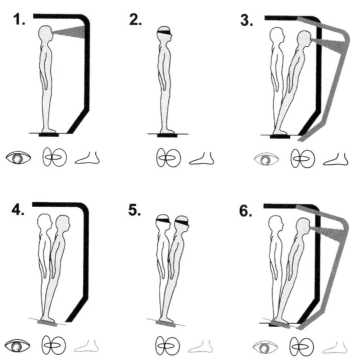

Fig. 2. Six testing conditions (1–6) for the Sensory Organization Test used with the Neuro-Com Smart Balance Master.

to directly follow the athlete's COG sway. During sway reference support surface conditions (4–6), the force plate tilts synchronously with the patients' A-P COG sway. Similarly, during sway referenced visual surround conditions (3, 6), the visual surround tilts synchronously with A-P COG sway. Sway referencing causes orientation of the support surface or surround to remain constant relative to body position. The SOT can assess patients' ability to ignore the inaccurate information from the sway referenced senses.

An overall composite equilibrium score describing a person's overall level of performance during all of the trials in the SOT is calculated, with higher scores being indicative of better balance performance. The composite score is the average of the following 14 scores: the condition 1 average score, the condition 2 average score, and the 3 equilibrium scores from each of the trials in conditions 3 to 6. The equilibrium scores from each of the trials represent a nondimensional percentage comparing the patients' peak amplitude of anterior-posterior sway to the theoretical anterior-posterior limit of stability. Additionally, relative differences between the equilibrium scores of various conditions are calculated using ratios to reveal specific information about each of the sensory systems involved with maintaining balance. For example, a vestibular ratio is computed by using scores attained in condition 5 (eyes closed, sway referenced platform) and condition 1 (eyes open, fixed platform). This ratio indicates the relative reduction in postural stability when visual and somatosensory inputs are simultaneously disrupted. Condition 4:Condition 1 represents the visual ratio, and Condition 2:Condition 1 represents the somatosensory ratio. These ratios are useful in identifying sensory integration problems.

Results of several studies using the SOT in concussed athletes have identified sensory interaction and balance deficits that typically resolve within 3 to 5 days after injury.[7,38–41] Cavanaugh and colleagues,[42,43] concluded that when applying approximate entropy techniques to the SOT data, athletes balance deficits can be shown to persist longer than 3 to 4 days, even among athletes with no signs of unsteadiness on the standard SOT analysis. The investigators concluded that approximate entropy provides a theoretically distinct, valuable measurement alternative that appears to provide unique insights and may prove useful for reducing uncertainty in the return-to-play decision.

In general, these studies indicate that the regions of the brain responsible for coordinating the sensory modalities (thalamus and its interconnective pathways to the cerebral cortex) may be initially disrupted following concussive injury. These studies also suggest that the sensory system most often affected following concussion is the vestibular system (**Fig. 3**).[7] If a person has difficulty balancing under conditions in which sensory systems have been altered, it can be hypothesized that they are unable to ignore altered environmental conditions and therefore select a motor response based on the altered environmental cues, which could potentially predispose them to further injury should they return to participation while experiencing sensory interaction problems.

There are 2 possible mechanisms for vestibular dysfunction following cerebral concussion: (1) the peripheral receptors themselves may be damaged and provide inaccurate senses of motion or (2) the brain centers responsible for central integration of vestibular, visual, and somatosensory information may be impaired. Mallinson and Longridge[25] found evidence of central integration balance deficits and subtle peripheral vestibular deficits when comparing SOT and electronystagmography results in subjects with mild head injury from an associated whiplash injury. These findings suggest that various combinations of peripheral and central deficits may be the cause of balance deficits in athletes with concussion. An additional factor that surfaced from

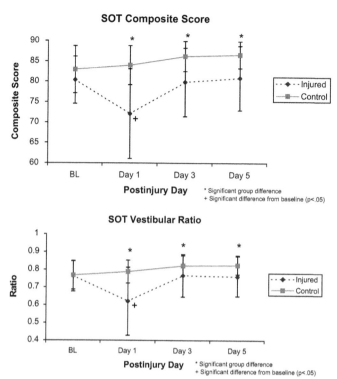

Fig. 3. Composite Score means (*top*) and vestibular ratio means (*bottom*) on the NeuroCom Smart Balance Master for 36 concussed and 36 control subjects across test sessions (Preseason through day 5 after injury). Higher scores represent better performance. (*From* Guskiewicz KM, Ross SE, Marshall SW. Postural stability and neuropsychological deficits after concussion in collegiate athletes. J Athl Train 2001;36:263–73; with permission.)

the author's research is the possibility that concentration and attention impairments identified on day 1 after injury could be a contributing factor to decreased postural stability. Future research should focus on this potential relationship.

Both the modified CTSIB and SOT require sophisticated force plate systems that provide a way to challenge and alter information sent to the various sensory systems. Although the aforementioned studies suggest that force platform sway measures provide valuable information in making return to play decisions following concussion, there is still a question of practicality and accessibility for the sports medicine clinician.

LOW-TECHNOLOGY (CLINICAL) BALANCE ASSESSMENT FOLLOWING SPORT-RELATED CONCUSSION

In an attempt to provide a more cost-effective, yet quantifiable method of assessing balance in athletes, the Balance Error Scoring System (BESS) was developed by researchers at the University of North Carolina at Chapel Hill. This clinical balance test can be performed on the sideline, with the use of only a stopwatch and a piece of medium-density foam (Power Systems Airex Balance Pad 81,000, Knoxville, TN, USA). Testing involves 3 different stances (double, single, and tandem) completed twice, once while on a firm surface and once on the foam, for a total of 6 trials (**Fig. 4**). Athletes are asked to assume the required stance by placing their hands on

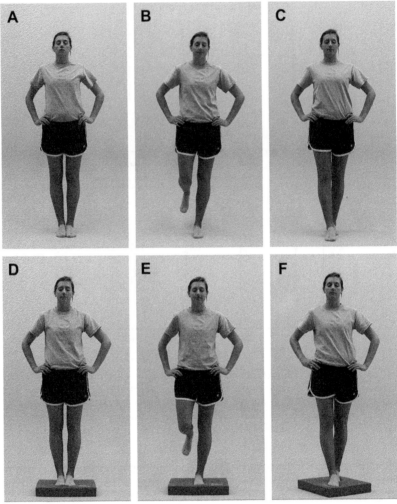

Fig. 4. Balance Error Scoring System performed on firm surface (*A–C*) and foam surface (*D–F*).

the iliac crests and upon eye closure, the 20-second test begins. During the single leg stances, subjects are asked to maintain the contralateral limb in 20° to 30° of hip flexion and 40° to 50° of knee flexion. Additionally, the athlete is asked to stand quietly and as motionless as possible in the stance position, keeping their hands on the iliac crests and eyes closed. The single-limb stance tests are performed on the nondominant foot. This same foot is placed toward the rear on the tandem stances. Patients are told that upon losing their balance, they are to make any necessary adjustments and return to the testing position as quickly as possible. Performance is scored by adding 1 error point for each error committed (**Box 1**). Trials are considered to be incomplete if the athlete is unable to sustain the stance position for longer than 5 seconds during the entire 20-second testing period. These trials are assigned a standard maximum error score of 10.

Box 1
Balance error scoring system

Errors

    Hands lifted off iliac crests

    Opening eyes

    Step, stumble, or fall

    Moving hip into more than 30° of flexion or abduction

    Lifting forefoot or heel

    Remaining out of testing position for more than 5 seconds

The BESS score is calculated by adding 1 error point for each error committed during each of the 6 (20 seconds) trials.

The BESS, which has been described as a rapid, easy-to-administer, and inexpensive clinical balance test, has identified postconcussion deficits in several studies.[2,4,7,40,45] McCrea and colleagues[4] reported that BESS scores in concussed college football players changed from baseline on average by 5.7 points, when measured immediately following the game or practice in which the injury occurred. Notably, however, at 1 day after injury, their average BESS score was only 2.7 points greater than baseline. For most athletes, BESS performance returned to preseason baseline levels (average 12 errors) by 3 to 7 days after injury. In a large study of American collegiate football players, impairment on the BESS was seen in 36% of injured subjects immediately following concussion, compared with 5% of the control group. A total of 24% of injured subjects remained impaired on the BESS at 2 days after injury, compared with 9% by day 7 after injury. Sensitivity values for the BESS were highest at the time of injury (sensitivity 0.34). Specificity values for this instrument ranged from 0.91 to 0.96 across postinjury days 1 to 7.[2]

Significant correlations between the BESS and force platform sway measures with normal subjects have been established for 4 static balance tests (single-leg stance/firm surface, tandem stance/firm surface, double-leg stance/foam surface, single-leg stance/foam surface, and tandem stance/foam surface), with inter-rater reliability intraclass correlation coefficients ranging from 0.78 to 0.96.[46] Researchers have reported that BESS performance can be influenced by a number of factors, including the type of sport played,[47] a history of ankle injuries and ankle instability,[48] and exertion and fatigue.[49,50] Healthy athletes typically demonstrate a subtle learning (ie, practice) effect on the BESS when it is administered over brief retest intervals,[51,52] which should be considered when interpreting postinjury results during serial testing, and factoring in a practice effect if the test is being administered multiple times over a short period of time.

In comparison to the SOT scores on 36 concussed athletes previously mentioned (see **Fig. 3**), the BESS revealed a similar recovery curve (**Fig. 5**) when administered on the same day as the SOT.[7] Furthermore, the BESS is sensitive to the effects of concussion with and without the use of other brief screening instruments, such as a graded symptom checklist and the Standardized Assessment of Concussion (SAC).[2] However, when used in combination with a graded symptom checklist and the SAC, the BESS is more sensitive and specific for accurately classifying injured and noninjured athletes during the acute postinjury phase.[2,4]

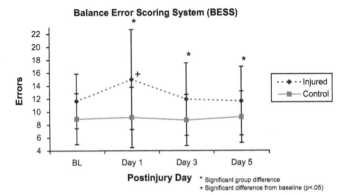

Fig. 5. Balance Error Scoring System means (± standard deviation; combined errors on all 6 trials) for 36 injured and 36 control subjects across test sessions (preseason through day 5 after injury). Lower scores represent better performance. (*From* Guskiewicz KM, Ross SE, Marshall SW. Postural stability and neuropsychological deficits after concussion in collegiate athletes. J Athl Train 2001;36:263–73; with permission.)

DUAL-TASK, VIRTUAL REALITY, AND GAIT ASSESSMENT FOLLOWING TBI

More contemporary, and perhaps functional, approaches for identifying postural instability and movement dysfunction following TBI have focused on gait and balance assessment in a virtual environment or during conditions of divided attention (dual task). Researchers[53,54] have identified alternative approaches to using SOT as the balance portion of a dual task with attention divided between the *balance* task of the SOT and a *cognitive* task given either verbally or visually while taking the SOT. This assessment method may have utility in the sports medicine setting, but must first be validated using concussed athletes. It may also have utility as a method of rehabilitation for athletes recovering from postconcussion syndrome.

Other researchers have experimented with virtual environments for assessing an athlete's ability to react and respond to environmental stimuli.[55,56] Slobounov and colleagues[55] tested balance in concussed athletes at days 3, 10, and 30 after injury. Subjects were exposed to a virtual reality image of the room moving. Standard balance testing recovered by day ten, but responses to visual field motion remained abnormal at day thirty despite subjective symptoms and neuropsychological testing having returned to baseline levels. A follow-up study by the same group[57] identified residual postural abnormality in subjects recovering from mTBI while assessing virtual time-to-contact measures, which essentially assesses the dynamic properties of postural control in a 3-dimensional space. The researchers concluded that residual deficits of balance become more prominent when concussed individuals are exposed to more demanding conflicting visual scenes. Other contemporary methods have focused more on gait analysis as a means to identify motor dysfunctions following mTBI. Parker and colleagues[58] examined college athletes who had sustained concussion and performed neuropsychological testing and gait stability testing postinjury days 2, 5, 14, and 28. Gait was assessed as a single-task, and then while completing a simple mental task (dual task). A persistent significant difference was noted in the dual-task gait assessment at day 28, although not in the single-task or isolated neuropsychological assessment. A similar study recently conducted by Catena and colleagues[59] found that level walking with a concurrent verbal cognitive task was able to distinguish between individuals with concussion and those without concussion immediately following concussive injury. The concussed individuals walked more slowly and more conservatively (reduced sagittal plan movement of body's center of mass). By day 6 after injury, attention had recovered to the point at which the divided task was no longer effective in perturbing balance in those with concussion, and it appeared that the concussed subjects had recovered. By day 14 after injury, a more conservative control of mediolateral center of mass was observed in the concussed group during a more challenging task involving obstacle crossing. The authors concluded that although this work was preliminary, the information someday could lead to clinically executable dynamic balance control tests after concussion.

In summary, preliminary findings involving contemporary assessment techniques suggest that in challenging cases, difficult tasks combining divided attention and motor challenges may be more sensitive for identifying deficits in otherwise healthy active athletes. The clinical significance of altered response to virtual reality environments or dual-task gait assessments is intriguing. However, their clinical utility has yet to be established. These dual-task paradigms may also be useful in developing rehabilitation programs for athletes recovering from postconcussion syndrome.

SUMMARY

Balance assessment, whether through the use of a force plate or a clinical balance test, such as the BESS, is useful in identifying neurologic impairment in athletes following concussion. In many cases, this impairment lasts only a few days after injury; however, in a small number of cases in which there are lingering vestibular issues, the deficits can last significantly longer. In such cases, balance/vestibular training may be indicated for assuring a full return to activity for the athlete. Clinicians should realize that *balance* is only one small piece of a large puzzle in the assessment of concussion and may not be affected in every concussed athlete. With repeated testing, there is a subtle practice effect with both the BESS and SOT, so the absence of this improvement in concussed athletes should be considered in the interpretation.

Many of the concussion management consensus statements used by sports medicine clinicians recommend the inclusion of objective balance assessment as part of a comprehensive injury evaluation and follow-up. The new "Zurich Guidelines," which resulted from the *Third International Conference on Concussion in Sport*,[1] include, as part of its standardized concussion assessment tool (SCAT2), a systematic balance assessment similar to that of the BESS. The SCAT2 uses the first 3 trials (firm conditions) of the BESS, and errors are recorded in the same way. It is recommended that whenever possible, the BESS, in its entirety (including the foam conditions), be completed for assessing clinical balance of concussed athletes. To ensure best use and interpretation of the BESS or any other metric of postural stability for clinical management of concussion, postinjury scores should be compared with a preseason baseline score. Finally, it is important to recognize that although symptom severity, neurocognitive function, and postural stability are often affected initially following concussion, they are not necessarily related or even affected to the same degree. Thus, a comprehensive concussion assessment plan includes assessment of all these domains.

REFERENCES

1. McCrory H, Meeuwisse W, Johnson K, et al. Consensus statement on concussion in sport: the 3rd international conference on concussion in sport held in Zurich, November 2008. Br J Sports Med 2009;43:76–84.

2. McCrea M, Barr WB, Guskiewicz K, et al. Standard regression-based methods for measuring recovery after sport-related concussion. J Int Neuropsychol Soc 2005; 11:58–69.
3. Guskiewicz KM, Bruce SL, Cantu RC, et al. National athletic trainers' association position statement: management of sport-related concussion. J Athl Train 2004; 39:280–97.
4. McCrea M, Guskiewicz KM, Marshall SW, et al. Acute effects and recovery time following concussion in collegiate football players: the NCAA concussion study. JAMA 2003;290:2556–63.
5. Notebaert AJ, Guskiewicz KM. Current trends in athletic training practice for concussion assessment and management. J Athl Train 2005;40:320–5.
6. McCrea M, Hammeke T, Olsen G, et al. Unreported concussion in high school football players. Clin J Sport Med 2004;14(1):13–7.
7. Guskiewicz KM, Ross SE, Marshall SW. Postural stability and neuropsychological deficits after concussion in collegiate athletes. J Athl Train 2001;36:263–73.
8. Guskiewicz KM. Postural stability assessment following concussion: one piece of the puzzle. Clin J Sport Med 2001;11:182–9.
9. Hellebrant F, Braun G. The influence of sex and age on the postural sway of man. Am J Phys Anthropol 1939;24:347–59.
10. Sugano H, Takeya T. Measurement of body movement and its clinical applications. Jpn J Physiol 1970;20:296–308.
11. Shumway-Cook A, Horak F. Assessing the influence of sensory interaction on balance. Phys Ther 1986;66:1548–50.
12. Jansen E, Larsen R, Mogens B. Quantitative romberg's test: measurement & computer calculations of postural stability. Acta Neurol Scand 1982;66:93–9.
13. Nashner L. Adaptation of human movement to altered environments. Trends Neurosci 1982;5:358–61.
14. Guyton A. Textbook of medical physiology. Philadelphia: WB Saunders Co; 1986. p. 1610–5.
15. Vander A, Sherman J, Luciano D. Human physiology: the mechanisms of body function. 5th edition. New York: McGraw-Hill, Inc; 1990.
16. Nashner L, Black F, Wall C. Adaptation to altered support and visual conditions during stance: patients with vestibular deficits. J Neurosci 1982;2:536–44.
17. Horstmann G, Dietz V. The contribution of vestibular input to the stabilization of human posture: a new experimental approach. Neurosci Lett 1988;95: 179–84.
18. Dietz V, Horstmann G, Berger W. Significance of proprioceptive mechanisms in the regulation of stance. Prog Brain Res 1989;80:419–23.
19. Dornan J, Fernie G, Holliday P. Visual input: it's importance in the control of postural sway. Arch Phys Med Rehabil 1918;59:586–91.
20. Nashner L, Berthoz A. Visual contribution to rapid motor responses during postural control. Brain Res 1978;150:403–7.
21. Diener H, Dichgans J, Guschlbauer B, et al. The significance of proprioception on postural stabilization as assessed by ischemia. Brain Res 1984;296:103–9.
22. Norre M. Sensory interaction testing in platform posturography. J Laryngol Otol 1993;107:496–501.
23. Ingersoll C, Armstrong C. The effects of closed-head injury on postural sway. Med Sci Sports Exerc 1992;24:739–42.
24. Geurts AC, Ribbers GM, Knoop JA, et al. Identification of static and dynamic postural instability following traumatic brain injury. Arch Phys Med Rehabil 1996;77:639–44.

25. Mallinson AI, Longridge NS. Dizziness from whiplash and head injury: differences between whiplash and head injury. Am J Otol 1998;19(6):814–8.
26. Wober C, Oder W, Kollegger H, et al. Posturographic measurement of body sway in survivors of severe closed head injury. Arch Phys Med Rehabil 1993;74: 1151–6.
27. Greenwald BD, Cifu DX, Marwitz JH, et al. Factors associated with balance deficits on admission to rehabilitation after traumatic brain injury: a multicenter analysis. J Head Trauma Rehabil 2001;16:238–52.
28. Rinne MB, Pasanen ME, Vartiainen MV, et al. Motor performance in physically well-recovered men with traumatic brain injury. J Rehabil Med 2006;38:224–9.
29. Kaufman KR, Brey RH, Chou LS, et al. Comparison of subjective and objective measurements of balance disorders following traumatic brain injury. Med Eng Phys 2006;28:234–9.
30. Campbell M, Parry A. Balance disorder and traumatic brain injury: preliminary findings of a multi-factorial observational study. Brain Inj 2005;19:1095–104.
31. Gagnon I, Forget R, Sullivan SJ, et al. Motor performance following a mild traumatic brain injury in children: an exploratory study. Brain Inj 1998;12:843–53.
32. Arcan M, Brull M, Najenson T, et al. FGP assessment of postural disorders during the process of rehabilitation. Scand J Rehabil Med 1977;9:165–8.
33. Mauritz K, Dichgans J, Hufschmidt A. Quantitative analysis of stance in late cortical cerebellar atrophy of the anterior lobe and other forms of cerebellar ataxia. Brain 1979;102:461–82.
34. Rubin AM, Woolley SM, Dailey VM, et al. Postural stability following mild head or whiplash injuries. Am J Otol 1995;16:216–21.
35. Guskiewicz KM, Weaver NL, Padua DA, et al. Epidemiology of concussion in collegiate and high school football players. Am J Sports Med 2000;28(5):643–50.
36. Shaw N. The neurophysiology of concussion. Prog Neurobiol 2002;67(4):281.
37. Guskiewicz KM, Perrin DH, Gansneder BM. Effect of mild head injury on postural stability in athletes. J Athl Train 1996;31(4):300–6.
38. Guskiewicz KM, Riemann BL, Perrin DH, et al. Alternative approaches to the assessment of mild head injury in athletes. Med Sci Sports Exerc 1997;29(Suppl 7): S213–21.
39. Mrazik M, Ferrara MS, Peterson CL, et al. Injury severity and neuropsychological and balance outcomes of four college athletes. Brain Inj 2000;14(10):921–31.
40. Riemann BL, Guskiewicz KM. Effects of mild head injury on postural stability as measured through clinical balance testing. J Athl Train 2000;35:19–25.
41. Peterson CL, Ferrara MS, Mrazik M, et al. Evaluation of neuropsychological domain scores and postural stability following cerebral concussion in sports. Clin J Sport Med 2003;13:230–7.
42. Cavanaugh JT, Guskiewicz KM, Giuliani C, et al. Detecting altered postural control after cerebral concussion in athletes without postural instability. Br J Sports Med 2005;39(11):805–11.
43. Cavanaugh JT, Guskiewicz KM, Stergiou N. A nonlinear dynamic approach for evaluating postural control: new directions of the management of sport-related cerebral concussion. Sports Med 2005;35(11):935–50.
44. Register-Mihalik JK, Mihalik JP, Guskiewicz KM. Balance deficits after sports-related concussion in individuals reporting posttraumatic headache. Neurosurgery 2008;63:76–80 [discussion: 80–2].
45. Broglio SP, Puetz TW. The effect of sport concussion on neurocognitive function, self-report symptoms and postural control: a meta-analysis. Sports Med 2008;38: 53–67.

46. Riemann BL, Guskiewicz KM, Shields EW. Relationship between clinical and force plate measures of postural stability. J Sport Rehabil 1999;8:71–82.
47. Bressel E, Yonker JC, Kras J, et al. Comparison of static and dynamic balance in female collegiate soccer, basketball, and gymnastics athletes. J Athl Train 2007; 42:42–6.
48. Docherty CL, Valovich McLeod TC, Shultz SJ. Postural control deficits in participants with functional ankle instability as measured by the balance error scoring system. Clin J Sport Med 2006;16:203–8.
49. Susco TM, Valovich McLeod TC, Gansneder BM, et al. Balance recovers within 20 minutes after exertion as measured by the balance error scoring system. J Athl Train 2004;39:241–6.
50. Wilkins JC, Valovich McLeod TC, Perrin DH, et al. Performance on the balance error scoring system decreases after fatigue. J Athl Train 2004;39:156–61.
51. Valovich McLeod TC, Perrin DH, Guskiewicz KM, et al. Serial administration of clinical concussion assessments and learning effects in healthy young athletes. Clin J Sport Med 2004;14:287–95.
52. Valovich TC, Perrin DH, Gansneder BM. Repeat administration elicits a practice effect with the balance error scoring system but not with the standardized assessment of concussion in high school athletes. J Athl Train 2003;38:51–6.
53. Broglio SP, Tomporowski PD, Ferrara MS. Balance performance with a cognitive task: a dual-task testing paradigm. Med Sci Sports Exerc 2005;37:689–95.
54. Ross LM, Register-Mihalik JK, Mihalik JP, et al. Effects of a single task vs. a dual task paradigm on cognition and balance in healthy subjects: a feasibility and reliability study. J Sport Rehabil, in press.
55. Slobounov S, Tutwiler R, Sebastianelli W, et al. Alteration of postural responses to visual field motion in mild traumatic brain injury. Neurosurgery 2006;59:134–9 [discussion: 134–9].
56. Mihalik JP, Kohli L, Whitton MC. Do the physical characteristics of a virtual reality device contraindicate its use for balance assessment? J Sport Rehabil 2008; 17(1):38–49.
57. Slobounov S, Cao C, Sebastianelli W, et al. Residual deficits from concussion as revealed by virtual time-to-contact measures of postural stability. Clin Neurophysiol 2008;119:281–9.
58. Parker TM, Osternig LR, van Donkelaar P, et al. Recovery of cognitive and dynamic motor function following concussion. Br J Sports Med 2007;41:868–73 [discussion: 873].
59. Catena RD, van Donkelaar P, Chou L. Different gait tasks distinguish immediate vs. long-term effects of concussion on balance control. J Neuroeng Rehabil 2009;6:25.

The Role of Neuroimaging in Sport-Related Concussion

Sanjay P. Prabhu, MBBS, FRCR[a,b,*]

KEYWORDS

• Concussion • Neuroimaging • Sport-related

Individuals engaged in various sports and recreational physical activities are prone to injury. The Centers for Disease Control and Prevention estimates that approximately 1.1 million people with traumatic brain injury (TBI) are treated and released from emergency departments in the United States each year and an additional 235,000 are hospitalized for these injuries.[1] The most common TBI in athletes is concussion, a transient disturbance of neurologic function caused by trauma. Although the symptoms associated with concussion have been recognized for centuries, the term "post concussion syndrome" was described in the early part of the last century as the subjective posttraumatic syndrome caused by a direct blow to the head. Commonly, the course is self-limited, resolving usually within weeks of the incident. Indeed, 90% of athletes are symptom-free within 10 days.

The basis for the loss of consciousness following concussion has been variously hypothesized to result from changes in the reticular system (reticular theory), increased neuronal firing and cerebral excitability (convulsive theory), mechanical injury disrupting brain function (centripetal theory), and activation of cholinergic neurons resulting in suppression of behavioral responses (central to pontine cholinergic system theory), among others.[2] A number of changes, including alterations in neurotransmitter levels and disruption of neuronal membranes, have been described following traumatic injury to the brain.

Most concussive injuries are mild and resolve without long-standing sequelae. However, there is increasing evidence that concussion can affect cognitive function adversely and contribute to long-term disability in a proportion of patients. This

---

The author has nothing to disclose.
[a] Division of Neuroradiology, Department of Radiology, Children's Hospital Boston, 300 Longwood Avenue, Boston, MA 02115, USA
[b] Harvard Medical School, 25 Shattuck Street, Boston, MA 02115, USA
* Corresponding author. Department of Radiology, Children's Hospital Boston, 300 Longwood Avenue, Boston, MA 02115.
E-mail address: sanjay.prabhu@childrens.harvard.edu

Clin Sports Med 30 (2011) 103–114
doi:10.1016/j.csm.2010.09.003
0278-5919/11/$ – see front matter © 2011 Elsevier Inc. All rights reserved.

problem is particularly significant in the young athlete. A number of studies indicate that concussion can have long-term sequelae including poor attention span, headache, impaired memory, behavioral problems, and learning difficulties.[3]

The challenge faced by the clinician taking care of this population is to determine when an athlete is fit to return to play and predict what long-term damage could result from single or repeated episodes of mild traumatic brain injury (mTBI). Among the dangers of returning too early to the sporting activity is the second-impact syndrome, which can be fatal. A number of guidelines have been proposed to help the sports medicine professional in this scenario. However, formulation of these guidelines has been hampered by a lack of objective tools to measure the structural damage to the brain and determine the pace of neurophysiological recovery in an individual case. Imaging studies have been evaluated as a tool with the potential to objectively assess damage resulting from TBI and develop individual-specific recovery plans. Most of the data available pertain to mild to moderate TBI in general, but are relevant to the injured athlete.

NEUROIMAGING FOLLOWING MILD TBI—AN OVERVIEW

With the advent of ultrafast multislice computed tomography (CT) scanners, CT imaging can be completed in seconds and is still the modality of choice in emergency departments to look for macroscopic abnormalities associated with acute sports-related brain trauma. Magnetic resonance imaging (MRI) has greater contrast resolution than CT and can detect structural abnormalities earlier than CT. However, until recently, it has not been used in the acute setting because of its susceptibility to metal and motion-related artifact, incompatibility with certain life-support equipment within the scanner environment, long scan times, and decreased sensitivity in detecting skull fractures. These limitations have been addressed in the past decade. Scan times have become shorter and MRI-compatible equipment has been developed. In light of these developments, MRI is emerging as a possible alternative to CT in the acute setting. However, at present, in most institutions, the first imaging study performed in a patient with TBI is a CT scan. MRI is reserved for follow-up neuroimaging.

Traditionally, sequences used for the MRI have been designed to look at macroscopic structural damage. Newer sequences have been developed that have the potential to increase the sensitivity of MRI to detect both structural and functional abnormalities associated with TBI in the acute setting and subsequently in the period of rehabilitation. These newer techniques include susceptibility-weighted imaging, arterial spin labeling, diffusion-weighted imaging (DWI), diffusion tensor imaging (DTI), functional MRI (fMRI), magnetic resonance spectroscopy (MRS), and magneto-encephalography (MEG). Quantitative MRI techniques like voxel-based morphometry (VBM) and brain segmentation algorithms also hold promise in objectively assessing changes following TBI. Advances in positron emission tomography (PET) and development of hybrid techniques like PET/MRI also have the potential to increase our understanding of changes in the microstructure and electrochemical alterations in the brain parenchyma following trauma. The use of these new techniques are especially relevant in cases where conventional CT and MRI sequences are unable to detect a macroscopic structural abnormality in the brain. Using these techniques, recent studies have looked at the brain that is "structurally normal" on conventional imaging, but manifests clinically as reduced responsiveness in the acute setting and delayed functional response on follow-up neuropsychological evaluation.

This article discusses some of the newer techniques and addresses their use in the acute setting and explores their potential role in long-term follow-up after mild to moderate TBI. Also addressed are the challenges faced before some of these newer techniques can be incorporated into routine clinical management of the injured athlete.

NEW TECHNIQUES IN NEUROIMAGING FOLLOWING BRAIN TRAUMA

The newer techniques described in this article can be broadly divided into structural and functional techniques (**Table 1**).

Susceptibility-Weighted Imaging

Improvements in gradient echo imaging methods have increased our ability to detect the susceptibility-related effects of shear-related hemorrhagic injury. Susceptibility-weighted imaging (SWI) uses the paramagnetic property of blood products and increases visibility of microhemorrhages by accentuating signal dropout by rapid spin dephasing. SWI is extremely sensitive to iron and blood products and detects microhemorrhages where conventional MRI fails (**Fig. 1**). Similar to gradient echo images, SWI detects hemorrhage at all stages, because iron remains even after the fluid from blood is reabsorbed.

The technical aspects and clinical applications of SWI have been elaborated in detail by various investigators.[4,5] SWI is best used at higher field strengths, as the TE (time to echo) is much longer at low fields and acquisitions need to be longer. In addition, at higher field strengths, isotropic in-plane resolution can be obtained and the signal-to-noise ratio (SNR) is higher. The use of even higher field strengths can increase the resolution and SNR significantly. Another advantage of SWI over conventional gradient echo sequences is the ability to differentiate between hemorrhage and calcium and visualize vessel connectivity and microbleed location in relation to the vasculature and other structures in the brain. SWI is routinely used in the author's practice as part of the routine imaging protocol in patients with TBI, both at presentation and follow-up examinations. Automated and semi-automated methods of counting number of hemorrhages on SWI images have been described, but are not used routinely in the author's clinical practice.

In spite of its ability to detect intraparenchymal injury, the exact role of microhemorrhages on SWI images in determining prognosis is not completely clear. Most studies so far have indicated that the number and volume of SWI hemorrhagic lesions measured using automated methods in the injured brain may correlate with specific neuropsychological deficits on long-term follow-up.[6] Another study concluded that SWI findings rarely discriminated by outcome, when compared with T2-weighted and fluid-attenuated inversion-recovery (FLAIR) imaging.[7] It is important to point out that the foci of microhemorrhages in patients with TBI do not correlate directly with

Table 1
Newer techniques in neuroimaging following traumatic brain injury

Structural Techniques	Functional Techniques
Susceptibility-weighted imaging (SWI)	Magnetic resonance spectroscopy (MRS)
Diffusion-weighted imaging (DWI)	Arterial spin labeling (ASL)
Diffusion tensor imaging (DTI)	Magnetoencephalography (MEG)
Quantitative MRI techniques (eg, segmentation and voxel-based morphometry)	Single-emission computed tomography (SPECT) and positron emission tomography (PET)
	PET/MRI
	Functional MRI (fMRI)

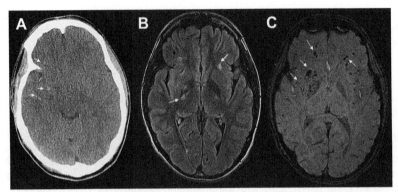

Fig. 1. Susceptibility-weighted imaging: 16-year-old right-handed male who suffered a head injury while stunt riding a bike in an indoor park. (*A*) CT performed on day of admission shows small hyperdense acute hemorrhagic foci in the right temporal and inferior frontal lobe. (*B*) Axial FLAIR image on day 5 after injury shows foci of hyperintensity in the right temporal and both inferior frontal lobes indicating areas of white matter injury. (*C*) Axial SWI shows multiple foci of hypointensity, significantly greater than seen on the CT and FLAIR images, thereby indicating the true extent of the abnormality.

the neurologic impairment; instead, these are likely markers of a more severe injury and may indicate diffuse axonal injury (DAI).

Another study investigated the impact of the field strengths of the magnets on the depiction of traumatic microbleeds by T2*-weighted gradient echo MRI. This group concluded that, in clinical practice, MRI at 1.5 T seems to be adequate for this purpose in most cases. Based on their findings, they recommended that MRI at 3 T may be appropriate if there is a strong clinical suspicion of DAI, despite unremarkable routine MRI, and possibly if evidence of DAI is sought after a long interval from trauma.[8]

There is room for improvement in the technical aspects of acquiring the SWI sequence, such as standardization across scanner manufacturers, reducing acquisition times, and decreasing artifact around the skull base and improving acquisition in the spine.

Diffusion-Weighted Imaging and Diffusion Tensor Imaging

Diffusion-weighted imaging (DWI) and apparent diffusion coefficient (ADC) maps have been used for lesion detection and as a predictor of outcome in adults with TBI. Few studies, however, have been reported in children.[9] The intracellular accumulation of water that occurs in cytotoxic edema is expressed as a reduction in the ADC (**Fig. 2**A).

Diffusion tensor imaging (DTI) provides measures of white matter integrity in the brain by tracking axonal tracts and their projections in the brain.[10,11] The first premise of DTI is that white matter tracts follow orderly paths in anteroposterior, lateral, and craniocaudal directions. The second principle used for DTI is the principle of anisotropy, which states that the diffusion rate of water molecules is dependent on the direction and integrity of the white matter tracts in a particular direction. Fractional anisotropy (FA) is a scalar value between 0 and 1 that describes the degree of anisotropy of a diffusion process. A value of 0 means that diffusion is isotropic, ie, free diffusion in all directions, and a value of 1 indicates that diffusion occurs only along one axis and is fully restricted along all other directions. Therefore, FA is a measure used in diffusion tensor imaging that is thought to reflect fiber density and integrity, axonal diameter, and myelination in white matter. Color coding the various axonal projections as a 2-dimensional representation produces a color FA map (**Fig. 3**A). The most commonly used convention for color

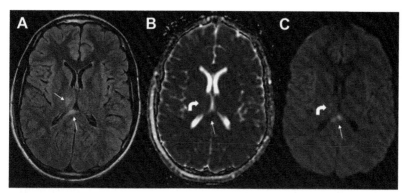

Fig. 2. Utility of diffusion-weighted imaging: 16-year-old male who sustained a TBI during a motocross competition when he fell while attempting to flip his bike in the air. MRI performed on day 3 after the accident. (*A*) Axial FLAIR image shows areas of hyperintensity in the splenium of the corpus callosum and right thalamus (*arrows*). (*B*) ADC map shows areas of decreased signal intensity (*arrows*) in the callosal splenium and right thalamus, thereby suggesting that the changes seen on FLAIR images is an acute process. (*C*) Trace diffusion image confirms restricted diffusion in the splenium (*arrows*). Note that the change in the right thalamus is of high signal intensity on the ADC map (*curved arrow*), indicating that this is an older injury.

coding the FA map is as follows: green represents anterior-posterior pathways, red color represents lateral pathways, and blue represents the craniocaudal pathways. These 2-dimensional maps can be used to track various axonal tracts of interest in a 3-dimensional (3D) representation, termed diffusion tractography (**Fig. 3**B). Specific tracts of interest following trauma include the corpus callosum, longitudinal fasciculus, cingulum bundle, and uncinate fasciculus.[12,13]

Recent studies have shown that there is significantly greater fractional anisotropy as a result of reduced radial diffusivity in the corpus callosum and several left hemisphere tracts following mTBI. The role of DTI has been studied in adults and adolescents.[14–16]

One such study was aimed at determining whether frontal white matter diffusion abnormalities can help predict acute executive function impairment after mild TBI.[14]

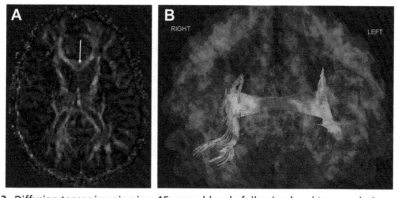

Fig. 3. Diffusion tensor imaging in a 15-year-old male following head trauma during snowboarding. (*A*) Color fractional anisotropy map displayed using the "red, green, blue" convention described in the text. (*B*) Same data reconstructed to provide a 3D tractography image that can be further analyzed to evaluate the integrity of each of the major tracts in the brain.

Based on DTI and standardized neuropsychological assessments, the investigators concluded that impaired executive function following mTBI is associated with axonal injury involving the dorsolateral prefrontal cortex.

In a similar study of acute mTBI involving adolescents, increased fractional anisotropy and decreased apparent diffusion coefficient and radial diffusivity correlated with the more intense post concussion symptoms and emotional distress that were seen in the mTBI group compared with the controls.[17] The role of DWI and ADC for outcome prediction has also been studied following pediatric TBI. One such study found that average total brain ADC value alone had the greatest ability to predict outcome, correctly predicting outcome in 84% of cases.[9] It is interesting that preliminary longitudinal data suggest that apparent diffusion coefficient and fractional anisotropy may normalize, at least partially, in several white matter tracts following a single-episode mTBI. These findings indicate that cytotoxic edema may be present during the semi-acute phase of mTBI and damage to axons affecting the intracellular ionic milieu, reflected as abnormal diffusion values.[16] These alterations may serve as potential biomarkers of recovery following brain injury. What is particularly relevant in this discussion of sports-related concussion is whether there is a more lasting change following repeated trauma. This question has not been addressed in large studies. The most attractive feature of this finding is that it is applicable even in brain regions that appear normal on conventional imaging. Early identification of young athletes at high risk for poor outcome may assist in aggressive clinical management following trauma.

In summary, DTI appears to have the potential to be more sensitive than conventional imaging methods in detecting subtle, but clinically relevant, changes following mTBI and may be critical in redefining the diagnosis, prognosis, and management of these patients.

Quantitative MRI (Segmentation and Voxel-based Morphometry)

The differences in the MRI signal intensity of the gray and white matter permits segmentation of the brain parenchyma into 2 separate compartments. Similarly, the extra-axial spaces and the ventricles filled with cerebrospinal fluid (CSF) can also be separated. This segmentation enables volume calculation of the 3 different tissue-CSF compartments because the slice thickness of the scan and the distance between slices are known.[18] Such measurements enable accurate determination of qualitative and quantitative changes in specific brain areas following mild to moderate trauma.[19,20] One of the measures studied in patients following TBI is the ventricle-to-brain ratio (VBR). This ratio is the total volume of the ventricles divided by the total brain volume. Increased VBR indicates increasing atrophy, and is directly related to the severity of injury. It is reflective of global changes but may disproportionately reflect white matter volume loss compared with that of gray matter.[21]

Voxel-based morphometry (VBM) is a method of voxel-by-voxel analysis of 3D MRI data. In subjects following TBI, VBM has been used to look for sites where major differences occur in subjects with TBI compared with age-matched control subjects without damage. Voxel density in the gray and white matter is plotted on a standard 3D surface plot of the brain. In a study in young patients following moderate to severe brain injury, differences have been shown in the frontal and temporal regions, more so in the gray matter.[22] At present, VBM is a research tool that is not used in routine clinical practice in the author's center.

Magnetic Resonance Spectroscopy

Magnetic resonance spectroscopy (MRS) has long been used as a noninvasive method to measure concentrations of various compounds in the brain within a sampled region. Use of higher field strengths has increased our ability to accurately determine concentrations of a broader range of metabolites including neurotransmitters like glutamate, glutamine, gamma-amino butyric acid, and glycine. The value of MRS has been clearly documented in acute ischemic injury with the presence of lactate, an indicator of anaerobic metabolism, consistent with energy substrate depletion.[23]

More recently, the role of MRS in the evaluation of patients with TBI has been studied by a number of groups.[24–26] Preliminary findings in one study indicated significantly lower levels of gray matter glutamine and higher levels of white matter creatine (Cr) in subjects with mTBI relative to healthy controls.[26] Furthermore, Cr levels were predictive of executive function and emotional distress in the combined groups, thereby suggesting that change in levels of Cr, a critical component of the brain's energy metabolism, and glutamate, the brain's major neurotransmitter, may occur following mTBI. Moreover, the different pattern of results for gray and white matter suggests tissue-specific metabolic responses to mTBI. In a study of patients with severe TBI, supratentorial and infratentorial fractional anisotropy (FA), N-acetylaspartate-to-creatine (NAA/Cr) ratio in the pons, thalamus, and insula clearly separated the unfavorable outcome, favorable outcome, and control groups, with no overlap. Unfavorable outcome was predicted with up to 86% sensitivity and 97% specificity and these values were better than those obtained with DTI or MRS alone. These findings led the investigators to suggest that FA and NAA/Cr ratios hold potential as quantitative outcome-prediction tools at the subacute phase of TBI.[27]

In spite of the results of such studies, the evidence for MRS in prognostication is not yet sufficient for use in routine clinical practice in all patients undergoing MRI for evaluation of TBI.[28] The yield of applying newer techniques of obtaining and analyzing the MRS, like multivoxel acquisition and 2-dimensional correlation spectroscopy (2D-COSY), needs to be evaluated in the follow-up of athletes following brain injury.[29]

Magnetoencephalography and TBI

Magnetoencephalography (MEG) is a noninvasive modality used to measure the neuromagnetic fields generated by activation of neurons. These fields are transmitted to the scalp and measured using sensors on the surface, generating data similar to standard encephalogram (EEG) data, but with fewer artifacts and better spatial resolution. Unlike other functional MRI techniques, MEG has the ability to detect rapid changes in neuronal activity, and this makes it possible to separate out the different components of a complex cognitive task like word comprehension. Small studies have looked at the use of MEG in TBI.[30,31] These studies suggest a role for MEG in the evaluation of patients with TBI, especially in conjunction with other modalities. At present, MEG is available in only a few centers across the world because of its relatively high cost. However, its increasing use in other conditions, such as epilepsy, may make this technique mainstream in the near future.

Arterial Spin Labeling

Perfusion MRI can be performed noninvasively by labeling the hydrogen nuclei of the intravascular arterial water using 1 or 2 radiofrequency pulses. These pulses invert the longitudinal magnetization of arterial blood just upstream of the region of interest. This causes modification of the measurable magnetization and T1 relaxation time of the labeled blood. During acquisition, the signal obtained includes the measurable magnetization of the region of interest to which is added the magnetization from the labeled blood pool present in the explored volume. A second unlabeled acquisition serves as a reference to calculate the perfusion images. The advantage of being able to assess perfusion and cerebral blood flow (CBF) without use of intravenous contrast medium and the relatively rapid acquisition times make it an attractive technique for use in the emergency care setting.

One study has demonstrated the hemodynamic impairment that can occur and persist in patients with mTBI, the extent of which is more severe in thalamic regions and correlates with neurocognitive dysfunction during the extended course of disease.[32] A more recent study demonstrated that in addition to global CBF reduction in subjects with TBI, there is more prominent regional hypoperfusion in the posterior cingulate cortices, the thalami, and multiple locations in the frontal cortices.[33] Diffuse injury was mainly associated with reduced CBF in the posterior cingulate cortices and the thalami, where the greatest volume losses were detected. In contrast, hypoperfusion in superior and middle frontal cortices was associated with focal lesions. These results suggest that structural lesions, both focal and diffuse, are the main contributors to the absolute CBF alterations found in chronic TBI and that CBF alterations as measured by the arterial spin labeling technique may serve as a tool to assess functioning neuronal volume.[33]

SPECT, PET, and PET/MRI

Available data suggest that single-photon emission computed tomography (SPECT) in cases of mTBI may show lesions where no abnormalities are seen on structural imaging. This may be helpful in explaining the cause of persistent behavioral changes. However, some lesions seen on structural scans are not detected with SPECT. It has been suggested that an initial negative SPECT after TBI may be predictive of good clinical outcome, but the utility of an abnormal scan for prognostication is less clear.[34]

Cerebral ischemia is believed to be an important mechanism of secondary neuronal injury following TBI. Flow defects on the cerebral blood flow on positron emission tomography (PET) imaging have been shown to indicate areas of irreversible tissue damage (necrosis) in the chronic stage. Interestingly, the area of hypoperfusion surrounding the lesion partly resulted in tissue necrosis, but a large part of the hypoperfused tissue survived in the chronic stage.[35] Based on these findings, it can be hypothesized that there is some degree of impaired cerebral blood flow and metabolism around the area of contusion even in the subacute stage after TBI. The use of PET for studying cerebral blood flow is limited in the emergency setting by the logistics of moving the patient to the scanning area and tracer availability at short notice.

The development of an integrated PET/MR prototype system for brain imaging is the latest step in the evolution of PET. Early experience with this new imaging system suggests that MRI-based attenuation correction is feasible and high-resolution MRI and PET data can be fused without significant loss of performance of either imaging modality.[36] PET/MR combination might attain wider clinical application if the technology becomes cost-effective and more data emerge on its advantages compared with other modes of imaging. In the emergency setting, the drawbacks of this technique are similar to PET and MRI, with regard to logistics of getting the patient to the scanner and getting the tracer into the patient at the appropriate time.

Functional MRI and TBI

Functional brain imaging identifies patterns of brain activation associated with specific cognitive or behavioral events. Neuronal function is inferred in functional MRI (fMRI) by the blood oxygen level dependent (BOLD) signal, which reflects magnetic field inhomogeneities caused by changes in the oxygenation state of hemoglobin. Neural activation results in a local increase in cerebral blood flow to the area out of proportion to the cerebral oxygen consumption, thereby resulting in net reduction in the amount of deoxyhemoglobin. The paramagnetic property of deoxyhemoglobin as opposed to the diamagnetic property of oxygenated hemoglobin is responsible for the field inhomogeneities. The resultant BOLD signal is dependent upon the changes in cerebral blood flow, cerebral blood volume, and cerebral oxygen consumption.[34] The data obtained are reconstructed using statistical packages and co-registered with a structural MRI. At present, fMRI is used primarily as a research tool in the area of TBI. Although it is possible to obtain functional MRI studies on existing scanners with a few modifications, the analysis of the scans requires considerable expertise, both in the reconstruction and interpretation of the data. Further, there is a need for standardization of the activation tasks used in fMRI studies. Most fMRI tasks need the subject to perform an active task, thereby limiting its use to alert and cooperative patients. More recently, an emerging area of fMRI is aimed at mapping resting state connectivity or the default mode network.[37,38] Resting state networks refers to the temporal coherence between different brain regions indicated by spontaneous blood-oxygen-level dependent fluctuations in the absence of any active task performance, ie, when the brain is "at rest." It is debatable whether this reflects consciously directed mental activity at rest or, alternatively, constitutes an intrinsic property of functional brain organization persisting in the absence of consciousness. Alterations in the resting state connectivity have been reported to occur in various forms of brain injury and may be especially relevant in light of the reticular theory invoked to explain the loss of consciousness following concussion.[2]

Currently available data indicate that the activation patterns in subjects following TBI may have significant differences compared with controls when performing cognitive activation tasks.[39] Changes have been reported in the right parietal and right dorsolateral frontal regions in performing a working memory task compared with control subjects after TBI within 1 month following injury.[40] The same group showed that the response to higher processing tasks in TBI suggested that these subjects do not have actual deficits in working memory ability, but they lose the ability to recruit additional neural resources during these tasks. They suggest that disturbances in catecholamine-mediated neural pathways that are needed for working memory function may be disrupted in these patients. Interestingly, when performing so-called "go-stop" tasks that require either a specific response to be made or no response depending on the stimulus, subjects with history of mTBI show reduced activation in the prefrontal cortex when no response was required and in the cingulate region when a response was indicated.[41,42] These changes may explain behavior and decisions made by the athlete on and off the field.

SUMMARY

Some of the newer techniques described in this article are being increasingly used in the clinical assessment of patients following mild to moderate TBI. Other techniques are used in research, but may have clinical relevance, which needs to be proven by large-scale, well-designed studies that demonstrate a clear benefit in scanning these patients. Specifically, there is a need for large studies with a special emphasis on the effects of repeated head trauma in the young athlete. This is especially relevant in cases where conventional imaging does not demonstrate a macroscopic abnormality. The emphasis has to shift from identifying structural abnormalities on imaging studies to understanding the functional changes in the brain that may explain the long-term neuropsychological effects of concussion and mTBI.

REFERENCES

1. Langlois JA, Rutland-Brown W, Wald MM. The epidemiology and impact of traumatic brain injury: a brief overview. J Head Trauma Rehabil 2006;21(5):375–8.
2. Shaw NA. The neurophysiology of concussion. Prog Neurobiol 2002;67(4): 281–344.
3. Buzzini SR, Guskiewicz KM. Sport-related concussion in the young athlete. Curr Opin Pediatr 2006;18(4):376–82.
4. Haacke EM, Mittal S, Wu Z, et al. Susceptibility-weighted imaging: technical aspects and clinical applications, part 1. AJNR Am J Neuroradiol 2009;30(1): 19–30.
5. Barnes SR, Haacke EM. Susceptibility-weighted imaging: clinical angiographic applications. Magn Reson Imaging Clin N Am 2009;17(1):47–61.
6. Babikian T, Freier MC, Tong KA, et al. Susceptibility weighted imaging: neuropsychologic outcome and pediatric head injury. Pediatr Neurol 2005;33(3):184–94.
7. Chastain CA, Oyoyo U, Zipperman M, et al. Predicting outcomes of traumatic brain injury by imaging modality and injury distribution. J Neurotrauma 2009; 26(8):1183–96.
8. Scheid R, Ott DV, Roth H, et al. Comparative magnetic resonance imaging at 1.5 and 3 tesla for the evaluation of traumatic microbleeds. J Neurotrauma 2007; 24(12):1811–6.
9. Galloway NR, Tong KA, Ashwal S, et al. Diffusion-weighted imaging improves outcome prediction in pediatric traumatic brain injury. J Neurotrauma 2008; 25(10):1153–62.
10. Wakana S, Jiang H, Nagae-Poetscher LM, et al. Fiber tract-based atlas of human white matter anatomy. Radiology 2004;230(1):77–87.
11. Jellison BJ, Field AS, Medow J, et al. Diffusion tensor imaging of cerebral white matter: a pictorial review of physics, fiber tract anatomy, and tumor imaging patterns. AJNR Am J Neuroradiol 2004;25(3):356–69.
12. Niogi SN, Mukherjee P, Ghajar J, et al. Extent of microstructural white matter injury in postconcussive syndrome correlates with impaired cognitive reaction time: a 3T diffusion tensor imaging study of mild traumatic brain injury. AJNR Am J Neuroradiol 2008;29(5):967–73.
13. Rutgers DR, Toulgoat F, Cazejust J, et al. White matter abnormalities in mild traumatic brain injury: a diffusion tensor imaging study. AJNR Am J Neuroradiol 2008; 29(3):514–9.
14. Lipton ML, Gulko E, Zimmerman ME, et al. Diffusion-tensor imaging implicates prefrontal axonal injury in executive function impairment following very mild traumatic brain injury. Radiology 2009;252(3):816–24.
15. Chu Z, Wilde EA, Hunter JV, et al. Voxel-based analysis of diffusion tensor imaging in mild traumatic brain injury in adolescents. AJNR Am J Neuroradiol 2010;31(2):340–6.
16. Mayer AR, Ling J, Mannell MV, et al. A prospective diffusion tensor imaging study in mild traumatic brain injury. Neurology 2010;74(8):643–50.
17. Wilde EA, McCauley SR, Hunter JV, et al. Diffusion tensor imaging of acute mild traumatic brain injury in adolescents. Neurology 2008;70(12):948–55.
18. Bigler ED, Tate DF. Brain volume, intracranial volume, and dementia. Invest Radiol 2001;36(9):539–46.
19. Hofman PA, Stapert SZ, van Kroonenburgh MJ, et al. MR imaging, single-photon emission CT, and neurocognitive performance after mild traumatic brain injury. AJNR Am J Neuroradiol 2001;22(3):441–9.

20. MacKenzie JD, Siddiqi F, Babb JS, et al. Brain atrophy in mild or moderate traumatic brain injury: a longitudinal quantitative analysis. AJNR Am J Neuroradiol 2002;23(9):1509–15.

21. Garnett MR, Cadoux-Hudson TA, Styles P. How useful is magnetic resonance imaging in predicting severity and outcome in traumatic brain injury? Curr Opin Neurol 2001;14(6):753–7.

22. Gale SD, Baxter L, Roundy N, et al. Traumatic brain injury and grey matter concentration: a preliminary voxel based morphometry study. J Neurol Neurosurg Psychiatry 2005;76(7):984–8.

23. Mader I, Rauer S, Gall P, et al. (1)H MR spectroscopy of inflammation, infection and ischemia of the brain. Eur J Radiol 2008;67(2):250–7.

24. Ashwal S, Holshouser B, Tong K, et al. Proton MR spectroscopy detected glutamate/glutamine is increased in children with traumatic brain injury. J Neurotrauma 2004;21(11):1539–52.

25. Cohen BA, Inglese M, Rusinek H, et al. Proton MR spectroscopy and MRI-volumetry in mild traumatic brain injury. AJNR Am J Neuroradiol 2007;28(5):907–13.

26. Gasparovic C, Yeo R, Mannell M, et al. Neurometabolite concentrations in gray and white matter in mild traumatic brain injury: a 1H-magnetic resonance spectroscopy study. J Neurotrauma 2009;26(10):1635–43.

27. Tollard E, Galanaud D, Perlbarg V, et al. Experience of diffusion tensor imaging and 1H spectroscopy for outcome prediction in severe traumatic brain injury: preliminary results. Crit Care Med 2009;37(4):1448–55.

28. Greer DM. Multimodal magnetic resonance imaging for determining prognosis in patients with traumatic brain injury—promising but not ready for primetime. Crit Care Med 2009;37(4):1523–4.

29. Ziegler A, Gillet B, Beloeil JC, et al. Localized 2D correlation spectroscopy in human brain at 3 T. MAGMA 2002;14(1):45–9.

30. Lewine JD, Davis JT, Sloan JH, et al. Neuromagnetic assessment of pathophysiologic brain activity induced by minor head trauma. AJNR Am J Neuroradiol 1999;20(5):857–66.

31. Lewine JD, Davis JT, Bigler ED, et al. Objective documentation of traumatic brain injury subsequent to mild head trauma: multimodal brain imaging with MEG, SPECT, and MRI. J Head Trauma Rehabil 2007;22(3):141–55.

32. Ge Y, Patel MB, Chen Q, et al. Assessment of thalamic perfusion in patients with mild traumatic brain injury by true FISP arterial spin labelling MR imaging at 3T. Brain Inj 2009;23(7):666–74.

33. Kim J, Whyte J, Patel S, et al. Resting CBF alterations in chronic traumatic brain injury: an arterial spin labeling perfusion fMRI study. J Neurotrauma 2010;27(8):1399–411.

34. Silver JM, McAllister TW, Yudofsky SC. Textbook of traumatic brain injury. 1st edition. Washington, DC: American Psychiatric Pub; 2005.

35. Kawai N, Nakamura T, Tamiya T, et al. Metabolic disturbance without brain ischemia in traumatic brain injury: a positron emission tomography study. Acta Neurochir Suppl 2008;102:241–5.

36. Hofmann M, Steinke F, Scheel V, et al. MRI-based attenuation correction for PET/MRI: a novel approach combining pattern recognition and atlas registration. J Nucl Med 2008;49(11):1875–83.

37. Martuzzi R, Ramani R, Qiu M, et al. Functional connectivity and alterations in baseline brain state in humans. Neuroimage 2009;49(1):823–34.

38. Greicius MD, Supekar K, Menon V, et al. Resting-state functional connectivity reflects structural connectivity in the default mode network. Cereb Cortex 2009;19(1):72–8.

39. Lovell MR, Pardini JE, Welling J, et al. Functional brain abnormalities are related to clinical recovery and time to return-to-play in athletes. Neurosurgery 2007; 61(2):352–9 [discussion: 359–60].

40. McAllister TW, Saykin AJ, Flashman LA, et al. Brain activation during working memory 1 month after mild traumatic brain injury: a functional MRI study. Neurology 1999;53(6):1300–8.

41. Christodoulou C, DeLuca J, Ricker JH, et al. Functional magnetic resonance imaging of working memory impairment after traumatic brain injury. J Neurol Neurosurg Psychiatry 2001;71(2):161–8.

42. Easdon C, Levine B, O'Connor C, et al. Neural activity associated with response inhibition following traumatic brain injury: an event-related fMRI investigation. Brain Cogn 2004;54(2):136–8.

Medical Therapies for Concussion

William P. Meehan III, MD[a,b],*

KEYWORDS

- Concussion • Mild traumatic brain injury • Head injury
- Trauma • Injury • Sports

Although concussion is a common sports injury, there are few published data on effective treatments. Many current recommendations are based on anecdotal evidence and consensus. Even when the search is expanded beyond the realm of sports, to include all forms of concussive brain injury, data remain scarce. The following article reviews the current recommendations for the management of sport-related concussion and some of the previously studied, potential therapies for the signs and symptoms of concussive brain injury in general. It is not an exhaustive review of all possible candidates for therapy, but rather a discussion of some of the more common recommendations, common therapies, and potential medications with the most published data available.

The terms concussion and mild traumatic brain injury are used interchangeably. However, concussions are not always mild. Exactly when a mild traumatic brain injury becomes moderate is unclear. Most often, the difference between mild, moderate, and severe traumatic brain injury is determined by the Glasgow Coma Scale at the time of injury.[1] However, the acute characteristics of concussion do not consistently predict recovery time. At some point, if symptoms and deficits in cognitive function persist, the patient originally believed to have mild traumatic brain injury should be considered to have more significant injury. This review discusses therapies investigated for the treatment of functional traumatic brain injury as a whole, not solely those initially labeled as mild.

PHYSICAL AND COGNITIVE REST

Current guidelines recommend physical and cognitive rest as the mainstays for treating sport-related concussion.[2] Physical rest is straightforward and understood by

Funding/support: This manuscript was supported by the National Institutes of Health through a T32 Award to Dr Meehan (T32 HD040128–06A1).

The author reports no conflicts of interest.

[a] Sports Concussion Clinic, Division of Sports Medicine, Department of Orthopedics, Children's Hospital Boston, 319 Longwood Avenue, Boston, MA 02115, USA

[b] Division of Emergency Medicine, Department of Medicine, Children's Hospital Boston, 300 Longwood Avenue, Boston, MA 02115, USA

* Corresponding author. Sports Concussion Clinic Division of Sports Medicine, Children's Hospital Boston, 319 Longwood Avenue, Boston, MA 02115.

E-mail address: william.meehan@childrens.harvard.edu

most athletes. To achieve physical rest, athletes are removed, not only from activities that place them at risk of further contact to the head but also from other strenuous aerobic activities and resistance training, such as running, ice skating, weight lifting, and so forth. Once athletes are symptom free at rest, they are returned to play in a graded, stepwise fashion. If they develop symptoms as they progress through these return-to-play stages, they return to the previous level at which they were symptom free for a period of time before attempting to progress again.[3] This recommendation is based mainly on anecdotal evidence and consensus. However, some investigators have begun to study the role of physical activity during recovery, starting with the safety of light exercise on a treadmill.[4]

Cognitive rest is more difficult. To achieve cognitive rest, athletes minimize activities that require concentration and attention, such as reading, schoolwork, video games, text messaging, working online, and playing games that require concentration, such as Scrabble or chess. For some athletes, school attendance and academic workloads need to be adjusted.[3] Again, this recommendation is based on mostly anecdotal evidence and consensus.

Studies have revealed that athletes who sustain sport-related concussions have quantitative deficits in their cognitive function compared with their preseason, baseline function.[5–8] Young scholar-athletes' academic performance depends largely on memory and processing speed. As a result, their grades are likely to be affected during recovery. Therefore, academic accommodations should be considered during recovery from a concussion.[9] This may help injured athletes preserve their grades, in addition to facilitating cognitive rest during the academic year.

Majerske and colleagues[10] studied the effect of overall activity, combining both physical and cognitive activity, on symptoms and neurocognitive performance during concussion recovery. Their results suggest that high levels of overall activity may interfere with recovery, whereas more moderate levels may be acceptable, or even beneficial. However, the investigators point out that the retrospective nature of the study leaves it vulnerable to a confounder: athletes with milder injuries may have been more likely to engage in activity than those with major injuries. Thus, those engaging in moderate activity may have started with a less severe injury than those engaging in minimal activity. Nevertheless, their findings indicate the need for further investigation into the effects of activity on concussion recovery.

EDUCATION

Unlike a fracture, laceration, or other structural injury, concussion can be difficult to recognize both by the athlete[11,12] and by the athlete's family members, friends, teammates, classmates, work colleagues, schoolteachers, employers, and so forth.[13] The signs, symptoms, cognitive sequelae, and time course of recovery after a concussion are often unfamiliar to the patient. Moreover, because concussed athletes have no cast, or scar, or other visible signs of injury, the legitimacy of their injury is often questioned by those around them. Thus, education regarding the typical recovery process of concussive brain injury is one of the main functions of clinicians caring for athletes with sport-related concussions. This education has been shown to improve symptoms.[14–16] Ponsford and colleagues[17] studied 202 adults after mild traumatic brain injury. Patients were separated into 2 groups. The intervention group, seen 1 week after injury, underwent neuropsychological assessment, and was given a booklet of information about the symptoms of concussion, the likely time course of recovery, and suggested coping strategies. This group underwent follow-up evaluation at 3 months after the injury. The nonintervention group was given the standard emergency department information and treatment, and was also evaluated at 3 months after the injury. The intervention group reported fewer symptoms at their 3 month follow-up than the nonintervention group. A similar study by many of the same investigators was performed in pediatric patients. Again the intervention group reported fewer symptoms at the 3-month follow-up.[18]

MEDICATIONS

Most athletes who sustain a sport-related concussion have spontaneous resolution of their symptoms, recovery of their balance, and return of their cognitive function in a period of days to weeks.[3,19–21] However, some people who sustain concussive brain injury have a prolonged recovery.[3] The following interventions might be considered for these patients.

The evidence for many of the medications discussed in this article is equivocal.[14,22] Many of the data are of low quality, without large, double-blind, randomized controlled trials.[23] Many of the studies include patients with more severe injuries than are typically seen in sports. Each therapy is associated with potential adverse effects. In many cases, the therapies described are off-label. It is the author's firm belief that pharmacologic treatment of sport-related concussions should be considered only if the following 3 conditions are met:

1. The athlete's symptoms have exceeded the typical recovery period for a sport-related concussion.
2. The symptoms are negatively affecting the patient's life to such a degree that the possible benefit of treatment outweighs the potential risks of the medication being considered.
3. The clinician caring for the athlete is knowledgeable and experienced in the assessment and management of sport-related concussion or concussive brain injury in general.

No effective pharmacologic treatment has been shown to speed recovery from traumatic brain injury.[24] As a result, no standard approach exists.[25,26] The heterogeneity of injury forces, mechanisms, and postinjury signs and symptoms makes such a therapy a distant goal.[23] However, medications are used in treating the signs and symptoms of concussion.[27]

Previous literature has grouped the symptoms after a sport-related concussion into 4 general categories[28]:

1. Sleep disturbance
2. Somatic (mostly headache)
3. Emotional
4. Cognitive.

Because the medications chosen often depend on the symptoms experienced by the affected athlete, they are organized by those symptoms.

SLEEP DISTURBANCE

Complaints of sleep disturbance are common following concussion.[29,30] The management of sleep disturbance should include, and perhaps start with, a discussion of sleep hygiene.[13,31,32] Today's athletes are exposed to constant stimulation. Their bedrooms are often filled with televisions, stereos, video games, mobile phones, and computers. They are constantly bombarded with social messages online or via text messaging. Eliminating these distractions from the bedroom, and lying down to rest in a quiet, dark room, helps the athlete to fall asleep. Simply turning these stimuli off does not suffice, because the mere presence of a computer, or a to-do list, date book, or planner, can often trigger stress and anxiety regarding the tasks that lay ahead, particularly in athletes who are often competitive and highly motivated. In addition, those with sleep disturbance should be counseled to avoid, or at least minimize, caffeine, nicotine, and alcohol use, as well as daytime naps.[31]

Medications may also be helpful. Melatonin is an endogenous hormone produced primarily by the pineal gland from serotonin. Its production and secretion are increased during times of darkness, and maintained only at low levels during the daylight hours.[33] It is nontoxic and safe,[34,35] making it an ideal candidate for assisting with sleep. In addition, there is some evidence that it may have other beneficial roles in recovery from traumatic brain injury.[35] It is the author's choice for first-line therapy for sleep disturbance following sport-related concussion. Trazodone, a serotonin reuptake inhibitor, is a commonly used agent to treat sleep disturbance after traumatic brain injury, and is sometimes mentioned as first-line therapy.[13] Although benzodiazepines seem to be a logical choice, most experts recommend avoiding them because of their negative effects on arousal and cognition.[13] Other therapies that may be considered include zolpidem, tricyclic antidepressants, psychotherapy, phototherapy, and chronotherapy.[31]

SOMATIC

Headaches are common after sustaining a concussion.[13,30,36] Headache is the most common symptom reported after concussion,[37,38] and sport-related concussion specifically.[19,39] As every clinician who manages concussions can attest, postconcussive headaches can be difficult to treat. There seems to be an inverse relationship between the severity of head trauma and the occurrence of posttraumatic headaches.[37,40–42] Although the use of analgesics, such as ibuprofen, may be beneficial in the short-term, rebound headaches are common and can complicate treatment and recovery.[37,41,42] Therefore, their frequent use should be discouraged. Posttraumatic headaches are often categorized according to the International Headache Society classification system to tailor treatment.[41–43] Most patients who develop headaches after trauma have tension-type headache or migraines.[37,41,43,44]

Antidepressants are commonly used to treat posttraumatic headaches.[27] Amitriptyline has been studied specifically for treating posttraumatic headaches, and has shown some success.[14,38,44–46] In a retrospective review of 23 patients treated with amitriptyline for headaches after sustaining a head injury, 90% made an excellent or good recovery.[45] However, not all investigators have seen such an effect.[47] Because amitriptyline can be used to treat tension-type headaches and migrainelike headaches, the most common forms of posttraumatic headaches,[38,41,43] it is often an ideal choice. It has been recommended for posttraumatic headaches that are not otherwise categorized.[41] Furthermore, its sedative effects can help those suffering from sleep disturbance after a concussion in addition to treating their headaches.[42] Therefore, it is commonly used by the author to treat athletes with persistent headaches after sustaining a sport-related concussion.

β-Blockers, calcium channel blockers, valproic acid, topiramate, triptans, dihydroergotamine, and gabapentin, have all been discussed as potential medical therapies for persistent headaches after concussion and may make reasonable choices in the appropriate circumstances.[41,42,44,48,49]

In addition to pharmacologic therapy, biofeedback, physical therapy, trigger point injections, and psychotherapy may also be considered, either as primary or adjunctive treatments, for persistent posttraumatic headaches.[37,42,44]

Headaches after concussion can persist for months, years, or, in rare cases, never remit.[41] It is often unclear in such cases, especially when all other signs and symptoms of concussion have resolved, whether a patient is still recovering from a concussion or has a new, daily, persistent headache, perhaps triggered at the time of injury.[41] Such situations make return-to-play decisions difficult.

EMOTIONAL

Emotional symptoms are commonly reported after traumatic brain injury,[30] in particular depression.[13,50] In athletes, the injury itself, as well as the restrictions placed on their physical and cognitive activity during the recovery phase, may lead to depression. Because the duration of symptoms from sport-related concussion is usually short, the author believes that depressive symptoms in these cases are best managed conservatively, with coping strategies, the support of family and friends, and counseling by a trained psychologist. However, there may be cases for which these interventions do not suffice and medical therapies should be considered. Tricyclic antidepressants and serotonin reuptake inhibitors are recommended as options in the treatment of traumatic brain injury–related depression.[13,51,52] The prescription of these medications is best left to those providers with experience in managing depression.

Sertraline has been studied in the setting of traumatic brain injury and has been shown to not only treat depression, but perhaps offer cognitive benefits as well.[22,53] In a study of patients with depression after traumatic brain injury, Fann and colleagues[53] conducted a single-blind placebo run-in trial of sertraline. They showed not only a significant change in depression scores but also improvements in psychomotor speed, memory, and general cognitive efficiency. Other serotonin reuptake inhibitors, such as citalopram and fluoxetine, have also been studied.[22,54] Studies of amitriptyline suggest that, although it is useful in treating primary depression, it may be less effective in treating depression following traumatic brain injury.[50,51]

COGNITIVE

Cognitive symptoms, such as difficulties with memory, difficulties with concentration, and slowed processing speed, are common complaints after concussive brain injury.[30,51] The advent of computerized neuropsychological testing, and its spreading use among athletes who sustain sport-related concussions, have revealed quantitative deficits in cognitive function after injury.[6–8] Certain strategies to help preserve cognitive function have been proposed.

Cognitive Rehabilitation

There is little evidence to suggest that cognitive rehabilitation is effective for treating the effects of a concussion.[14] Given the short duration of signs and symptoms following sport-related concussions,[3,19–21] the routine use of cognitive rehabilitation in the management of sport-related concussions is unnecessary and of doubtful benefit. However, there may be cases of prolonged recovery in which its use is considered. Although conflicting evidence exists, some studies suggest that certain aspects of cognitive performance may be enhanced by focused rehabilitation.[55–57]

Medications

Medications are commonly used in treating the neurobehavioral sequelae of traumatic brain injury.[51] As the effects of most sport-related concussions resolve quickly, the routine use of these medications is unnecessary. However, in cases of prolonged recovery, for which the main complaints are cognitive in nature, particularly if the athlete has quantifiable cognitive deficits, a trial of pharmacologic agents may be considered.

The role of methyphenidate after traumatic brain injury has been investigating more than most other cognitive agents.[13,22,23,58–65] There is evidence, including randomized controlled trials, to support the use of methylphenidate in the setting of traumatic brain injury.[13,22,58–60,66] It is recommended to treat deficits in attention and speed of processing, and as an option for treating deficiencies in general cognitive functioning.[51]

In a randomized, double-blind, placebo-controlled trial, Whyte and colleagues[59] showed an improvement in the speed of performance on 5 attention tasks in patients given methylphenidate compared with controls given placebo. Plenger and colleagues[58] conducted a randomized, double-blind, placebo-controlled trial on 23 patients with complicated mild to moderately severe traumatic brain injury. They found that patients given methylphenidate scored significantly better on their disability rating scale and on tests of attention and motor performance at a 30 day follow-up appointment than subjects given placebo.

However, not all studies have shown such effects.[22] Williams and colleagues[60] studied pediatric patients who sustained mild to severe traumatic brain injury in a double-blind, placebo-controlled trial and found no significant differences between patients taking methylphenidate and those taking placebo. However, this study included only 10 patients and may have been inadequately powered to detect any potential benefit. Some clinicians are reluctant to use methylphenidate after traumatic brain injury because of its potential for lowering seizure thresholds.[22] As with all medications discussed in this review, the decision to start methylphenidate should be undertaken cautiously, after careful consideration of the individual athlete's sequelae, the possible benefits of medication, and the associated risks of medication.

Amantadine is a dopaminergic agent with possible N-methyl-D-aspartate antagonist effects.[67] The role of amantadine after traumatic brain injury has been investigated,[22,23,51,65–69] with several studies suggesting that amantadine is safe in this setting and may improve aspects of cognitive function.[23,65,68–71] In a study of 22 patients with mild, moderate, and severe traumatic brain injury, Kraus and colleagues[68] showed improvements in executive function as well as an increase in glucose metabolism in the prefrontal cortex on positron emission tomography in patients taking amantadine. However, results are mixed. In a randomized, double-blind, placebo-controlled trial, Schneider and colleagues[72] found no significant difference on neuropsychological measurements between subjects taking amantadine and those taking placebo. However, the investigators acknowledge that, given their small sample size, the study may not have been powered adequately.

Amantadine has shown some efficacy in pediatric patients.[23,73,74] In a retrospective, case-controlled study of 54 pediatric patients, Green and colleagues[73] concluded that amantadine was safe and well-tolerated after traumatic brain injury and lead to subjective improvement as well as significant increases in Ranchos Los Amigos scores. Similarly, Beers and colleagues[74] studied the effects of amantadine in pediatric patients after traumatic brain injury and concluded that the medication was safe in this setting. Their results suggested that cognition may be improved with amantadine, but differences were not statistically significant.

To a lesser extent, several other medications have been investigated as potential therapies for the cognitive sequelae of traumatic brain injury. These medications include doenpezil,[75–80] rivastigmine,[52,81] cytidine diphosphoryl choline,[82] fluoxetine,[83] sertraline,[53] pramiracetam,[51] bromocriptine,[51] and atomoxetine.[22]

Most patients with sport-related concussion recover quickly. Therefore, the potential benefits of many of the therapies discussed earlier are outweighed by the potential risks. However, in patients whose recoveries are prolonged and are associated with significant, negative effects on their quality of life, medical therapies should be considered. Sport-related concussions are distinct, in some respects, from other forms of traumatic brain injury. They generally involve low-force mechanisms. They occur in athletes whose personality traits, overall health, and moods likely differ from the general population. They are often recurrent, because athletes are usually anxious to return to the high-risk activity during which the injury was sustained. Further research conducted specifically in patients who sustain sport-related concussions would provide guidance on how these patients are best managed.

REFERENCES

1. Lee LK. Controversies in the sequelae of pediatric mild traumatic brain injury. Pediatr Emerg Care 2007;23:580–3 [quiz: 584–6].
2. McCrory P, Meeuwisse W, Johnston K, et al. Consensus statement on concussion in sport–the 3rd International Conference on Concussion in Sport held in Zurich, November 2008. J Sci Med Sport 2009;12:340–51.
3. McCrory P, Meeuwisse W, Johnston K, et al. Consensus statement on concussion in sport: the 3rd International Conference on Concussion in Sport held in Zurich, November 2008. J Athl Train 2009;44:434–48.
4. Leddy JJ, Kozlowski K, Donnelly JP, et al. A preliminary study of subsymptom threshold exercise training for refractory post-concussion syndrome. Clin J Sport Med 2010;20:21–7.
5. Collins MW, Grindel SH, Lovell MR, et al. Relationship between concussion and neuropsychological performance in college football players. JAMA 1999;282:964–70.
6. Lovell MR, Collins MW, Iverson GL, et al. Recovery from mild concussion in high school athletes. J Neurosurg 2003;98:296–301.
7. Schatz P, Pardini JE, Lovell MR, et al. Sensitivity and specificity of the ImPACT Test Battery for concussion in athletes. Arch Clin Neuropsychol 2006;21:91–9.
8. Van Kampen DA, Lovell MR, Pardini JE, et al. The "value added" of neurocognitive testing after sports-related concussion. Am J Sports Med 2006;34:1630–5.
9. McCrory P, Collie A, Anderson V, et al. Can we manage sport related concussion in children the same as in adults? Br J Sports Med 2004;38:516–9.
10. Majerske CW, Mihalik JP, Ren D, et al. Concussion in sports: post-concussive activity level, symptoms and neurocognitive performance. J Athl Train 2008; 43(3):265–74.
11. Gerberich SG, Priest JD, Boen JR, et al. Concussion incidences and severity in secondary school varsity football players. Am J Public Health 1983;73:1370–5.
12. McCrea M, Hammeke T, Olsen G, et al. Unreported concussion in high school football players: implications for prevention. Clin J Sport Med 2004;14:13–7.
13. Arciniegas DB, Anderson CA, Topkoff J, et al. Mild traumatic brain injury: a neuropsychiatric approach to diagnosis, evaluation, and treatment. Neuropsychiatr Dis Treat 2005;1:311–27.
14. Comper P, Bisschop SM, Carnide N, et al. A systematic review of treatments for mild traumatic brain injury. Brain Inj 2005;19:863–80.
15. Salazar AM. Impact of early intervention on outcome following mild head injury in adults. J Neurol Neurosurg Psychiatr 2002;73:239.
16. Wade DT, King NS, Wenden FJ, et al. Routine follow up after head injury: a second randomised controlled trial. J Neurol Neurosurg Psychiatr 1998;65:177–83.
17. Ponsford J, Willmott C, Rothwell A, et al. Impact of early intervention on outcome following mild head injury in adults. J Neurol Neurosurg Psychiatr 2002;73:330–2.

18. Ponsford J, Willmott C, Rothwell A, et al. Impact of early intervention on outcome after mild traumatic brain injury in children. Pediatrics 2001;108:1297–303.

19. Guskiewicz KM, McCrea M, Marshall SW, et al. Cumulative effects associated with recurrent concussion in collegiate football players: the NCAA concussion study. JAMA 2003;290:2549–55.

20. Iverson GL, Brooks BL, Collins MW, et al. Tracking neuropsychological recovery following concussion in sport. Brain Inj 2006;20:245–52.

21. Guskiewicz KM, Ross SE, Marshall SW. Postural stability and neuropsychological deficits after concussion in collegiate athletes. J Athl Train 2001;36:263–73.

22. Chew E, Zafonte RD. Pharmacological management of neurobehavioral disorders following traumatic brain injury–a state-of-the-art review. J Rehabil Res Dev 2009;46:851–79.

23. Tenovuo O. Pharmacological enhancement of cognitive and behavioral deficits after traumatic brain injury. Curr Opin Neurol 2006;19:528–33.

24. Beauchamp K, Mutlak H, Smith WR, et al. Pharmacology of traumatic brain injury: where is the "golden bullet". Mol Med 2008;14:731–40.

25. Zafonte R, Friedewald WT, Lee SM, et al. The citicoline brain injury treatment (CO-BRIT) trial: design and methods. J Neurotrauma 2009;26:2207–16.

26. Mittenberg W, Burton DB. A survey of treatments for post-concussion syndrome. Brain Inj 1994;8:429–37.

27. Mittenberg W, Canyock EM, Condit D, et al. Treatment of post-concussion syndrome following mild head injury. J Clin Exp Neuropsychol 2001;23:829–36.

28. Reddy CC. A treatment paradigm for sports concussion. Brain Injury Professional 2004;4:24–5.

29. Kapural M, Krizanac-Bengez L, Barnett G, et al. Serum S-100beta as a possible marker of blood-brain barrier disruption. Brain Res 2002;940:102–4.

30. Paniak C, Reynolds S, Phillips K, et al. Patient complaints within 1 month of mild traumatic brain injury: a controlled study. Arch Clin Neuropsychol 2002;17:319–34.

31. Rao V, Rollings P. Sleep disturbances following traumatic brain injury. Curr Treat Options Neurol 2002;4:77–87.

32. Zafonte RD, Fichtenberg NL. Sleep disturbance in traumatic brain injury: pharmacologic options. NeuroRehabilitation 1996;7:189–95.

33. Ganong WF. Review of medical physiology. 19th edition. Stamford (CT): Appleton and Lange; 1999.

34. Samantaray S, Das A, Thakore NP, et al. Therapeutic potential of melatonin in traumatic central nervous system injury. J Pineal Res 2009;47:134–42.

35. Maldonado MD, Murillo-Cabezas F, Terron MP, et al. The potential of melatonin in reducing morbidity-mortality after craniocerebral trauma. J Pineal Res 2007;42:1–11.

36. Faux S, Sheedy J. A prospective controlled study in the prevalence of posttraumatic headache following mild traumatic brain injury. Pain Med 2008;9:1001–11.

37. Packard RC. Epidemiology and pathogenesis of posttraumatic headache. J Head Trauma Rehabil 1999;14:9–21.

38. Weiss HD, Stern BJ, Goldberg J. Post-traumatic migraine: chronic migraine precipitated by minor head or neck trauma. Headache 1991;31:451–6.

39. Guskiewicz KM, Weaver NL, Padua DA, et al. Epidemiology of concussion in collegiate and high school football players. Am J Sports Med 2000;28:643–50.

40. Couch JR, Bearss C. Chronic daily headache in the posttrauma syndrome: relation to extent of head injury. Headache 2001;41:559–64.

41. Lenaerts ME, Couch JR. Posttraumatic headache. Curr Treat Options Neurol 2004;6:507–17.

42. Lane JC, Arciniegas DB. Post-traumatic Headache. Curr Treat Options Neurol 2002;4:89–104.
43. Haas DC. Chronic post-traumatic headaches classified and compared with natural headaches. Cephalalgia 1996;16:486–93.
44. Lew HL, Lin PH, Fuh JL, et al. Characteristics and treatment of headache after traumatic brain injury: a focused review. Am J Phys Med Rehabil 2006;85:619–27.
45. Tyler GS, McNeely HE, Dick ML. Treatment of post-traumatic headache with amitriptyline. Headache 1980;20:213–6.
46. Label L. Treatment of post-traumatic headaches: maprotiline or amitriptyline? Neurology 1991;41(Suppl 1):247.
47. Saran A. Antidepressants not effective in headache associated with minor closed head injury. Int J Psychiatry Med 1988;18:75–83.
48. Packard RC. Treatment of chronic daily posttraumatic headache with divalproex sodium. Headache 2000;40:736–9.
49. McBeath JG, Nanda A. Use of dihydroergotamine in patients with postconcussion syndrome. Headache 1994;34:148–51.
50. Dinan TG, Mobayed M. Treatment resistance of depression after head injury: a preliminary study of amitriptyline response. Acta Psychiatr Scand 1992;85:292–4.
51. Warden DL, Gordon B, McAllister TW, et al. Guidelines for the pharmacologic treatment of neurobehavioral sequelae of traumatic brain injury. J Neurotrauma 2006;23:1468–501.
52. Silver JM, Koumaras B, Meng X, et al. Long-term effects of rivastigmine capsules in patients with traumatic brain injury. Brain Inj 2009;23:123–32.
53. Fann JR, Uomoto JM, Katon WJ. Cognitive improvement with treatment of depression following mild traumatic brain injury. Psychosomatics 2001;42:48–54.
54. Silver JM, McAllister TW, Arciniegas DB. Depression and cognitive complaints following mild traumatic brain injury. Am J Psychiatry 2009;166:653–61.
55. Tsaousides T, Gordon WA. Cognitive rehabilitation following traumatic brain injury: assessment to treatment. Mt Sinai J Med 2009;76:173–81.
56. Cicerone KD. Remediation of "working attention" in mild traumatic brain injury. Brain Inj 2002;16:185–95.
57. Ho MR, Bennett TL. Efficacy of neuropsychological rehabilitation for mild-moderate traumatic brain injury. Arch Clin Neuropsychol 1997;12:1–11.
58. Plenger PM, Dixon CE, Castillo RM, et al. Subacute methylphenidate treatment for moderate to moderately severe traumatic brain injury: a preliminary double-blind placebo-controlled study. Arch Phys Med Rehabil 1996;77:536–40.
59. Whyte J, Hart T, Schuster K, et al. Effects of methylphenidate on attentional function after traumatic brain injury. A randomized, placebo-controlled trial. Am J Phys Med Rehabil 1997;76:440–50.
60. Williams SE, Ris MD, Ayyangar R, et al. Recovery in pediatric brain injury: is psychostimulant medication beneficial? J Head Trauma Rehabil 1998;13:73–81.
61. Kaelin DL, Cifu DX, Matthies B. Methylphenidate effect on attention deficit in the acutely brain-injured adult. Arch Phys Med Rehabil 1996;77:6–9.
62. Whyte J, Hart T, Vaccaro M, et al. Effects of methylphenidate on attention deficits after traumatic brain injury: a multidimensional, randomized, controlled trial. Am J Phys Med Rehabil 2004;83:401–20.
63. Lee H, Kim SW, Kim JM, et al. Comparing effects of methylphenidate, sertraline and placebo on neuropsychiatric sequelae in patients with traumatic brain injury. Hum Psychopharmacol 2005;20:97–104.
64. Siddall OM. Use of methylphenidate in traumatic brain injury. Ann Pharmacother 2005;39:1309–13.

65. Napolitano E, Elovic EP, Qureshi AI. Pharmacological stimulant treatment of neurocognitive and functional deficits after traumatic and non-traumatic brain injury. Med Sci Monit 2005;11:RA212–20.
66. Sivan M, Neumann V, Kent R, et al. Pharmacotherapy for treatment of attention deficits after non-progressive acquired brain injury. A systematic review. Clin Rehabil 2010;24:110–21.
67. Meythaler JM, Brunner RC, Johnson A, et al. Amantadine to improve neurorecovery in traumatic brain injury-associated diffuse axonal injury: a pilot double-blind randomized trial. J Head Trauma Rehabil 2002;17:300–13.
68. Kraus MF, Smith GS, Butters M, et al. Effects of the dopaminergic agent and NMDA receptor antagonist amantadine on cognitive function, cerebral glucose metabolism and D2 receptor availability in chronic traumatic brain injury: a study using positron emission tomography (PET). Brain Inj 2005;19:471–9.
69. Leone H, Polsonetti BW. Amantadine for traumatic brain injury: does it improve cognition and reduce agitation? J Clin Pharm Ther 2005;30:101–4.
70. Sawyer E, Mauro LS, Ohlinger MJ. Amantadine enhancement of arousal and cognition after traumatic brain injury. Ann Pharmacother 2008;42:247–52.
71. Williams SE. Amantadine treatment following traumatic brain injury in children. Brain Inj 2007;21:885–9.
72. Schneider WN, Drew-Cates J, Wong TM, et al. Cognitive and behavioural efficacy of amantadine in acute traumatic brain injury: an initial double-blind placebo-controlled study. Brain Inj 1999;13:863–72.
73. Green LB, Hornyak JE, Hurvitz EA. Amantadine in pediatric patients with traumatic brain injury: a retrospective, case-controlled study. Am J Phys Med Rehabil 2004;83:893–7.
74. Beers SR, Skold A, Dixon CE, et al. Neurobehavioral effects of amantadine after pediatric traumatic brain injury: a preliminary report. J Head Trauma Rehabil 2005;20:450–63.
75. Walker W, Seel R, Gibellato M, et al. The effects of donepezil on traumatic brain injury acute rehabilitation outcomes. Brain Inj 2004;18:739–50.
76. Morey CE, Cilo M, Berry J, et al. The effect of aricept in persons with persistent memory disorder following traumatic brain injury: a pilot study. Brain Inj 2003; 17:809–15.
77. Whelan FJ, Walker MS, Schultz SK. Donepezil in the treatment of cognitive dysfunction associated with traumatic brain injury. Ann Clin Psychiatry 2000;12:131–5.
78. Masanic CA, Bayley MT, VanReekum R, et al. Open-label study of donepezil in traumatic brain injury. Arch Phys Med Rehabil 2001;82:896–901.
79. Kaye NS, Townsend JB 3rd, Ivins R. An open-label trial of donepezil (aricept) in the treatment of persons with mild traumatic brain injury. J Neuropsychiatry Clin Neurosci 2003;15:383–4 [author reply: 384–5].
80. Zhang L, Plotkin RC, Wang G, et al. Cholinergic augmentation with donepezil enhances recovery in short-term memory and sustained attention after traumatic brain injury. Arch Phys Med Rehabil 2004;85:1050–5.
81. Tenovuo O. Central acetylcholinesterase inhibitors in the treatment of chronic traumatic brain injury-clinical experience in 111 patients. Prog Neuropsychopharmacol Biol Psychiatry 2005;29:61–7.
82. Levin HS. Treatment of postconcussional symptoms with CDP-choline. J Neurol Sci 1991;103(Suppl):S39–42.
83. Horsfield SA, Rosse RB, Tomasino V, et al. Fluoxetine's effects on cognitive performance in patients with traumatic brain injury. Int J Psychiatry Med 2002;32: 337–44.

The Female Athlete: The Role of Gender in the Assessment and Management of Sport-Related Concussion

Tracey Covassin, PhD, ATC[a],*, RJ Elbin, PhD[b]

KEYWORDS

- Concussion • Gender differences • Females • Symptoms

Recent estimates from the Centers for Disease Control and Prevention indicate that sport and recreational traumatic brain injuries (TBIs) have increased from 300,000 per year[1] to approximately 1.6 million to 3 million per year in the United States.[2] This trend suggests that concussions are a growing problem that affects athletes at both the high school and collegiate level. An increase in female participation in sport shows that there are currently more than 178,000 women participating on National Collegiate Athletic Association (NCAA) teams[3] and approximately 3 million women playing organized high school sports.[4] These trends have provided an impetus for researchers to examine differences between the genders, which might affect the assessment and management of sport-related concussion. Therefore, this article addresses the role of gender in the assessment and management of sport-related concussion.

GENDER DIFFERENCES IN THE EPIDEMIOLOGY OF SPORT-RELATED CONCUSSIONS

Several researchers have identified differences in the incidence of sport-related concussion among collegiate athletes of different genders. Covassin and colleagues[5] examined NCAA injury data from 1997 to 2000 and found collegiate female athletes to

The authors have nothing to disclose.

[a] Department of Kinesiology, Michigan State University, 105 Im Sport Circle, East Lansing, MI 48824, USA

[b] Department of Kinesiology, Leisure, and Sport Science, East Tennessee State University, PO Box 70654, Johnson City, TN 37614, USA

* Corresponding author.

E-mail address: covassin@msu.edu

Clin Sports Med 30 (2011) 125–131

doi:10.1016/j.csm.2010.08.001

0278-5919/11/$ – see front matter. Published by Elsevier Inc.

sportsmed.theclinics.com

be at a higher risk of concussions occurring in games than collegiate male athletes. Specifically, women's soccer (2.09/1000 athlete exposure [AE]) and basketball (0.74/1000AE) had a higher injury rate than men's soccer (1.36/1000AE) and basketball (0.48/1000AE).[5] Hootman and colleagues[6] recently summarized 16 years (1988–2004) of NCAA injury data and reported concussions accounted for a higher injury rate in women's ice hockey (0.91/1000AE), soccer (0.41/1000AE), and basketball (0.22/1000AE) than men's ice hockey (0.41/1000AE), soccer (0.28/1000AE), and basketball (0.16/1000AE). Women's ice hockey may be misleading because data were collected only for 3 years (2000–2003) for this sport versus 16 years for the other sports.[6] According to these data, it appears that female collegiate athletes are at a higher risk for concussion than male collegiate athletes.

There are only a few studies published that have examined gender differences on incidence rates for sport-related concussion in high school athletes. One of the first studies to examine concussion at the high school level was conducted in the 1990s by Powell and Barber-Foss.[7] Similar to the epidemiologic trends observed at the collegiate level, in high school sports played by both sexes, girls had a slightly higher game injury rate than boys. Specifically, girl's soccer (0.71/1000AE), basketball (0.42/1000AE), and softball (0.13/1000AE) had a higher game injury rate for concussions than boy's soccer (0.57/1000AE), basketball (0.28/1000AE), and baseball (0.12/1000AE). A more recent investigation by Gessel and colleagues[8] reported that concussions accounted for a higher game injury rate in high school girls' sports (soccer, 0.97/1000AE; basketball, 0.60/1000AE) than in high school boys' sports (soccer, 0.59/1000AE; basketball, 0.11/1000AE). It appears that the incidence rates of concussion differ by gender at both the collegiate and high school levels.

Numerous explanations have been proposed to account for female athletes being more at risk for concussion than male athletes. Studies have found that women have a decreased head-neck segment mass compared with male athletes, which could result in greater angular acceleration to the head after a concussive impact.[9–13] College-age women have been found to have approximately 43% less head-neck segment mass compared with college-age men.[10] Researchers have also suggested that female soccer players have a larger ball-to-head size ratio than men, possibly predisposing them to concussion.[13,14] Moreover, female athletes have decreased neck strength and neck girth compared with male athletes.[10,11,15] Tierney and colleagues[10] reported that female collegiate students showed 49% less neck strength and 30% less neck girth compared with male collegiate students. Similarly, Garces and colleagues[15] reported that male collegiate students had 30% to 40% more strength in cervical extensors and flexors than female collegiate students. Mansell and colleagues[16] investigated an 8-week cervical resistance training program on neck girth, cervical strength, and head-neck segment dynamic stabilization in collegiate soccer players. Although the neck girth and strength were increased in female soccer players, there were no gender-related differences in head-neck segment dynamic stabilization during a force application (ie, weight) in collegiate soccer players.

It is currently debated whether estrogen, the primary female sex hormone, has a detrimental or a neuroprotective effect with regard to concussion. Animal models have shown that estrogen treatment before experimentally induced brain injury (eg, fluid percussion brain injury) has protective effects for male rats but detrimental effects for female rats.[17] One reason may be that estrogen acts as a neuroprotector because of the hormone's lipid antioxidant properties.[18] There is limited research published on the role that estrogen may have on the risk of concussion.

Studies have also found that female athletes tend to report more concussion symptoms than male athletes.[19] This disparity in self-reporting of concussion symptoms could be because of the nature of the male sport environment, especially in contact and collision sports (eg, football, wrestling, hockey) in which the incidence of concussion is highest. Male athletes are under constant pressure to play through pain, to show their masculinity and their toughness. They are oftentimes praised for their courage and rewarded when playing through pain and injury. In contrast, studies have found that female athletes are more concerned about their future health than male athletes.[20] These interesting differences between the male and female sport environments may explain the observed differences in the self-reporting of concussion symptoms between genders.

DIFFERENCES IN SPORT-RELATED CONCUSSION OUTCOMES BETWEEN GENDERS

Gender differences in cognitive function have been well documented. Specifically, women perform better on tasks involving verbal memory and perceptual motor speed, whereas men perform better on tasks of visuospatial ability.[21] These differences have also been documented by neurocognitive measures commonly used for managing concussion.[22–24] Covassin and colleagues[24] reported that at the college level, women performed higher on verbal memory than men, whereas men showed higher visual memory scores than women. These results warrant consideration of differences between genders in cognitive performance after concussion.

Several researchers have suggested that female athletes present more concussion symptoms acutely and take a longer period to recover from concussions[19,25,26] than male athletes.[19] Broshek and colleagues[19] found that, in high school and college athletes, concussed women displayed slower reaction times and greater total symptoms than concussed males. When excluding sports that require the use of a helmet (football), women were twice as likely as men to exhibit cognitive impairments.[19] These findings were among the first to suggest that sport-related concussion may affect athletes differently based on gender. However, athletes in this study represent significantly fewer women (28%) than men (72%), which may limit the generalizability of these findings. Nonetheless, more recent studies have also highlighted gender differences in sport-related concussion outcomes.

Covassin and colleagues[26] found gender differences in neurocognitive performance in concussed collegiate athletes. Specifically, female concussed athletes showed significantly lower scores on visual memory than male concussed athletes. In a more recent study, Colvin and colleagues[25] found that concussed collegiate female soccer players showed significantly slower reaction times and higher total symptom scores than concussed male soccer players.

Differences based on gender have also been found in the reporting of postconcussion symptoms. Female athletes tend to have a greater number of and more prolonged symptoms than male athletes.[19,27,28] Preiss-Farzanegan and colleagues[28] reported that women who incurred a sport-related mild TBI reported increased symptoms, particularly with regard to headache, dizziness, fatigue, and poor concentration, when compared with men. In a meta-analysis by Farace and Alves,[27] women who incurred a TBI had a worse outcome on 85% of measured variables, primarily symptoms, including headache, dizziness, anxiety, fatigue, and poor memory and concentration, than men.

Differences in the reporting of postconcussion symptoms between concussed male and female athletes have been attributed to neuroanatomical factors, organizational (cerebral) variability, hormonal discrepancies, and sports environment/social differences.[19] de Courten-Myers[29] reported that men had a greater number of cortical neuronal densities, whereas women had a greater area of neuropil (ie, containing unmyelinated neuronal processes). Esposito and colleagues[30] found that women have a greater cerebral blood flow rate coupled with a higher basal rate of glucose metabolism. These 2 differences could yield a more exacerbated neurometabolic cascade (ionic fluxes followed by hypoglycolysis) after concussion.[31] In addition, the decrease in cerebral blood flow and increase in metabolic demands caused by brain injury may interact with the already increased metabolic demands in women.[19]

There has long been a debate in the literature as to whether estrogen has a detrimental or a protective effect on concussion outcome. If estrogen has a deleterious effect, it may be because of receptor-mediated alterations in energy metabolism[17] or estrogen-potentiating neuronal response to excitatory amino acid.[32] Emerson and colleagues[17] found that estrogen improves neurologic outcome after a TBI in male rats but shows detrimental effects in female rats. In contrast, Kupina and colleagues[33] found that estrogen had a neuroprotective effect because female mice demonstrated a better outcome than male mice after experimental brain injury. Specifically, male mice had a 20% mortality rate, whereas no deaths were recorded among female mice. Most research exploring the protective or deleterious effects that hormones may have on brain injury outcome has been conducted using animal models. Continued research in this area in humans is warranted.

CONSIDERING GENDER DIFFERENCES IN THE ASSESSMENT AND MANAGEMENT OF SPORT-RELATED CONCUSSION

The assessment and management of sport-related concussion has seen vast improvement over the past decade. Results from empirical studies have increased the knowledge and awareness of sport-related concussion. As a result, management strategies for this injury have been refined, benefiting both sports-medicine professionals and injured athletes. More specifically, this progress has seen the suggested abolishment of historically used concussion grading scales, improved diagnostic methods, individual case management recommendations, and the use of computerized neurocognitive test batteries.[34,35]

The management of sport-related concussion continues to be a germane issue for clinicians and researchers alike. Until recently, determining the status of a concussed athlete was primarily a subjective decision made by sports medicine professionals. It is now recommended that the assessment and management of sport-related concussion take on a multifaceted approach that consists of various measures that may include a sideline mental status examination, a postural stability assessment, and a neurocognitive test battery.[36] These measures, used in conjunction with symptom inventories, offer clinicians a wide variety of information on the status of recovery of the concussed athlete. When implemented with the recommended pre- and posttest methodology, these measures add objectivity to concussion assessment and management.[37]

Gender differences in the risk, symptoms, and recovery should be considered when assessing and managing a concussed athlete. The incidence of sport-related concussion in high school and collegiate populations may be higher for female athletes in basketball, ice hockey, and soccer.[5,6] Therefore, health care professionals, coaches, athletes, and parents need to pay close attention to female athletes who incur a direct or indirect blow to the head, especially in the aforementioned sports. Moreover, sports medicine professionals need to pursue concussion evaluation with the same due diligence for female athletes as for male athletes.

Disparities in the reporting of concussion symptoms between male and female athletes should be a consideration when managing a concussion. Female concussed athletes report more symptoms of dizziness, fatigue, concentration, and lightheaded-ness than male concussed athletes.[19,28] Female soccer players who report headache symptoms 1 week postconcussion have greater cognitive impairments than athletes who do not report headache symptoms. In the general population, women have a higher incidence of headaches than men.[38] Moreover, women have almost double the prevalence of migraine headaches compared with men.[25,39–41] Recently, researchers have found that concussed athletes who display migraine headache symptoms take longer periods to recovery postinjury.[42,43] This predilection toward migraines may translate to a longer recovery time for female athletes.

Preliminary studies suggest that female athletes take longer periods to recover from a concussion than male athletes,[19,25,26] including on measures of reaction time[25] and visual memory.[26] More specifically, female concussed athletes may take up to 7 days longer to recover from a concussion than male concussed athletes. As a result of these preliminary studies, clinicians should be aware of varying recovery time from concussion between male and female athletes.

SUMMARY

The detection and management of concussion in sport continue to be an important issue for sports medicine professionals. Advancements in the knowledge of this injury continue to reshape concussion management to ensure the well-being and safety of athletes. Recent studies suggest that the risk and recovery from sport-related concussion may vary between male and female athletes, with women having a higher risk of sustaining a concussion and taking a longer time to recover than men. Therefore, sports medicine professionals should not assume that the recovery from concussion is uniform in both male and female athletes. However, more research is warranted on concussed female athletes, particularly studies examining mechanism, symptoms, and recovery time.

REFERENCES

1. Thurman D, Guerrero J. Trends in hospitalization associated with traumatic brain injury. JAMA 1999;282:954–7.
2. CDC. Nonfatal traumatic brain injuries from sports and recreation activities—United States, 2001–2005. MMWR Morb Mortal Wkly Rep 2007;56:733–7.
3. DeHaas DM. 1981-82-2007-08 NCAA sports sponsorship and participation rates report. Indianapolis (IN): National Collegiate Athletic Association; 2009.
4. NFHSA. Participation in high school sports increases again; confirms NFHS commitment to stronger leadership. Indianapolis (IN): National Federation of State High School Associations; 2008.
5. Covassin T, Swanik C, Sachs M. Sex differences and the incidence of concussions among collegiate athletes. J Athl Train 2003;38:238–44.
6. Hootman J, Dick R, Agel J. Epidemiology of collegiate injuries for 15 sports: summary and recommendations for injury prevention initiatives. J Athl Train 2007;42:311–9.
7. Powell JW, Barber-Foss KD. Traumatic brain injury in high school athletes. JAMA 1999;282:958–63.
8. Gessel LM, Fields SK, Collins CL, et al. Concussions among United States high school and collegiate athletes. J Athl Train 2007;42:495–503.
9. Plagenhoef S, Evans F, Abdelnour T. Anatomical data for analyzing human motion. Res Q Exerc Sport 1983;54:169–78.

10. Tierney RT, Sitler MR, Swanik B, et al. Gender differences in head-neck segment dynamic stabilization during head acceleration. Med Sci Sports Exerc 2005;37: 272–9.
11. Kreighbaum E, Barthels K. Biomechanics: a qualitative approach for studying human movement. Needham Heights (MA): Allyn & Bacon; 1996.
12. Barth JT, Freeman JR, Broshek DK, et al. Acceleration-deceleration sport-related concussion: the gravity of it all. J Athl Train 2001;36:253–6.
13. Schneider K, Zernicke RF. Computer simulation of head impact: Estimation of head-injury risk during soccer heading. International Journal of Sport Biomechanics 1988;4:358–71.
14. Barnes B, Cooper L, Kirkendall D, et al. Concussion history in elite male and female soccer players. Am J Sports Med 1998;26:433–8.
15. Garces G, Medina L, LMilutinovic P, et al. Normative database of isometric cervical strength in a healthy population. Med Sci Sports Exerc 2002;33:464–70.
16. Mansell J, Tierney R, Sitler M, et al. Resistance training and head-neck segment dynamic stabilization in male and female collegiate soccer players. J Athl Train 2005;40:310–9.
17. Emerson CS, Headrick JP, Vink R. Estrogen improves biochemical and neurologic outcome following traumatic brain injury in male rats, but not females. Brain Res 1993;608:95–100.
18. Hall E, Pazara K, Linseman K. Sex differences in postischemic neuronal necrosis in gerbils. J Cereb Blood Flow Metab 1991;11:292–8.
19. Broshek DK, Kaushik T, Freeman JR, et al. Sex differences in outcome following sports-related concussion. J Neurosurg 2005;102:856–63.
20. Granito VJ. Psychological aspects of athletic injury: themes and gender differences. Dissertation Abstracts International: Section B: the Sciences and Engineering 2000;61:530.
21. Weiss E, Kemmler G, Eberhard A, et al. Sex differences in cognitive functions. Pers Individ Dif 2003;35:863–75.
22. Barr W. Neuropsychological testing of high school athletes: preliminary norms and test-retest indices. Arch Clin Neuropsychol 2003;18:91–101.
23. Brown C, Guskiewicz K, Bleiberg J. Athlete characteristics and outcome scores for computerized neuropsychological assessment: a preliminary analysis. J Athl Train 2007;42:515–23.
24. Covassin T, Swanik C, Sachs M, et al. Sex differences in baseline neuropsychological function and concussion symptoms of collegiate athletes. Br J Sports Med 2006;40:923–7 [discussion: 927].
25. Colvin A, Mullen J, Lovell M, et al. The role of concussion history and gender in recovery from soccer-related concussion. Am J Sports Med 2009;37: 1699–704.
26. Covassin T, Schatz P, Swanik B. Sex differences in neuropsychological function and post-concussion symptoms of concussed collegiate athletes. Neurosurgery 2007;61:345–51.
27. Farace E, Alves W. Do woman fare worse? A meta-analysis of gender differences in traumatic brain injury outcomes. J Neurosurg 2000;93:539–45.
28. Preiss-Farzanegan S, Chapman B, Wong T, et al. The relationship between gender and postconcussion symptoms after sport-related mild traumatic brain injury. Phys Med Rehabil 2009;1:245–53.
29. de Courten-Myers GM. The human cerebral cortex: gender differences in structure and function. J Neuropathol Exp Neurol 1999;58:217–26.

30. Esposito G, Van Horn JD, Weinberger DR, et al. Gender differences with cerebral blood flow as a function of cognitive state with PET. J Neurol Med 1996;37: 559–64.
31. Giza C, Hovda D. The neurometabolic cascade of concussion. J Athl Train 2001; 36:228–35.
32. Smith S. Estrogen administration increases neuronal responses to excitatory amino acids as a long-term effect. Brain Res 1989;503(2):354–7.
33. Kupina NC, Detloff MR, Bobrowski WF, et al. Cytoskeletal protein degradation and neurodegeneration evolves differently in males and females following experimental head injury. Exp Neurol 2003;180:55–73.
34. Aubry M, Cantu R, Dvorak J, et al. Summary and agreement statement of the 1st international symposium on concussion in sport, Vienna 2001. Clin J Sport Med 2002;12:6–11.
35. McCrory P, Johnston K, Meeuwisse W, et al. Summary and agreement statement of the 2nd International conference on concussion in sport, Prague 2004. Br J Sports Med 2005;39:196–204.
36. Guskiewicz KM, Bruce SL, Cantu R, et al. National athletic trainers' association position statement: management of sports-related concussion. J Athl Train 2004;39:280–97.
37. Lovell MR, Collins MW, Bradley J. Return to play following sports-related concussion. Clin Sports Med 2004;23:421–41, ix.
38. Silberstein S, Young W. Headache and facial pain. In: Goetz G, editor. Textbook of clinical neurology. Philadelphia: Saunders Company; 2007. p. 1247–54.
39. Launer L, Terwindt G, Ferrari M. The prevalence and characteristics of migraine in a population-based cohort: the GM study. Neurology 1999;53:537–42.
40. Lipton R, Diamond S, Reed M, et al. Migraine diagnosis and treatment: results from the American migraine study II. Headache 2001;41:638–45.
41. Lipton R, Stewart W, Diamond S, et al. Prevalence and burden of migraine in the United States: data from the American migraine study. Headache 2002;41: 646–57.
42. Lau B, Lovell MR, Collins MW, et al. Neurocognitive and symptom predictors of recovery in high school athletes. Clin J Sport Med 2009;19:216–21.
43. Mihalik J, Stump J, Collins MW, et al. Posttraumatic migraine characteristics in athletes following sports-related concussion. J Neurosurg 2005;102:850–5.

The Pediatric Athlete: Younger Athletes with Sport-Related Concussion

William P. Meehan III, MD[a,b,*], Alex M. Taylor, PsyD[a,c], Mark Proctor, MD[d]

KEYWORDS

- Concussion • Mild traumatic brain injury • Head injury
- Trauma • Injury • Sports

Most athletes involved in organized sports participation are pediatric athletes.[1] Approximately 25% of pediatric concussions presenting to emergency departments occur during athletic activity.[2] Fortunately, much of the published medical investigations were conducted in high-school and college athletes, therefore offering physicians some insight into the mechanisms, signs, symptoms, assessment, and management of a pediatric athlete who sustains a sport-related concussion (SRC).

Very little data regarding SRC, however, have been published in pre–high-school-aged athletes.[3] This situation is concerning because the human brain continues to develop into young adulthood. The effects of concussive brain injury on the developing brain are not well understood. There is both scientific and clinical evidence that traumatic brain injury (TBI) in children differs from that in adults. In addition, children and adults differ in the role played by sports participation in their lives, the amount of knowledge they are expected to acquire on a daily basis, and the frequency with which their cognitive function is assessed or tested.[4] Therefore, the recommendations

---

Funding/Support: This article was supported by the NIH through a T32 Award to Dr Meehan (T32 HD040128-06A1).

The authors report no conflicts of interest.

[a] Sports Concussion Clinic, Division of Sports Medicine, Department of Orthopedics, Children's Hospital Boston, 319 Longwood Avenue, Boston, MA 02115, USA

[b] Division of Emergency Medicine, Department of Medicine, Children's Hospital Boston, Boston, MA, USA

[c] Department of Neurology, Children's Hospital Boston, Boston, MA, USA

[d] Department of Neurosurgery, Children's Hospital Boston, Boston, MA, USA

* Corresponding author. Sports Concussion Clinic, Division of Sports Medicine, Children's Hospital Boston, 319 Longwood Avenue, Boston, MA 02115.

E-mail address: william.meehan@childrens.harvard.edu

for managing young athletes with concussion differ from those of adults. This article discusses the differences between pediatric and adult athletes who sustain SRCs.

EPIDEMIOLOGY

Concussion accounts for approximately 9% of all high-school athletic injuries.[5] The rates of SRCs are highest in contact and collision sports.[5–7] Most athletes engaged in such sports are younger than 19 years,[1] making concussion a major concern for clinicians caring for young athletes. Of all pediatric concussions presenting to the emergency departments, approximately 25% occur during sports.[2] Many athletes with SRCs do not present to an emergency department or seek medical attention.[7–9] Surveys of the general population suggest that a higher percentage of concussions are due to athletics, with some studies suggesting that more than 85% of concussions in 16- to 34-year-old people are related to sports.[10]

MECHANISM/BIOMECHANICS

The biomechanics of concussive injury differs between adult and pediatric patients. Factors including differences in relative size of the head compared with the rest of the body, brain water content, vasculature, degree of myelination, and shape of the skull account for the biomechanical differences.[3,4,11,12]

Concussion is caused primarily by a rotational acceleration of the brain.[13–15] Clinicians have hypothesized that increasing both the cervical muscle strength and tone at the time of impact can reduce the risk of concussion by increasing the effective mass of the head, which becomes more of a unit with the rest of the body as the neck muscles strengthen. This, in turn, reduces the resultant acceleration for a given force.[1,16] This difference in neck strength has biomechanical effects, shown both experimentally in animals and clinically in children.[17] Recent evidence supports this hypothesis.[18] Given the relatively weak cervical muscle strength compared with their older counterparts, younger athletes might be at increased risk for concussion when hit with the same magnitude of force. Of course, as other investigators have pointed out, this same decrease in muscle strength may result in less force delivered by the striking athlete at the time of injury, thereby decreasing the risk of injury.[5]

Countering this hypothesis, biomechanicians have demonstrated that greater force is required to cause similar concussive injury in smaller brains than in larger brains with greater mass.[11,17] Thus, it has been suggested that children symptomatic after a concussion have sustained greater force than an adult with similar postconcussive symptoms.[4] This would suggest that the weaker neck muscles and larger head may be a more important issue than the overall small size of the athlete because these weaker forces are disproportionately applied to the brain.

Clinically, the different effects of age on head injury have been investigated. An analysis by Berney and colleagues[19] revealed that children younger than 3 years sustained head injuries associated with lower energy mechanisms and more skull fractures, subdural hematomas, and early seizures than their older counterparts. They were also less likely to lose consciousness than older children. Those children aged 3 to 9 years sustained head injuries after higher energy mechanisms, were more likely to lose consciousness, were more often comatose, had less subdural hemorrhages, and had more significant cerebral edema. Injuries sustained by children older than 9 years were more like adult injuries with high energy mechanisms and more extradural hematomas. These age-dependent injury patterns warrant further investigation into the possible differences in concussive brain injury between patients of varying ages.

PATHOPHYSIOLOGY

Pediatric and adult brains are in different phases of development, with the child's brain growing and needing to acquire high volumes of new learning at a much faster pace. The pathophysiological response to TBI also differs between the mature and developing brain.[12,20–22] Clinically, a syndrome of delayed deterioration after a lucid period without a focal structural injury has been described in children (sometimes referred to as "talk and die"); it is not often seen in adults.[23–25] Another possible example of different responses to concussive brain injury between adult and pediatric patients is second impact syndrome, which has been described exclusively in teenagers and young adults.[26–30]

Diffuse brain swelling after TBI is more common in pediatric patients and results from mechanisms different from that of adults. Although the exact reasons for this swelling are not known, differences in glutamate receptor expression, expression of aquaporin 4 by microglia, and brain water content may play a role.[12] Increased vulnerability to oxidative stress, differences in dopaminergic activity, vascular response to injury, and susceptibility of glutamate receptors between the developing and fully developed brain may also play a role in the difference in responses to TBI between adult and pediatric patients.[12,31]

The possibility that the mechanisms, forces, biomechanics, and pathophysiological responses to concussive brain injury differ between adults and children needs to be further explored, because such differences could change the assessment and management of pediatric athletes who sustain SRCs.

UNDERREPORTING

The assessment and management of pediatric concussion is further complicated by the lack of injury reporting. In a 1983 study of football players in Minnesota high schools, 29% of athletes who sustained a concussion were not examined by anyone at all. Only 22% were examined by medical personnel. The remainder were attended to by a coach, parent, or teammate.[9] More recent research suggests that underreporting continues. A 2004 study published by McCrea and colleagues[8] revealed that only 47.3% of high-school football players report their injuries. Similar findings have been reported in other sports, including female athletics.[32] Underreporting of concussion is not exclusive to pediatric athletes.[33,34] However, pediatric athletic organizations are less likely to have a formal organized approach to concussion management, including preseason balance error scores, computerized neuropsychological testing, and dedicated personnel with concussion training, such as team physicians, athletic trainers, and neuropsychologists. This inherent lack of personnel and resources results in further reliance on self-reporting of symptoms in younger athletes, making underreporting more of an issue in pediatrics than in adult sports medicine.

ASSESSMENT

As mentioned earlier, younger athletes are often managed without the benefit of dedicated athletic trainers, team physicians, and neuropsychologists. Therefore, many of those athletes who seek medical care after a concussion are managed by primary care physicians who often do not have expertise in concussive brain injury or access to needed resources. In a 2006 survey of primary care physicians, many were unaware of published guidelines for the management of SRCs.[35] This lack of awareness likely reflects a lack of medical training in concussion management and the relatively small proportion of patients presenting to the primary care physician for concussions when compared with other issues such as asthma, infectious illnesses, obesity.

NEUROPSYCHOLOGICAL EVALUATION OF THE PEDIATRIC ATHLETE

In high-school, college, and professional athletes, neuropsychological evaluation has been shown to be useful in the management of concussion. Defined as the applied science of brain-behavior relationships, neuropsychology involves objective assessment of cognitive, social, and emotional functioning. Data are used to identify individual strengths and weaknesses, make differential diagnoses, and plan appropriate interventions within environmental and developmental contexts.[3,36–38] Sports medicine first recognized the utility of neuropsychological testing in the mid-1980s when the testing was used as part of a 4-year prospective study of mild TBI in college athletes.[39] A total of 2350 football players were evaluated with brief paper-and-pencil neuropsychological measures both pre- and postseason. Head-injured athletes were also evaluated 24 hours, 5 days, and 10 days after the injury. Compared with noninjured controls and their own preseason baseline performance, the concussed group demonstrated cognitive deficits for up to 10 days postinjury.

Subsequent studies have confirmed these findings, revealing several areas particularly sensitive to head injury: executive functioning, speed of information processing, attention, and memory.[40–53] Results suggest that recovery typically occurs within 2 to 14 days, although some patients demonstrate significantly longer recovery times.[40–43,45–52,54] There is also evidence that injured athletes who no longer report symptoms demonstrate worse performance on neurocognitive measures than uninjured controls, suggesting that there may be subtle deficits beyond the reported symptoms.[45] Neuropsychological testing is also sensitive enough to diagnose SRC, even in the absence of reported symptoms.[44,48,50,55,56] Given these findings, the use of neuropsychological testing has been endorsed by experts in SRC.[57–59] Neuropsychological testing can be especially useful for younger athletes to assist with planning academic interventions.[59]

Studies examining outcomes from SRC in younger athletes are more limited. Initial findings, however, are consistent with more severe TBI research, which suggests that recovery may be age related, with younger athletes faring worse. Results from an investigation that compared concussed college and high-school athletes with uninjured controls found that high-school athletes take longer to recover than college athletes, despite reporting lower numbers of previous concussions and less severe in-season injuries.[60] In addition, a study of 2141 high-school athletes found that up to 23% of the concussed athletes continued to demonstrate difficulties on cognitive tasks 3 weeks after injury.[61] In contrast, in a 6-year prospective study involving the National Football League (NFL) only 1.6% of the concussed participants took more than 14 days to recover.[62] In a subset of the NFL players who underwent baseline neuropsychological evaluations and then completed a second evaluation within a few days after concussion, there was no statistically significant decline on any traditional paper-and-pencil measures of neuropsychological functioning.[62] These data contrast findings of studies examining younger athletes, suggesting that age and developmental factors play a role in recovery from concussive brain injury.

Because an increasing number of sports organizations recognized the utility of neuropsychological assessment in managing SRCs, the limitations of traditional testing (paper and pencil) became evident. Most notably, the cost and availability of trained neuropsychologists to administer and interpret data for large organizations seemed prohibitive and led to the development and increased use of computer-based neuropsychological testing. Computer-based testing is more efficient, allowing for entire teams to be tested in a single session. Computers also provide a more accurate measurement of cognitive function, such as reaction time and speed of information processing. This added precision may increase the validity of test results in detecting subtle changes in neurocognitive functioning. In addition, computerized testing allows for the randomization of test stimuli, which should improve reliability across multiple administration periods by minimizing practice effects.[63]

Several computer-based tests exist at present, including Immediate Post-Concussion Assessment and Cognitive Testing (ImPACT Applications, Inc, Pittsburgh, PA, USA), CogSport (CogState Ltd, Melbourne, Victoria, Australia), Concussion Resolution Index (HeadMinder, Inc, New York, NY, USA), and Automated Neurocognitive Assessment Metrics (US Department of Defense). Many present guidelines recommend that baseline neuropsychological assessment be administered before the start of the season. This model allows athletes to serve as their own controls and aids in the interpretation of data in light of preexisting or contextual factors that have been shown to affect neuropsychological performance. With some exceptions, normative samples of computerized tests used to manage SRCs are based on older athletes and are therefore less generalizable to children. Ongoing research to develop and validate cognitive tests for children has shown the potential for increased clinical application with this population.[53,64]

In younger athletes, testing must be considered in the context of brain maturation and individual abilities. Rapid brain development, which continues through adolescence, may affect neuropsychological performance. Improvement in cognitive performance is likely, as new skills and abilities are acquired.[1,4,38,64] In one study examining neuropsychological testing among high-school athletes, older students performed better than their younger peers, reflecting improvements in cognitive function with age and development.[65] Thus, more frequent baseline testing is necessary in younger athletes because their baseline function changes with age.

Developmental disorders including learning disabilities or attention-deficit/hyperactivity disorder can also affect neuropsychological functioning. Research has shown more severe cognitive sequelae in college football players diagnosed with a learning disability.[43] Students with self-reported academic problems also perform worse on some baseline measures of functioning.[66] There is some evidence that girls experience more significant neuropsychological difficulties after SRC.[67–69] Other factors that may affect cognitive functioning include sleep deprivation, anxiety, and depression.[38,70]

The neuropsychological literature has also documented the effect of motivation on performance. In forensic settings, symptoms or deficits may be exaggerated. In athletes, secondary gains such as the benefit of academic accommodations may negatively affect performance.[37] Moreover, intentional suboptimal performance on baseline tests, with the hope of showing less deterioration after injury, has been documented in college athletes.[71] This area warrants further investigation. Careful consideration should be given to performing and interpreting neuropsychological tests, given the multiple factors that may affect performance in the developing child.

Given that some athletes deny symptoms and younger children may have difficulty verbalizing cognitive problems, objective neuropsychological data can aid return-to-play decisions. A score significantly lower than baseline or, in the absence of baseline testing, lower than premorbid estimates of functioning may reflect ongoing sequelae and preclude return to play. Acute findings can also help determine appropriate management strategies. In pediatric populations, neuropsychological assessment while the athlete remains symptomatic is useful in determining the appropriate academic accommodations.[38,59] In all cases, neuropsychological testing should not be used as a stand-alone measure but as part of a comprehensive assessment that includes a clinical interview, evaluation of symptoms, overall medical history, and physical examination.

Although there is some evidence that a history of concussion is associated with neuropsychological impairment, data concerning the long-term effects of repetitive concussions vary. The number or severity of previous injuries has not been shown to conclusively predict long-term sequelae.[43,47,72–75] In general, studies of athletes with a history of concussion suggest an increased risk of sustaining additional concussions, worse on-field presentations with subsequent concussions, slowed recoveries, and greater acute changes in memory performance. In the extreme cases, such as boxing, findings suggest that the extent of neuropsychological impairments may be associated with the number of bouts fought.[76] The likely relationship between exposure and outcome argues for conservative management of the pediatric athlete.

Many physicians do not have easy access to neuropsychological testing. In one study, only 16% of respondents reported they could reliably access neuropsychological testing within 1 week of injury.[35] Because the most recent guidelines refer to neuropsychological testing as the cornerstone of concussion management,[58] it seems that even those aware of recent management strategies will often not have access to the needed resources to follow such guidelines. Furthermore, most of the assessments available, both symptom scales and neurocognitive assessments, have been researched in older athletes, leading to concerns over the appropriateness of the assessments in younger patients.[53] Although the utility of most currently available computerized measures in the youngest athletes is limited, specific pediatric versions are in development. These measures, and more traditional neuropsychological measures, are useful not only in assisting return-to-play decisions but also in guiding targeted academic accommodations for younger athletes by providing practitioners with objective evidence to support their treatment plans.

RECOVERY

Most athletes recover from SRCs in a relatively short period.[47,59,77,78] However, studies have shown longer recovery times in younger athletes than in older athletes.[59] In a study using neuropsychological testing to track the recovery of high-school athletes compared with college athletes, Field and colleagues[60] have reported a protracted rate of recovery in the high-school athletes,[50] which may be related to age-dependent brain physiology.

Experimental models of concussion reporting a temporal window of vulnerability after trauma also suggest that the developing brain may be more susceptible to injury during the acute recovery phase.[22,64,79,80] Research examining more severe pediatric head injury has shown a relationship between age and outcome. Rather than the younger brain being more "plastic" and thus better able to recover from injury, current theory suggests that early insult may have a significant impact on later development.[36,81–83] Long-term sequelae have been documented in younger children with acquired brain injury. In research involving TBI, insult occurring during infancy and preschool age is associated with worse outcomes than injury sustained in later childhood or adolescence. Undeveloped or developing skills are presumed to be particularly vulnerable.[81,82,84,85] Moreover, contextual factors, including access to care and academic demands, may affect recovery in younger individuals.[3,38,53,59]

Furthermore, there is some evidence that concussive injuries sustained early in life may have minimal effect on already established cognitive skills but may significantly delay the development of future skills.[83,86] Obviously, this effect is much more of a concern for the developing mind of a child than the fully developed mind of an adult athlete.

MANAGEMENT

Although much of the management of pediatric athletes who sustain SRC is at present similar to that of adults, there are some differences worth noting. As mentioned earlier, the mind of the pediatric athlete is still developing. Cognitive function continues to increase. Therefore, baseline testing should occur more frequently in younger athletes,[4,87] and the clinician should be more sensitive to the relative vulnerability of the child's brain than with the adult. Because younger athletes require longer recovery times, more conservative return-to-play decisions should be considered for them.[3,4,58,60,88–91] The American Academy of Pediatrics recommends conservative management of concussion.[92]

Although cognitive function is compromised after concussion in both adult and pediatric athletes, younger athletes are unique because their cognitive function is constantly being assessed and tested in school. Furthermore, their cognitive performance is graded, and those grades are placed in their permanent academic records. There is the potential for greater secondary consequences of concussion in children, in whom social and academic progress rely on normal growth and development.[3,4,84,85] Many of their future opportunities, such as college acceptance and employment, are based, in part, on their grades, which must be considered in their management. Academic accommodations should be put in place to help attenuate any effects their injury might otherwise have on their grades during recovery.[3,4,59]

SUMMARY

TBI affects the developing brain differently than the fully developed brain. The specific effects of concussion on the developing brain are still being elucidated through clinical and scientific investigation. As compared with adults, clinicians should expect longer recovery times for younger patients after a concussion. Given the daily cognitive demands placed on school-aged athletes, concussion management in this age group should include, when available, neuropsychological assessment and appropriate academic planning. Given the increased vulnerability, ongoing development, and contextual factors that have the potential to complicate recovery from concussion in children, more conservative management is warranted.

REFERENCES

1. Buzzini SR, Guskiewicz KM. Sport-related concussion in the young athlete. Curr Opin Pediatr 2006;18(4):376–82.
2. Browne GJ, Lam LT. Concussive head injury in children and adolescents related to sports and other leisure physical activities. Br J Sports Med 2006;40(2):163–8.
3. Kirkwood MW, Yeates KO, Wilson PE. Pediatric sport-related concussion: a review of the clinical management of an oft-neglected population. Pediatrics 2006; 117(4):1359–71.
4. McCrory P, Collie A, Anderson V, et al. Can we manage sport related concussion in children the same as in adults? Br J Sports Med 2004;38(5):516–9.

5. Gessel LM, Fields SK, Collins CL, et al. Concussions among United States high school and collegiate athletes. J Athl Train 2007;42(4):495–503.
6. Koh JO, Cassidy JD, Watkinson EJ. Incidence of concussion in contact sports: a systematic review of the evidence. Brain Inj 2003;17(10):901–17.
7. Tommasone BA, Valovich McLeod TC. Contact sport concussion incidence. J Athl Train 2006;41(4):470–2.
8. McCrea M, Hammeke T, Olsen G, et al. Unreported concussion in high school football players: implications for prevention. Clin J Sport Med 2004;14(1):13–7.
9. Gerberich SG, Priest JD, Boen JR, et al. Concussion incidences and severity in secondary school varsity football players. Am J Public Health 1983;73(12):1370–5.
10. Gordon KE, Dooley JM, Wood EP. Descriptive epidemiology of concussion. Pediatr Neurol 2006;34(5):376–8.
11. Goldsmith W, Plunkett J. A biomechanical analysis of the causes of traumatic brain injury in infants and children. Am J Forensic Med Pathol 2004;25(2):89–100.
12. Bauer R, Fritz H. Pathophysiology of traumatic injury in the developing brain: an introduction and short update. Exp Toxicol Pathol 2004;56(1–2):65–73.
13. Denny-Brown D, Russell R. Experimental cerebral concussion. Brain 1941;64:93–164.
14. Holbourn A. Mechanics of head injury. Lancet 1943;2(2):438–41.
15. Ommaya AK, Gennarelli TA. Cerebral concussion and traumatic unconsciousness. Correlation of experimental and clinical observations of blunt head injuries. Brain 1974;97(4):633–54.
16. Tysvaer AT. Head and neck injuries in soccer. Impact of minor trauma. Sports Med 1992;14(3):200–13.
17. Ommaya AK, Goldsmith W, Thibault L. Biomechanics and neuropathology of adult and paediatric head injury. Br J Neurosurg 2002;16(3):220–42.
18. Mihalik JP, Blackburn JT, Greenwald RM, et al. Collision type and player anticipation affect head impact severity among youth ice hockey players. Pediatrics 2010;125(6):e1394–401.
19. Berney J, Favier J, Froidevaux AC. Paediatric head trauma: influence of age and sex. I. Epidemiology. Childs Nerv Syst 1994;10(8):509–16.
20. McKeever CK, Schatz P. Current issues in the identification, assessment, and management of concussions in sports-related injuries. Appl Neuropsychol 2003;10(1):4–11.
21. Prins ML, Hovda DA. Developing experimental models to address traumatic brain injury in children. J Neurotrauma 2003;20(2):123–37.
22. Giza CC, Hovda DA. The neurometabolic cascade of concussion. J Athl Train 2001;36(3):228–35.
23. Sakas DE, Whittaker KW, Whitwell HL, et al. Syndromes of posttraumatic neurological deterioration in children with no focal lesions revealed by cerebral imaging: evidence for a trigeminovascular pathophysiology. Neurosurgery 1997;41(3):661–7.
24. Schnitker MT. A syndrome of cerebral concussion in children. J Pediatr 1949;35(5):557–60.
25. Snoek JW, Minderhoud JM, Wilmink JT. Delayed deterioration following mild head injury in children. Brain 1984;107(Pt 1):15–36.
26. Centers for Disease Control and Prevention (CDC). Sports-related recurrent brain injuries–United States. MMWR Morb Mortal Wkly Rep 1997;46(10):224–7.
27. Cantu R. Second impact syndrome: a risk in any contact sport. Phys Sportsmed 1995;23(6):27.

28. Kelly JP, Nichols JS, Filley CM, et al. Concussion in sports. Guidelines for the prevention of catastrophic outcome. JAMA 1991;266(20):2867–9.
29. McCrory PR, Berkovic SF. Second impact syndrome. Neurology 1998;50(3): 677–83.
30. Saunders RL, Harbaugh RE. The second impact in catastrophic contact-sports head trauma. JAMA 1984;252(4):538–9.
31. Grundl PD, Biagas KV, Kochanek PM, et al. Early cerebrovascular response to head injury in immature and mature rats. J Neurotrauma 1994;11(2):135–48.
32. Williamson IJ, Goodman D. Converging evidence for the under-reporting of concussions in youth ice hockey. Br J Sports Med 2006;40(2):128–32 [discussion: 128–32].
33. Maroon JC. Concussion from the inside: the athlete's perspective. In: Bailes JE, Lovell MR, Maroon JC, editors. Sports-related concussion. St Louis (MO): Quality Medical Publishing, Inc; 1999. p. 231–51.
34. Delaney JS, Lacroix VJ, Leclerc S, et al. Concussions during the 1997 Canadian Football League season. Clin J Sport Med 2000;10(1):9–14.
35. Pleacher MD, Dexter WW. Concussion management by primary care providers. Br J Sports Med 2006;40(1):e2 [discussion: e2].
36. Kirkwood MW, Randolph C, Yeates KO. Returning pediatric athletes to play after concussion: the evidence (or lack thereof) behind baseline neuropsychological testing. Acta Paediatr 2009;98(9):1409–11.
37. Kirkwood MW, Kirk JW. The base rate of suboptimal effort in a pediatric mild TBI sample: performance on the medical symptom validity test. Clin Neuropsychol 2010;24(5):860–72.
38. Purcell L. What are the most appropriate return-to-play guidelines for concussed child athletes? Br J Sports Med 2009;43(Suppl 1):i51–5.
39. Barth JT, Alves WM, Ryan TV, et al. Mild head injuries in sports: neuropsychological sequelae and recovery of function. In: Levin HS, Eisenberg HM, Benton AL, editors. Mild head injury. New York: Oxford University Press; 1989. p. 257–75.
40. Barr WB, McCrea M. Sensitivity and specificity of standardized neurocognitive testing immediately following sports concussion. J Int Neuropsychol Soc 2001; 7(6):693–702.
41. Belanger HG, Vanderploeg RD. The neuropsychological impact of sports-related concussion: a meta-analysis. J Int Neuropsychol Soc 2005;11(4):345–57.
42. Chen JK, Johnston KM, Collie A, et al. A validation of the post concussion symptom scale in the assessment of complex concussion using cognitive testing and functional MRI. J Neurol Neurosurg Psychiatr 2007;78(11):1231–8.
43. Collins MW, Grindel SH, Lovell MR, et al. Relationship between concussion and neuropsychological performance in college football players. JAMA 1999; 282(10):964–70.
44. Erlanger D, Feldman D, Kutner K, et al. Development and validation of a web-based neuropsychological test protocol for sports-related return-to-play decision-making. Arch Clin Neuropsychol 2003;18(3):293–316.
45. Fazio VC, Lovell MR, Pardini JE, et al. The relationship between post concussion symptoms and neurocognitive performance in concussed athletes. NeuroRehabilitation 2007;22(3):207–16.
46. Geary EK, Kraus MF, Pliskin NH, et al. Verbal learning differences in chronic mild traumatic brain injury. J Int Neuropsychol Soc 2010;16(3):506–16.
47. Guskiewicz KM, McCrea M, Marshall SW, et al. Cumulative effects associated with recurrent concussion in collegiate football players: the NCAA concussion study. JAMA 2003;290(19):2549–55.

48. Lovell MR, Collins MW, Iverson GL, et al. Recovery from mild concussion in high school athletes. J Neurosurg 2003;98(2):296–301.
49. Macciocchi SN, Barth JT, Alves W, et al. Neuropsychological functioning and recovery after mild head injury in collegiate athletes. Neurosurgery 1996;39(3): 510–4.
50. McClincy MP, Lovell MR, Pardini J, et al. Recovery from sports concussion in high school and collegiate athletes. Brain Inj 2006;20(1):33–9.
51. McCrea M, Guskiewicz KM, Marshall SW, et al. Acute effects and recovery time following concussion in collegiate football players: the NCAA concussion study. JAMA 2003;290(19):2556–63.
52. McCrea M, Kelly JP, Randolph C, et al. Immediate neurocognitive effects of concussion. Neurosurgery 2002;50(5):1032–40 [discussion: 1040–2].
53. Gioia GA, Schneider JC, Vaughan CG, et al. Which symptom assessments and approaches are uniquely appropriate for paediatric concussion? Br J Sports Med 2009;43(Suppl 1):i13–22.
54. Erlanger D, Kaushik T, Cantu R, et al. Symptom-based assessment of the severity of a concussion. J Neurosurg 2003;98(3):477–84.
55. Erlanger D, Saliba E, Barth J, et al. Monitoring resolution of postconcussion symptoms in athletes: preliminary results of a web-based neuropsychological test protocol. J Athl Train 2001;36(3):280–7.
56. Van Kampen DA, Lovell MR, Pardini JE, et al. The "value added" of neurocognitive testing after sports-related concussion. Am J Sports Med 2006;34(10):1630–5.
57. Aubry M, Cantu R, Dvorak J, et al. Summary and agreement statement of the first international conference on concussion in sport, Vienna 2001. Recommendations for the improvement of safety and health of athletes who may suffer concussive injuries. Br J Sports Med 2002;36(1):6–10.
58. McCrory P, Johnston K, Meeuwisse W, et al. Summary and agreement statement of the 2nd international conference on concussion in sport, Prague 2004. Br J Sports Med 2005;39(4):196–204.
59. McCrory P, Meeuwisse W, Johnston K, et al. Consensus statement on concussion in sport: the 3rd international conference on concussion in sport held in Zurich, November 2008. J Athl Train 2009;44(4):434–48.
60. Field M, Collins MW, Lovell MR, et al. Does age play a role in recovery from sports-related concussion? A comparison of high school and collegiate athletes. J Pediatr 2003;142(5):546–53.
61. Collins M, Lovell MR, Iverson GL, et al. Examining concussion rates and return to play in high school football players wearing newer helmet technology: a three-year prospective cohort study. Neurosurgery 2006;58(2):275–86 [discussion: 275–86].
62. Pellman EJ, Lovell MR, Viano DC, et al. Concussion in professional football: neuropsychological testing–part 6. Neurosurgery 2004;55(6):1290–303 [discussion: 1303–5].
63. Collie A, Darby D, Maruff P. Computerised cognitive assessment of athletes with sports related head injury. Br J Sports Med 2001;35(5):297–302.
64. Lovell MR, Fazio V. Concussion management in the child and adolescent athlete. Curr Sports Med Rep 2008;7(1):12–5.
65. Hunt TN, Ferrara MS. Age-related differences in neuropsychological testing among high school athletes. J Athl Train 2009;44(4):405–9.
66. Iverson GL, Collins MW, Roberge M, et al. Final Program, 36th Annual Meeting International Neuropsychological Society. J Int Neuropsychol Soc 2008; 14(Suppl 1):i–292.

67. Broshek DK, Kaushik T, Freeman JR, et al. Sex differences in outcome following sports-related concussion. J Neurosurg 2005;102(5):856–63.
68. Covassin T, Schatz P, Swanik CB. Sex differences in neuropsychological function and post-concussion symptoms of concussed collegiate athletes. Neurosurgery 2007;61(2):345–50 [discussion: 350–1].
69. Covassin T, Swanik CB, Sachs M, et al. Sex differences in baseline neuropsychological function and concussion symptoms of collegiate athletes. Br J Sports Med 2006;40(11):923–7 [discussion: 927].
70. Grindel SH, Lovell MR, Collins MW. The assessment of sport-related concussion: the evidence behind neuropsychological testing and management. Clin J Sport Med 2001;11(3):134–43.
71. Bailey CM, Echemendia RJ, Arnett PA. The impact of motivation on neuropsychological performance in sports-related mild traumatic brain injury. J Int Neuropsychol Soc 2006;12(4):475–84.
72. Iverson GL, Gaetz M, Lovell MR, et al. Cumulative effects of concussion in amateur athletes. Brain Inj 2004;18(5):433–43.
73. Gronwall D, Wrightson P. Cumulative effect of concussion. Lancet 1975;2(7943): 995–7.
74. Iverson GL, Brooks BL, Lovell MR, et al. No cumulative effects for one or two previous concussions. Br J Sports Med 2006;40(1):72–5.
75. Broglio SP, Ferrara MS, Piland SG, et al. Concussion history is not a predictor of computerised neurocognitive performance. Br J Sports Med 2006;40(9):802–5 [discussion: 802–5].
76. Heilbronner RL, Bush SS, Ravdin LD, et al. Neuropsychological consequences of boxing and recommendations to improve safety: a national academy of neuropsychology education paper. Arch Clin Neuropsychol 2009;24(1):11–9.
77. Iverson GL, Brooks BL, Collins MW, et al. Tracking neuropsychological recovery following concussion in sport. Brain Inj 2006;20(3):245–52.
78. Guskiewicz KM, Ross SE, Marshall SW. Postural stability and neuropsychological deficits after concussion in collegiate athletes. J Athl Train 2001;36(3): 263–73.
79. Vagnozzi R, Signoretti S, Tavazzi B, et al. Hypothesis of the postconcussive vulnerable brain: experimental evidence of its metabolic occurrence. Neurosurgery 2005;57(1):164–71 [discussion: 164–71].
80. Vagnozzi R, Tavazzi B, Signoretti S, et al. Temporal window of metabolic brain vulnerability to concussions: mitochondrial-related impairment–part I. Neurosurgery 2007;61(2):379–88 [discussion: 388–9].
81. Anderson V, Catroppa C, Morse S, et al. Functional plasticity or vulnerability after early brain injury? Pediatrics 2005;116(6):1374–82.
82. Ewing-Cobbs L, Prasad MR, Landry SH, et al. Executive functions following traumatic brain injury in young children: a preliminary analysis. Dev Neuropsychol 2004;26(1):487–512.
83. Taylor HG, Alden J. Age-related differences in outcomes following childhood brain insults: an introduction and overview. J Int Neuropsychol Soc 1997;3(6): 555–67.
84. Ewing-Cobbs L, Barnes M, Fletcher JM, et al. Modeling of longitudinal academic achievement scores after pediatric traumatic brain injury. Dev Neuropsychol 2004;25(1–2):107–33.
85. Ewing-Cobbs L, Prasad MR, Kramer L, et al. Late intellectual and academic outcomes following traumatic brain injury sustained during early childhood. J Neurosurg 2006;105(4 Suppl):287–96.

86. Gronwall D, Wrightson P, McGinn V. Effect of mild head injury during the preschool years. J Int Neuropsychol Soc 1997;3(6):592–7.
87. Giza CC, Kolb B, Harris NG, et al. Hitting a moving target: Basic mechanisms of recovery from acquired developmental brain injury. Dev Neurorehabil 2009;12(5): 255–68.
88. Russo S. Sport-related concussion in the young athlete. Curr Opin Pediatr 2006; 18:376–82.
89. Bruce DA, Schut L, Sutton LN. Brain and cervical spine injuries occurring during organized sports activities in children and adolescents. Clin Sports Med 1982; 1(3):495–514.
90. Theye F, Mueller KA. "Heads up": concussions in high school sports. Clin Med Res 2004;2(3):165–71.
91. Collins M. New developments in the management of sports concussion. Curr Opin Orthop 2004;15:100–7.
92. Committee on Sports Medicine and Fitness. American academy of pediatrics: medical conditions affecting sports participation. Pediatrics 2001;107(5):1205–9.

Helmets and Mouth Guards: The Role of Personal Equipment in Preventing Sport-Related Concussions

Daniel H. Daneshvar, MA[a],*, Christine M. Baugh, AB[a],
Christopher J. Nowinski, AB[a,b], Ann C. McKee, MD[a],
Robert A. Stern, PhD[a], Robert C. Cantu, MD[a,b,c,d,e]

KEYWORDS

- Concussion • Equipment • Helmet • Headgear
- Mouth guard • Face shield • Sport

Because the brain is freely floating within the cerebrospinal fluid, it moves at a rate that is different from that of the skull in response to a collision.[1] This discrepancy can result in a collision between the brain and skull, either on the side of the impact, coup, or opposite the impact, contrecoup.[2] The high-speed deceleration associated with these impacts may also result in stretching of the long axons at the base of the brain, resulting in diffuse axonal injury.[3] Depending on the extent of these injuries, neurologic dysfunction may be observed.[4]

Every year, approximately 1.7 million people in the United States are hospitalized or die as a result of a traumatic brain injury (TBI).[5] These figures, however, are thought to

This work was supported by the Boston University Alzheimer's Disease Center NIA P30 AG13846, supplement 0572063345-5, the National Operating Committee on Standards for Athletic Equipment, the National Collegiate Athletic Association, the National Federation of State High School Associations, the American Football Coaches Association, and the Sports Legacy Institute.
The authors have nothing to disclose.
[a] Center for the Study of Traumatic Encephalopathy, Department of Neurology, Boston University School of Medicine, 72 East Concord Street, B7800, Boston, MA 02118, USA
[b] Sports Legacy Institute, PO Box 181225, Boston, MA 02118, USA
[c] Department of Neurosurgery, Boston University School of Medicine, 720 Harrison Avenue # 710, Boston, MA 02118, USA
[d] Department of Surgery, Emerson Hospital, John Cuming Building, Suite 820, 131 ORNAC, Concord, MA 01742, USA
[e] Neurologic Sports Injury Center, Department of Neurosurgery, Brigham and Women's Hospital, Boston, MA, USA
* Corresponding author.
E-mail address: ddanesh@bu.edu

Clin Sports Med 30 (2011) 145–163
doi:10.1016/j.csm.2010.09.006
0278-5919/11/$ – see front matter © 2011 Elsevier Inc. All rights reserved.

drastically underrepresent the total incidence of TBI, as many individuals with mild or moderate TBI do not seek medical care.[5,6] A portion of these brain injuries are considered concussions, meaning that a direct or indirect blow to the head, face, neck, or body results in an alteration of mental status or produces 1 or more of 25 recognized postconcussion symptoms.[7] It has been estimated that 1.6 million to 3.8 million of these concussions occur annually as a direct result of participation in athletics.[5,6,8] The changes in neurologic function associated with concussion often present rapidly and resolve spontaneously.[9] As such, many concussions are unreported and unrecognized by coaches, trainers, or the athletes themselves.[10–13] A further confounding factor resulting in underreporting the total incidence of concussions is the desire of the athlete to return to play.[14]

Most symptoms associated with concussions are transient; however, there are several ways in which concussions can have lasting symptoms. For example, in some cases of concussion, memory impairment has been shown to last for months.[4] Furthermore, postconcussion syndrome (PCS) may occur, especially in situations in which an athlete is not properly treated after a concussion. PCS presents with physical, cognitive, emotional, and behavioral symptoms that can take months or even years to resolve.[15,16] If an athlete returns to play before symptoms resolve, the athlete risks a rare but sometimes fatal event known as second impact syndrome.[17,18] In addition, repetitive concussive and subconcussive blows can cause chronic traumatic encephalopathy or chronic traumatic encephalomyelopathy.[19,20]

The importance of understanding and preventing these impacts is increasing because athletes have been getting bigger, faster, and stronger, leading to more forceful collisions, which are more likely to cause concussions.[21,22] The mechanisms underlying these concussions, as well as methods of prevention, have been investigated both in the laboratory and in the field. The simplest of these preventative measures seem to be rule changes, rule enforcement, and player and coach education.[10] In addition to these suggestions, equipment changes have been proposed in an attempt to help prevent concussions, including modifications of helmets and mouth guards. This equipment has been critical for injury prevention; helmets have been shown to protect against skull fracture, severe TBI, and death, whereas mouth guards protect against oral and dental injury.[23–25] However, the specific effects of helmets and mouth guards on concussion incidence and severity are less clear.

HELMETS AND HEADGEAR

Protective headgear and helmets decrease the potential for severe TBI after a collision by reducing the acceleration of the head on impact, thereby decreasing the brain-skull collision and the sudden deceleration-induced axonal injury.[26] The energy-absorbing material within a helmet accomplishes this by compressing to absorb force during the collision and slowly restoring to its original shape. This compression and restoration prolongs the duration of the collision and reduces the total momentum transferred to the head.[27] There is variation in helmet design based on the demands and constraints of each sport. Although helmets and headgear in most sports are good at mediating the high-impact collisions responsible for severe TBI, the question remains as to what extent the helmets and headgear of each sport are able to respond to the lower-impact collisions responsible for concussion.

American Football

Early helmets

There has been a great deal of focus on the protection afforded by helmets in football. The primary intent of early football helmets, first reported in use during an Army-Navy game in 1893 and constantly evolving throughout the 1900s, was to prevent cata-strophic head injury and the resultant morbidity and mortality.[28] These early helmets, then nothing more than leather padding, were slowly phased out as metal and plastics were added to provide additional protection. However, even these basic helmets were not required for college play until 1939 and were not mandated until 1940 for athletes in the National Football League (NFL).[28] Despite these innovations throughout the early twentieth century, the incidence of head injuries continued to increase, prompting the formation of the National Operating Committee on Standards for Athletic Equipment (NOCSAE) in 1969 to initiate research efforts for head protection and to implement the first football helmet safety standards in 1973.[29]

These initial NOCSAE guidelines, the framework of which are still in existence, were meant to develop a standard method for measuring a particular helmet's ability to endure the annual repetitive impacts associated with football in conditions as varied as freezing cold, driving rain, heavy snow, or high heat and humidity.[28,30] However, because football collisions at that time were responsible for cerebral hematoma, cervical fractures, and death, the primary concern was the helmet's response to the most acutely severe, linear, acceleration-inducing impacts, rather than its response to the wide range and types of force that could result in concussion.[31–33] Although this focus, along with rule changes, ultimately proved successful in decreasing the risk of head injury, the hard-shelled helmet that resulted may not be best suited for protecting against the lower forces that also include a component of rotational accel-eration, which are thought to cause most concussions.[23,27,34,35] Furthermore, there is evidence that newly proposed helmet-testing methods, meant to encourage the development of helmets better suited to protecting against concussions, may be less accurate than the current testing methods at simulating in vivo concussive impacts.[36]

Mechanism of concussion

Many studies have attempted to measure the forces associated with different types of head impacts. Whereas most early attempts relied on sensors housed within the helmet itself, modern studies have used sensors in contact with the athlete's head.[37,38] This use of sensors has proved more accurate, as helmet acceleration does not always accurately reflect the acceleration of the head itself.[39] These studies have helped develop a better understanding of the types of impacts associated with concussion.

One modern study, examining 19,224 high school football impacts during 55 prac-tices and 13 games, found that impacts to the top of the head were associated with the highest force and the shortest duration of impact, resulting in the largest head jerk.[40] Although these impacts to the top of the head are more associated with severe injuries to the cervical spinal cord, rotational acceleration is more closely linked to concussion.[41,42] Impacts to the front of the head resulted in the highest rotational acceleration and were the most frequent among the high schoolers.[40] A similar study of 72 collegiate football players found that these impacts to the top of the head were 10% less frequent and associated with 1g to 2g lower accelerations than lateral hits, perhaps reflecting improved tackling form or increased neck strength.[43] These find-ings, of fewer hits to the top of the head in collegiate athletes than in high school athletes, have been validated elsewhere and reported in studies of professional athletes as well.[27,44] Biomechanical reconstruction of recorded concussive impacts in NFL athletes underscore the large role that rotational acceleration plays in concus-sion, as well as the importance of neck strength in mitigating this rotation.[45] This method of experimentally replicating recorded collisions may provide additional information about the relationship between linear and angular head acceleration and injury outcome, resulting in better helmet designs.[26,45] However, more work is needed to ensure that these models properly replicate factors potentially influencing concussion, such as bracing, neck strength, and body tension.[46]

Helmet designs

Football helmets have evolved from little more than modest leather headgear to the modern designs incorporating metals, plastics, and rubber. Analyses revealed that helmets with pneumatic padding within suspension liners were most effective at absorbing the high-intensity impacts that were of early concern.[32,33] Modern football helmets incorporate similar features, with hard plastic exteriors housing materials of various stiffness to absorb the force of collision and an inflating system meant to ensure proper fit.[28] Football helmets incorporate these basic design elements in various ways, in an attempt to afford better protection to the wearer.

There are several basic designs commonly used in the NFL. One helmet design relies on a continuous tubelike inflatable air-fit system nested into a molded foam network consisting of 2 different types of foam with different absorptive properties, ethyl vinyl acetate and polyvinyl chloride nitrile rubber (vinyl nitrile). Front and back pads consist of similar inflatable systems. A second design uses die cut, rather than molded, foams placed into a case. This creates a laminar system of foam, into which air can be introduced to ensure proper fit. An interchangeable molded urethane front pad completes the system. A third design uses a different approach: although the air liner is similar to that in the second system, it is not incorporated into the foam components. Instead, a foam, molded ethyl vinyl acetate component with vinyl nitrile inserts, similar to helmet 1, separates the air-liner fit system from an inner shell of expanded polypropylene. In addition, the plastic outer shell is ventilated and lighter than in the previous 2 designs. A noninterchangeable vinyl nitrile front pad completes the padding.[28]

Helmet manufacturers have begun to design helmets specifically intended to protect against concussion. A description of several of these helmets is in **Table 1**. One such helmet incorporates distinct design features meant to improve energy attenuation in response to lateral blows. These features include an exterior shell extending anterior to and distal to traditional shell shapes along the wearer's mandible, increased offset from the interior surface of the shell to the wearer's head in this area, and a unique interior liner construction.[47] A newer helmet design creates air turbulence within specialized shock absorbers to allow for differential response to a wider range of impact levels.[48] However, the effect of these and other changes must be further studied, both in the laboratory and on the field.

Evaluating helmets

There have been few studies evaluating the effectiveness of different helmet designs in reducing concussions. These studies have tended to be nonrandomized, retrospective analyses and have suffered from the same general pitfalls including selection bias and overreliance on subject recollection. In addition, because the guidelines for concussion assessment were not easily available until recently, many studies relying on coaches and athletic trainers to diagnose concussions may have drastically underreported the total number of concussions because only the most severe injuries would have been counted.[49,50] Even after educational outreach efforts by the Centers for Disease Control and Prevention, the Sports Legacy Institute, and others, knowledge about current concussion guidelines remains an issue.[51,52] By reporting only on the relationship between helmets and the most severe concussive injuries, these types

Table 1
Overview of material and construction of newer football helmets as compared with an older helmet design

	Riddell			Schutt		Adams	Xenith
	Original VSR-4	New VSR-4	Revolution	Air Varsity Commander	DNA	Pro Elite	X1
Forehead Pad Crown Pad	Molded urethane VN + CF	Molded urethane VN	Molded urethane VN + CF	Dual density VN Comolded EVA and PE	Skydex + CF Skydex + CF	VN VN/EPP + EVA CF	All pads use unique Aware Flow shock absorbers in a shock bonnet
Back and Sides	VN + CF	VN	VN + CF	Comolded EVA and PE	Skydex + CF	VN/EPP + EVA CF	
Jaw Pads	Interchangeable thickness CF	Interchangeable thickness CF	VN + CF	VN + CF	VN + CF	Interchangeable thickness CF	Interchangeable thickness CF
Fit Adjustment	Crown, back, and sides padding encased in inflatable vinyl bladders	Crown, back, and sides padding encased in inflatable vinyl bladders	Crown, back, and sides padding encased in inflatable vinyl bladders	Halo-style tubular air bladder	Vinyl air bladder around CF	Vinyl air bladder covering crown, back, and sides	Fit seeker cable tightens the shock bonnet after chin straps are pulled tight. No pumps.

Abbreviations: CF, comfort foam; EPP, expanded polypropylene; EVA, ethylene vinyl acetate; PE, polyethylene; VN, vinyl nitrile.
Adapted from Viano DC, Pellman EJ, Withnall C, et al. Concussion in professional football: performance of newer helmets in reconstructed game impacts—Part 13. Neurosurgery 2006;59(3):595; with permission.

of studies risk ignoring the vast majority of concussions, which are in the mild to moderate range.[38] Studies relying on hospitalization data would have a similar bias.

Data collected by the National Athletic Injury/Illness Reporting System from a sample of high school and collegiate athletes during the 1975 to 1977 seasons showed no difference in concussion rate among 13 helmet designs. However, this study was hampered by poor concussion reporting, as a rate of only 1 concussion per 10,000 athlete exposures was reported, less than one-fourth the most conservative current rates.[53,54]

Data on helmet models used and occurrence of cerebral concussions during 5 seasons were collected from a representative sample of college football teams, consisting of a total of 8312 player-seasons and 618,596 athlete-exposures. Of the 10 models of football helmets included in the analyses, the Riddell M155 had a significantly lower-than-expected frequency of concussions, whereas the Bike Air Power had a significantly higher frequency of concussions.[55] However, the number of concussions was again less than half of current conservative estimates of concussion rates.[54] In addition, more than half of the athletic exposures in the 2 statistically significant helmet models were from schools with more than 97% of the same helmet type, exposing the study to a potential bias. Because the study relied on athletic trainer report and all but a few athletes at most schools had the same helmet type, differences in athletic trainer reporting could have had significant effects on the observed concussion rates for many of the athletes studied. To directly compare helmets, each school, and thus each athletic trainer, would have needed to have a mix of all 10 of the helmet types studied. The reported relationship is further obscured by there being a near-linear relationship between the number of athletic exposures and the rate of concussions reported; the helmets with the most exposures tended to have the highest rate of concussion exposure. This finding could be in part because of the fact that larger programs, with more athletes in total and more of the most popular helmet types, may have had staff better trained to recognize concussions.

Another study evaluated the effect of polyurethane helmet covers. During 3 seasons from 1992 to 1994, a total of 155 athletes identified as having purchased a polyurethane helmet cover in the previous year were surveyed relating to their concussion history in the seasons before and after using the device. Athletes who reported more concussions in the 4 years before adopting the cover also reported a higher rate of concussion reoccurrence while using the device.[56] These results reflect the findings of other studies, which report that players with a history of concussion are significantly more likely to suffer a new concussion than those with no previous history.[34,55] Therefore, the use of a polyurethane football helmet cover does not seem to provide additional protection against incurring concussions in the future. In a more recent study, one cohort of 1173 high school athletes given Riddell Revolution helmets were compared with 968 using standard helmets. All athletes were given a baseline immediate postconcussion assessment and cognitive testing (ImPACT) examination. During the next 3 years, whenever athletes experienced a potential concussive blow, they was assessed for concussive signs using the ImPACT test. During the course of the study, the concussion rate in athletes wearing the Revolution helmet was 5.3% compared with a concussion rate of 7.6% in athletes wearing the standard helmet [χ^2 (1, 2, 141) = 4.96, $P<.027$]. Athletes wearing the Revolution helmet seemed to have a 31% decreased relative risk for sustaining a diagnosed concussion compared with those who were not.[47] However, limitations in the study design diminish the strength of the findings. The players in the Revolution helmets had new helmets, whereas the standard helmets were of varying age, and helmets tend to become less effective over time. Because athletic trainers are often unaware of all but the most severe concussions, the results may have been influenced more by reporting rates of the high school staff than absolute differences in the risk of concussion. Furthermore, concussions were diagnosed by ImPACT instead of a combination of neurologic examination that includes balance testing. Finally, the study was funded by Riddell, and a Riddell employee was a lead author, which pose an obvious conflict of interest. Although there was a difference in the rate of concussion between the 2 groups, concussed athletes in the 2 groups did not differ significantly in the average number of days to recover and return to play after their concussions.

Baseball

Several new concussion-proof helmet designs have been proposed and are now being introduced into Major and Minor League Baseball, but their degree of effectiveness in preventing concussion has not yet been demonstrated in any epidemiologic study. However, the role of standard baseball helmets in preventing more serious head injuries has been well validated.[57]

Cycling

Helmets have long been shown to decrease the rates of head injury in cyclists.[58–61] However, there have been no studies evaluating the different bicycle helmet designs in response to concussive impacts.

Ice Hockey

Ice hockey, like football, is a helmeted sport associated with a significant risk of concussion. For aforementioned reasons, including an increased awareness of diagnostic criteria, the rate of diagnosed concussions has been increasing; nonetheless, helmets are largely responsible for protecting hockey players from the most catastrophic head injuries.[10,11,54] The introduction of ice hockey helmet standards and the proper use of helmets have resulted in a decrease in fatal and catastrophic head injuries but with an increase in the concussion rate.[62] Although this increase in rate is likely due in large part to better concussion awareness and recognition, aggressive play may also be responsible for this increase in rate.[63]

Concussions in hockey most commonly occur as a result of collision with an opponent or with the boards.[64] Measurements from sensors within the helmets of hockey players have found that the impacts sustained by hockey players are comparable in magnitude to those experienced by football linemen but occur at approximately one-third of the frequency.[38] Since helmets have been made mandatory in hockey, there has been little literature published comparing the protective effects of different hockey helmets. However, there is evidence that player flexion and anticipation before a collision decreases the risk of concussion, providing a potential avenue for future helmet design.[46] Newer helmet-testing methods have begun to take into account the rotational acceleration component involved in a collision, which better simulates concussive impacts.[35]

Lacrosse

In a recent study of athletic trainers, concussion was found to be the most common injury in lacrosse and was responsible for a high percentage of all injuries among boys (73%) and men (85%) than among girls (40%) and women (41%). In men, the primary injury mechanism was player-to-player contact, whereas in women, injuries primarily resulted from stick or ball contact.[65]

Although the rate of concussions has increased dramatically in many sports, some have argued that this observation in men's lacrosse may be, in part, explained by the introduction of a new helmet. One study compared the rate of concussion in the years immediately after the helmet's introduction (1996–1997 to 2003–2004) with that of the preceding years (1988–1989 to 1995–1996). In practices, the rate of concussion increased by 0.14 concussions per 1000 athletic-exposures (95% confidence interval [CI], 0.09, 0.19; P<.01). In games, the rate increased by 0.84 (95% CI, 0.52, 1.16; P<.01).[66] However, this increase is certainly due, in part, to improved detection and diagnosis of concussion during that time frame.

Rugby

Headgear in rugby consists of relatively sparse padding, and its use is not mandated. Therefore, the role of headgear in preventing concussion and head injuries can be more easily studied. In one prospective study of 294 players younger than 15 years, headgear was distributed to players. Over the course of the study, there were 1179 player-exposures with headgear and 357 without headgear. During this period, there were only 9 reported concussions, 7 of which occurred to players wearing headgear, 2 to those not wearing headgear. As a result, there was no evidence indicating a protective effect of headgear; in fact, these data showed that headgears have a nonsignificant deleterious effect.[67] However, as only concussions that were medically verified were reported, many minor concussions may have been unreported. Headgear use was not randomized, as athletes had the choice of whether or not to wear headgear. This choice produces a potential bias, as athletes more concerned about head injury are more likely to wear headgear; certainly a subset of these athletes had had prior concussions and was therefore more susceptible to having additional concussions. In another study of 304 rugby players, followed weekly, headgear was shown to have a nonsignificant protective effect on concussions but a significant protective effect on orofacial and scalp injuries.[68] However, only 22 concussions were recorded, and the study was not adequately powered to determine a suitable effect size. A survey-based study of 131 men's club rugby union participants from 8 university teams in the United States reported 76 total concussed athletes. Although 51% of the surveyed athletes were not wearing headgear, 76% of the concussed athletes reported not wearing headgear. The remaining who were concussed while wearing headgear reported that their concussions were less severe than those of the athletes not wearing headgear.[69]

However, in the most thorough study, 1493 participants from 4 rugby leagues (under 13, under 15, under 18, and under 20) were randomly assigned 1 of 2 types of headgear or no headgear and followed for 2 years. Although compliance to the random assignment was low, nearly half of all athletic exposures consisted of athletes wearing 1 of the 2 headgear types. Regardless, the use of these padded headgears did not affect the rate of concussion or the number of days missed because of concussion.[70]

These findings, which indicate that rugby headgear does not seem to have a protective effect in concussion prevention, correspond to laboratory findings indicating that headgear are maximally compressed at impacts far less intense than those likely to cause a concussion.[71] Because they are unable to absorb additional force well below the threshold at which concussions occur, they would not be expected to have a major effect on the incidence of concussion. However, this ceiling effect may be avoided in future headgear by methods such as modifying padding materials and increasing padding thickness.[72]

Besides the apparent lack of scientific justification supporting the use of rugby headgear for concussion prevention, additional barriers remain to widespread headgear adoption. Although athletes tend to report that headgear is beneficial, athletes in one survey commonly reported that the headgear caused discomfort and poor ventilation and was often grabbed by opponents during play.[69,73]

Soccer

Several studies have sought to measure the nature of impacts experienced by soccer players. Although soccer players experienced significantly fewer impacts per hour than high school football lineman or hockey players, each impact tended to be associated with higher accelerations; whereas 20% of impacts in soccer were more than 75g, approximately 5% of impacts were more than 75g in football lineman and hockey players.[38] However, the head-ball collisions that were studied are not the most common source of concussions in soccer. Most concussions in soccer occur during the act of heading as a result of head-head or head-arm collisions.[74] Another study following athletes for 3 years found that the most common site of impact in a concussion-causing collision was the temporal area of the head.[44] This finding supports those of other sports and underscores the importance of rotational acceleration in concussion.

There are various types of headgear proposed to limit the effect of concussion in soccer athletes. Although there have been nonrandomized studies of the effect of headgear on head injuries in soccer, there have been few analytic studies looking specifically at the role of headgear on concussion rate or severity,[44,75] which is a potential area of interest.

One retrospective anonymous online survey of youth soccer players, aged 12 to 17 years, studied the role of headgear on concussion symptoms. Of those eligible for the study, 216 athletes were included in the non–headgear-wearing group and 52 were included in the headgear-wearing group. This study was strengthened by the fact that it asked respondents not only how many concussions they had experienced in the prior season but also how many times they had experienced specific symptoms associated with concussions in response to a collision. About 7.2% of the athletes reported having experienced at least 1 concussion, whereas 47.8% reported having experienced concussive symptoms at least once. Athletes wearing headgear were significantly less likely to receive laceration to those areas of the scalp and face covered by the headgear. Although the group that chose to wear headgear reported having experienced more concussions before the study (42.3% had experienced at least 1 prior concussion and 26.9% had experienced more than 1, compared with 11.1% and 4.6%, respectively) and would therefore be expected to be more knowledgeable and at increased risk of having an additional concussion, it was found that not wearing headgear was associated with a 2.65 relative risk of concussion ($P<.0001$).[75] This finding might be explained in part by the fact that fewer athletes who wore headgear considered themselves to be a header (44.2% of those who wore headgear as compared with 51.4% of those who did not). Although this study is promising, it was not ideal because headgear use was nonrandomized and the retrospective study relied principally on information recollected by athletes at the end of the season. Although the anonymous nature of the survey did not allow follow-up questions of participants or verification of data, this is nonetheless a likely strength because many studies have found more accurate concussion data when athletes anonymously report their history. However, if all soccer players were to wear headgear, the effect on concussions may be complicated by risk compensation. Rule changes in football, hockey, and lacrosse have suggested that mandating headgear removes inhibitions to strike or risk strikes to the head because it reduces pain from scalp injuries and lacerations. If all players were to become accustomed to a playing style in which contact to the head was no longer off limits, the addition of headgear might result in an increase in the frequency of total collisions to the head and potentially increase the total number of concussions as well.

There is some evidence that the same headgear may not be appropriate for all athletes. One study evaluating heading kinematics found that women experienced higher acceleration than men when heading a ball.[76] Although most concussions do not occur as a result of head-ball interactions, these findings nonetheless indicate that gender differences may need to be accounted for in future headgear designs. Additional laboratory testing found that although headgear is unlikely to be effective in attenuating impact during head-ball collisions, it may decrease the impact of head-head collisions by nearly 33%.[77]

However, because there is a specific mechanism of injury associated with concussion, the simplest preventative strategy may not be newer equipment. As concussions typically occurred in both men and women as a result of contact while heading the ball, limiting this type of contact through rule changes may be appropriate.[4]

Skiing/Snowboarding

Observational studies have found that 12.1% of US skiers wear helmets.[78] However, from 1982 through 1998 at the Saint Anthony Central Hospital (Denver, CO, USA) level I trauma center only 3 of the total 1214 patients admitted for all ski-related head injuries were wearing a helmet.[79] Several studies argue that helmets may reduce risk of concussion by up to 60%.[80–83]

MOUTH GUARDS

During the 1960s and 1970s, the use of mouth guards was made mandatory in many sports, including football, ice hockey, lacrosse, field hockey, and boxing. The rationale for these rule changes was to provide additional protection against dental and orofacial injuries and to reduce a player's risk of concussion.[25,84] However, at that time, as well as now, there is little evidence that mouth guards provide protection against concussion.

American Football

There is interest in the possibility that better-designed mouth guards might help dissipate force, thereby reducing the magnitude of the impact. Because mouth guards are already mandatory equipment in football, there is an opportunity to evaluate the role of specific types of mouth guards in preventing concussion. There is some scientific rationale that custom-fit mouth guards might be more effective at measurably absorbing the force of impact.[85] A study of 28 high school and college football players suggested a decrease in the rate of concussion after the use of customized mandibular orthotics; however, this study was marked by several design flaws. Concussion rate before customized mandibular orthotics was measured by self-report, whereas concussion rate following orthotic use was calculated only based on concussions diagnosed by athletic trainers and coaches. Also, because all athletes were given orthotics, the observed decrease in the concussion rate could simply be an artifact of different styles or age of play; all athletes were necessarily older when using the custom orthotics than they were when using standard mouth guards. Finally, calculation of the rate of concussion before the use of custom orthotics was not limited to games, whereas only concussions occurring during games were counted after the use of custom orthotics.[86] No large study has been able to demonstrate a significant difference in the concussion rate depending on the type of mouth guard used. One study recruited 87 of a total of 114 Division 1 teams to participate in a study evaluating the effect of various mouth guard types on the rate of concussion. There was no statistically significant result between the different mouth guards.[87] These findings have since been replicated by other large, multicenter cohort studies.[88]

Basketball

Many are interested in the potential role of mouth guards in reducing the number of concussions in basketball. However, recent studies have found no significant differences in concussion rates between mouth guard users and nonusers.[89]

Ice Hockey

There has been some interest in the degree to which helmets, mouth guards, and visors affect concussions in athletes. There are several different hockey helmet designs that have been shown to decrease total impact experimentally; however, there have been no studies to determine their utility in reducing concussions.

Mouth guards are not mandatory in the National Hockey League (NHL) because there is a debate over the extent to which they reduce concussion incidence and severity. In a study of 1033 NHL athletes, the rate of concussion was 1.42 times greater in individuals who did not wear mouth guards compared with those who did. However, this difference was not statistically significant (95% CI, 0.90–2.25). Despite the nonsignificant finding regarding concussion rate, symptom severity was significantly decreased by the use of mouth guards. Symptom severity, measured using the modified McGill abbreviated concussion evaluation post-concussion symptom scale, was found to be significantly worse in athletes who were not wearing mouth guards than in those who were ($P<.01$).[90,91]

Rugby

In rugby, there is evidence that mouth guards protect against orofacial injuries, but a study of 304 rugby players followed weekly showed no significant effect of mouth guards on the incidence of concussions, although only 22 total concussions were observed.[68]

Soccer

One anonymous survey of 278 youth soccer players aged 12 to 17 years found no significant relationship between mouth guard use and the rate of concussion.[75]

OTHER EQUIPMENT
Facial Protection

During the 1970s, full facial protection was mandated by all organized youth ice hockey associations worldwide. However, several studies have shown no significant relationship between the use of visors and the concussion rate in high school, college, or NHL athletes.[91–94]

In junior A ice hockey, full faceguards were found to provide a 4.7 times reduction in eye injuries and a nonsignificant reduction in the rate of concussion from 12.2 to 2.9 concussions per 1000 player-hours compared with no faceguard.[94] However, this study was hampered by restricted data collection for playing time and injuries, which were only recorded during home games. Therefore, injuries from away games were not included in the analysis. Also, players younger than 18 years had to wear mandatory full facial protection, whereas players older than 18 years could choose to wear a full shield, half shield, or no shield.[95] Playing style might have influenced this decision, as players with riskier playing styles may have chosen to play without visors.

In university level ice hockey, the use of full faceguards was found to reduce the number of games missed because of concussion, but not the incidence of concussion, compared with the use of half faceguard.[93] Although the use of full face shields significantly reduced players' risk of sustaining a dental injury, there was no difference in the incidence of concussions between players wearing different shield types. However, players who sustained concussions while wearing half shields required significantly more time before returning to competition than players who sustained concussions wearing full face shields.[96] One potential explanation for this finding is helmet placement. Players wearing half shields may have been tilting their helmets back to allow for an unobstructed view below the visor, thereby getting a clearer view but resulting in improper helmet placement. Alternatively, the minor visual impairment from the half shield could have led to an increased number of hits that were not foreseen by the athlete and therefore may have led to a greater number of concussions. Improper helmet alignment would causes less padding on the forehead and a loose chin strap decreasing the protective effect of the helmet. Neither of the aforementioned studies compared the incidence of concussion in athletes with visors to those without. In professional hockey, the use of a visor did not significantly reduce the prevalence of concussions. Visor use did, however, lower the prevalence of eye and nonconcussion head injuries.[92]

There is some additional interest in the potential of facial protection to mitigate concussion in other sports. In biomechanical reconstructions of professional football concussive injuries, impacts to the facemask resulted in high rotational accelerations, likely because facemasks sit outside the helmet shell and thus have an increased radius of rotation from the base of the head.[45] This may help influence future helmet designs.

In baseball, some have proposed that faceguards may reduce the risk of concussion, although this has not yet been studied. In youth baseball, facemasks have been shown to reduce the incidence of oculofacial injury in a nonrandomized prospective cohort study.[97] Overall, faceguards are also associated with a reduced risk of facial injury.[98]

Baseball Balls

In baseball, softer balls have been shown to reduce the risk of head injury compared with standard balls, but this equipment has yet to be studied in light of concussions. Theoretical biomechanical studies have indicated that baseballs with a lower mass and less stiffness have a reduced potential for injury.[99] Laboratory studies have shown that reduced-impact balls are less likely to result in head injury and skull fracture.[100] In practice, softer baseballs have been found to yield a 28% reduction in the risk of injury.[24,98,101]

Playing Surfaces

As the speed of athletes increases, the momentum transfer and impact associated with their collisions increase. The surface on which athletes play affects the player's speed and may influence the rate of concussions. In general, synthetic surfaces are harder and result in faster speeds than natural ones.[34] Some studies have found that athletes playing on synthetic fields have a higher risk of injury.[102] Laboratory studies have found that different fields have different impact attenuation properties, which would certainly be expected to at least influence head-ground collisions.[103]

DISCUSSION

Several studies have provided biomechanical evidence that the use of specific headgear or helmets reduces the impact forces to the brain. However, in most sports, these results have not translated into observed differences in rate or severity of concussion.

For some sports in which contact with hard surfaces is possible, such as skiing, snow-boarding, and cycling, there is evidence that helmets greatly reduce the incidence of head injuries in general; therefore, helmets are an important part of injury prevention and should be recommended in these sports.[61,104–106]

Risk compensation is a complicating factor associated with helmet and headgear use. In many cases, protective equipment can lead to a false sense of security, result-ing in a more dangerous style of play.[107] Often, the helmet itself may be used to initiate contact. This tendency to promote a more reckless style of play may help explain the higher rate of injury in children and adolescents as compared with adults.[108]

In general, helmets work best when properly used. This means that the helmets must be sized appropriately and worn with all straps correctly fastened and all padding in the proper positioning. Problems arise when helmets are older, incorrectly sized, worn improperly, or when padding is underinflated. Inclement weather also has been shown to affect a helmet's ability to absorb impacts.[28] Neck strength may be important in minimizing the risk of concussion in response to an impact. Therefore, rule changes mandating neck strength training, education about proper tackling form including prohibiting spearing, and monitoring player fatigue is warranted.[45] Encouraging practices with limited contact may also be an appropriate way to limit concussive blows in football; however, some studies indicate that helmet-only prac-tices are associated with similar impacts as those experienced in full-contact play.[43]

Although mouth guards have been shown to be effective in preventing dental and orofacial injury, there is currently no evidence that standard or fitted mouth guards decrease the rate or severity of concussions in athletes.[85] The bulk of the evidence indicating a potential protective effect of mouth guards on concussion incidence has been based on a limited case series studies and retrospective, nonrandomized, cross-sectional surveys.[91] There is also evidence that mouth guard use does not result in any difference in neurocognitive test performance after concussion.[109] In sports such as hockey, there is no evidence that visors play a protective role in preventing or mitigating concussions.[91–94]

Many of the studies on the protective effect of equipment on concussive risk have been complicated by retrospective, nonrandomized study designs. Individuals may choose to wear specialized protective equipment based on previous injury history, which has been shown to increase risk of future injuries, or because of a risky playing style. The preponderance of evidence seems to indicate that helmets and mouth guards provide a significant benefit in protecting against many catastrophic head, neck, and orofacial injuries. However, there is not yet significant evidence to advocate their effectiveness in preventing concussion. Nonetheless, additional research is needed both in the laboratory to improve equipment design and on the field to verify findings epidemiologically. Although newer equipment remains a promising potential tool in minimizing concussion severity and incidence, other methods such as rule changes, improved concussion education, and proper coaching and training may prove more effective in the immediate future.

REFERENCES

1. Viano DC, Casson IR, Pellman EJ, et al. Concussion in professional football: brain responses by finite element analysis: part 9. Neurosurgery 2005;57(5): 891–916 [discussion: 891–916].
2. Drew LB, Drew WE. The contrecoup-coup phenomenon: a new understanding of the mechanism of closed head injury. Neurocrit Care 2004;1(3):385–90.

3. Meythaler JM, Peduzzi JD, Eleftheriou E, et al. Current concepts: diffuse axonal injury-associated traumatic brain injury. Arch Phys Med Rehabil 2001;82(10): 1461–71.
4. McCrory P, Meeuwisse W, Johnston K, et al. Consensus statement on concussion in sport–the 3rd international conference on concussion in sport, held in Zurich, November 2008. J Clin Neurosci 2009;16(6):755–63.
5. Faul M, Xu L, Wald MM, et al. Traumatic brain injury in the United States: emergency department visits, hospitalizations and deaths 2002–2006. Atlanta (GA): Centers for Disease Control and Prevention, National Center for Injury Prevention and Control; 2010.
6. Langlois JA, Rutland-Brown W, Wald MM. The epidemiology and impact of traumatic brain injury: a brief overview. J Head Trauma Rehabil 2006;21(5): 375–8.
7. Team Physician Consensus Statement. Concussion (mild traumatic brain injury) and the team physician: a consensus statement. Med Sci Sports Exerc 2006; 38(2):395–9.
8. Finkelstein E, Corso P, Miller T. The incidence and economic burden of injuries in the United States. New York: Oxford University Press; 2006.
9. Parker TM, Osternig LR, van Donkelaar P, et al. Recovery of cognitive and dynamic motor function following concussion. Br J Sports Med 2007;41(12): 868–73 [discussion: 873].
10. Cantu RC, Mueller FO. The prevention of catastrophic head and spine injuries in high school and college sports. Br J Sports Med 2009;43(13):981–6.
11. Mueller FO, Cantu RC. Catastrophic sport injury research 26th annual report: fall 1982–spring 2008. Chapel Hill (NC): National Center for Catastrophic Injury Research; 2008. Available at: http://www.unc.edu/depts/nccsi/AllSport.pdf. Accessed September 13, 2010.
12. Delaney JS, Lacroix VJ, Leclerc S, et al. Concussions among university football and soccer players. Clin J Sport Med 2002;12(6):331–8.
13. Field M, Collins MW, Lovell MR, et al. Does age play a role in recovery from sports-related concussion? A comparison of high school and collegiate athletes. J Pediatr 2003;142(5):546–53.
14. Yard EE, Comstock RD. Compliance with return to play guidelines following concussion in US high school athletes, 2005–2008. Brain Inj 2009;23(11): 888–98.
15. Barlow KM, Crawford S, Stevenson A, et al. Epidemiology of postconcussion syndrome in pediatric mild traumatic brain injury. Pediatrics 2010;126(2): e374–81.
16. Cantu RC, Register-Mihalik J, Guskiewicz KW. A retrospective analysis of 215 athletic moderate to severe concussions. J Phys Med Rehabil, in press.
17. Cantu R, Gean A. Second impact syndrome in a small SDH: an uncommon catastrophic result of repetitive head injury with a characteristic imaging appearance. J Neurotrauma 2010;27(9):50–7.
18. Cantu RC. Second-impact syndrome. Clin Sports Med 1998;17(1):37–44.
19. McKee AC, Gavett BE, Stern RA, et al. TDP-43 proteinopathy and motor neuron disease in chronic traumatic encephalopathy. J Neuropathol Exp Neurol 2010; 69(9):918–29.
20. McKee AC, Cantu RC, Nowinski CJ, et al. Chronic traumatic encephalopathy in athletes: progressive tauopathy after repetitive head injury. J Neuropathol Exp Neurol 2009;68(7):709–35.

21. Wennberg RA, Tator CH. National hockey league reported concussions, 1986–87 to 2001–02. Can J Neurol Sci 2003;30(3):206–9.
22. Barth JT, Freeman JR, Broshek DK, et al. Acceleration-deceleration sport-related concussion: the gravity of it all. J Athl Train 2001;36(3):253–6.
23. Cantu RC, Mueller FO. Brain injury-related fatalities in American football, 1945–1999. Neurosurgery 2003;52(4):846–52 [discussion: 852–3].
24. McIntosh AS, McCrory P. Preventing head and neck injury. Br J Sports Med 2005;39(6):314–8.
25. Using mouthguards to reduce the incidence and severity of sports-related oral injuries. J Am Dent Assoc 2006;137(12):1712–20 [quiz: 1731].
26. Newman JA, Beusenberg MC, Shewchenko N, et al. Verification of biomechanical methods employed in a comprehensive study of mild traumatic brain injury and the effectiveness of American football helmets. J Biomech 2005;38(7):1469–81.
27. Pellman EJ, Viano DC, Withnall C, et al. Concussion in professional football: helmet testing to assess impact performance–part 11. Neurosurgery 2006; 58(1):78–96 [discussion: 78–96].
28. Levy ML, Ozgur BM, Berry C, et al. Birth and evolution of the football helmet. Neurosurgery 2004;55(3):656–61 [discussion: 661–2].
29. Bennett T, editor. The NFL's official encyclopedic history of professional football. 2nd edition. New York: Macmillan; 1977. p. 1–391.
30. In: Stephens K, editor. Standard drop test method and equipment used in evaluating the performance characteristics of protective headgear. Overland Park (KS): National Operating Committee on Standards for Athletic Equipment (NOCSAE); 2004.
31. Robey JM, Blyth CS, Mueller FO. Athletic injuries. Application of epidemiologic methods. JAMA 1971;217(2):184–9.
32. Bishop PJ, Norman RW, Kozey JW. An evaluation of football helmets under impact conditions. Am J Sports Med 1984;12(3):233–6.
33. Myers TJ, Yoganandan N, Sances A Jr, et al. Energy absorption characteristics of football helmets under low and high rates of loading. Biomed Mater Eng 1993; 3(1):15–24.
34. Levy ML, Ozgur BM, Berry C, et al. Analysis and evolution of head injury in football. Neurosurgery 2004;55(3):649–55.
35. Kis M, Saunders F, ten Hove MW, et al. Rotational acceleration measurements–evaluating helmet protection. Can J Neurol Sci 2004;31(4):499–503.
36. Gwin JT, Chu JJ, Diamond SG, et al. An investigation of the NOCSAE linear impactor test method based on in vivo measures of head impact acceleration in American football. J Biomech Eng 2010;132(1):011006.
37. Reid SE, Tarkington JA, Epstein HM, et al. Brain tolerance to impact in football. Surg Gynecol Obstet 1971;133(6):929–36.
38. Naunheim RS, Standeven J, Richter C, et al. Comparison of impact data in hockey, football, and soccer. J Trauma 2000;48(5):938–41.
39. Manoogian S, McNeely D, Duma S, et al. Head acceleration is less than 10 percent of helmet acceleration in football impacts. Biomed Sci Instrum 2006; 42:383–8.
40. Broglio SP, Sosnoff JJ, Shin S, et al. Head impacts during high school football: a biomechanical assessment. J Athl Train 2009;44(4):342–9.
41. Rihn JA, Anderson DT, Lamb K, et al. Cervical spine injuries in American football. Sports Med 2009;39(9):697–708.
42. Broglio SP, Schnebel B, Sosnoff JJ, et al. The biomechanical properties of concussions in high school football. Med Sci Sports Exerc 2010;14(1):13–7.

43. Mihalik JP, Bell DR, Marshall SW, et al. Measurement of head impacts in collegiate football players: an investigation of positional and event-type differences. Neurosurgery 2007;61(6):1229–35 [discussion: 1235].

44. Scott Delaney J, Puni V, Rouah F. Mechanisms of injury for concussions in university football, ice hockey, and soccer: a pilot study. Clin J Sport Med 2006;16(2):162–5.

45. Viano DC, Casson IR, Pellman EJ. Concussion in professional football: biomechanics of the struck player–part 14. Neurosurgery 2007;61(2):313–27 [discussion: 327–8].

46. Mihalik JP, Blackburn JT, Greenwald RM, et al. Collision type and player anticipation affect head impact severity among youth ice hockey players. Pediatrics 2010;125(6):e1394–401.

47. Collins M, Lovell MR, Iverson GL, et al. Examining concussion rates and return to play in high school football players wearing newer helmet technology: a three-year prospective cohort study. Neurosurgery 2006;58(2):275–86 [discussion: 275–86].

48. Xenith. Xenith innovation. 2010. Available at: http://www.xenith.com/football/innovation/. Accessed September 23, 2010.

49. Covassin T, Elbin R 3rd, Stiller-Ostrowski JL. Current sport-related concussion teaching and clinical practices of sports medicine professionals. J Athl Train 2009;44(4):400–4.

50. Notebaert AJ, Guskiewicz KM. Current trends in athletic training practice for concussion assessment and management. J Athl Train 2005;40(4):320–5.

51. Sarmiento K, Mitchko J, Klein C, et al. Evaluation of the Centers for Disease Control and Prevention's concussion initiative for high school coaches: "Heads Up: Concussion in High School Sports". J Sch Health 2010;80(3):112–8.

52. Sawyer RJ, Hamdallah M, White D, et al. High school coaches' assessments, intentions to use, and use of a concussion prevention toolkit: centers for disease control and prevention's heads up: concussion in high school sports. Health Promot Pract 2010;11(1):34–43.

53. Clarke KS, Powell JW. Football helmets and neurotrauma–an epidemiological overview of three seasons. Med Sci Sports 1979;11(2):138–45.

54. Hootman JM, Dick R, Agel J. Epidemiology of collegiate injuries for 15 sports: summary and recommendations for injury prevention initiatives. J Athl Train 2007;42(2):311–9.

55. Zemper ED. Analysis of cerebral concussion frequency with the most commonly used models of football helmets. J Athl Train 1994;29(1):44–50.

56. Torg JS, Harris SM, Rogers K, et al. Retrospective report on the effectiveness of a polyurethane football helmet cover on the repeated occurrence of cerebral concussions. Am J Orthop (Belle Mead NJ) 1999;28(2):128–32.

57. Nicholls RL, Elliott BC, Miller K. Impact injuries in baseball: prevalence, aetiology and the role of equipment performance. Sports Med 2004;34(1):17–25.

58. Williams M. The protective performance of bicyclists' helmets in accidents. Accid Anal Prev 1991;23(2–3):119–31.

59. Thompson DC, Rivara FP, Thompson R. Helmets for preventing head and facial injuries in bicyclists. Cochrane Database Syst Rev 2000;2:CD001855.

60. Haileyesus T, Annest JL, Dellinger AM. Cyclists injured while sharing the road with motor vehicles. Inj Prev 2007;13(3):202–6.

61. Scheiman S, Moghaddas HS, Bjornstig U, et al. Bicycle injury events among older adults in Northern Sweden: a 10-year population based study. Accid Anal Prev 2010;42(2):758–63.

62. Biasca N, Wirth S, Tegner Y. The avoidability of head and neck injuries in ice hockey: an historical review. Br J Sports Med 2002;36(6):410–27.

63. Daly PJ, Sim FH, Simonet WT. Ice hockey injuries. A review. Sports Med 1990; 10(2):122–31.

64. Flik K, Lyman S, Marx RG. American collegiate men's ice hockey: an analysis of injuries. Am J Sports Med 2005;33(2):183–7.

65. Lincoln AE, Hinton RY, Almquist JL, et al. Head, face, and eye injuries in scholastic and collegiate lacrosse: a 4-year prospective study. Am J Sports Med 2007;35(2):207–15.

66. Dick R, Romani WA, Agel J, et al. Descriptive epidemiology of collegiate men's lacrosse injuries: national collegiate athletic association injury surveillance system, 1988–1989 through 2003–2004. J Athl Train 2007;42(2): 255–61.

67. McIntosh AS, McCrory P. Effectiveness of headgear in a pilot study of under 15 rugby union football. Br J Sports Med 2001;35(3):167–9.

68. Marshall SW, Loomis DP, Waller AE, et al. Evaluation of protective equipment for prevention of injuries in rugby union. Int J Epidemiol 2005;34(1):113–8.

69. Kahanov L, Dusa MJ, Wilkinson S, et al. Self-reported headgear use and concussions among collegiate men's rugby union players. Res Sports Med 2005;13(2):77–89.

70. McIntosh AS, McCrory P, Finch CF, et al. Does padded headgear prevent head injury in rugby union football? Med Sci Sports Exerc 2009;41(2):306–13.

71. McIntosh AS, McCrory P. Impact energy attenuation performance of football headgear. Br J Sports Med 2000;34(5):337–41.

72. McIntosh A, McCrory P, Finch CF. Performance enhanced headgear: a scientific approach to the development of protective headgear. Br J Sports Med 2004; 38(1):46–9.

73. Pettersen JA. Does rugby headgear prevent concussion? Attitudes of Canadian players and coaches. Br J Sports Med 2002;36(1):19–22.

74. Gessel LM, Fields SK, Collins CL, et al. Concussions among United States high school and collegiate athletes. J Athl Train 2007;42(4):495–503.

75. Delaney JS, Al-Kashmiri A, Drummond R, et al. The effect of protective headgear on head injuries and concussions in adolescent football (soccer) players. Br J Sports Med 2008;42(2):110–5 [discussion: 115].

76. Tierney RT, Higgins M, Caswell SV, et al. Sex differences in head acceleration during heading while wearing soccer headgear. J Athl Train 2008;43(6):578–84.

77. Withnall C, Shewchenko N, Gittens R, et al. Biomechanical investigation of head impacts in football. Br J Sports Med 2005;39(Suppl 1):i49–57.

78. Buller DB, Andersen PA, Walkosz BJ, et al. The prevalence and predictors of helmet use by skiers and snowboarders at ski areas in western North America in 2001. J Trauma 2003;55(5):939–45.

79. Levy AS, Hawkes AP, Hemminger LM, et al. An analysis of head injuries among skiers and snowboarders. J Trauma 2002;53(4):695–704.

80. Mueller BA, Cummings P, Rivara FP, et al. Injuries of the head, face, and neck in relation to ski helmet use. Epidemiology 2008;19(2):270–6.

81. Hagel BE, Pless IB, Goulet C, et al. Effectiveness of helmets in skiers and snowboarders: case-control and case crossover study. BMJ 2005;330(7486):281.

82. Cusimano MD, Kwok J. The effectiveness of helmet wear in skiers and snowboarders: a systematic review. Br J Sports Med 2010;44(11):781–6.

83. Sulheim S, Holme I, Ekeland A, et al. Helmet use and risk of head injuries in alpine skiers and snowboarders. JAMA 2006;295(8):919–24.

84. Heintz W. The case for mandatory mouth protectors. Phys Sportsmed 1975;3: 61–3.
85. Winters JE Sr. Commentary: role of properly fitted mouthguards in prevention of sport-related concussion. J Athl Train 2001;36(3):339–41.
86. Singh GD, Maher GJ, Padilla RR. Customized mandibular orthotics in the prevention of concussion/mild traumatic brain injury in football players: a preliminary study. Dent Traumatol 2009;25(5):515–21.
87. Wisniewski JF, Guskiewicz K, Trope M, et al. Incidence of cerebral concussions associated with type of mouthguard used in college football. Dent Traumatol 2004;20(3):143–9.
88. Barbic D, Pater J, Brison RJ. Comparison of mouth guard designs and concussion prevention in contact sports: a multicenter randomized controlled trial. Clin J Sport Med 2005;15(5):294–8.
89. Labella CR, Smith BW, Sigurdsson A. Effect of mouthguards on dental injuries and concussions in college basketball. Med Sci Sports Exerc 2002;34(1):41–4.
90. Benson BW, Meeuwisse WH. Ice hockey injuries. Med Sport Sci 2005;49: 86–119.
91. Benson BW, Hamilton GM, Meeuwisse WH, et al. Is protective equipment useful in preventing concussion? A systematic review of the literature. Br J Sports Med 2009;43(Suppl 1):i56–67.
92. Stevens ST, Lassonde M, de Beaumont L, et al. The effect of visors on head and facial injury in national hockey league players. J Sci Med Sport 2006;9(3): 238–42.
93. Benson BW, Rose MS, Meeuwisse WH. The impact of face shield use on concussions in ice hockey: a multivariate analysis. Br J Sports Med 2002; 36(1):27–32.
94. Stuart MJ, Smith AM, Malo-Ortiguera SA, et al. A comparison of facial protection and the incidence of head, neck, and facial injuries in Junior A hockey players. A function of individual playing time. Am J Sports Med 2002;30(1):39–44.
95. Asplund C, Bettcher S, Borchers J. Facial protection and head injuries in ice hockey: a systematic review. Br J Sports Med 2009;43(13):993–9.
96. Benson BW, Mohtadi NG, Rose MS, et al. Head and neck injuries among ice hockey players wearing full face shields vs half face shields. JAMA 1999; 282(24):2328–32.
97. Danis RP, Hu K, Bell M. Acceptability of baseball face guards and reduction of oculofacial injury in receptive youth league players. Inj Prev 2000;6(3):232–4.
98. Marshall SW, Mueller FO, Kirby DP, et al. Evaluation of safety balls and faceguards for prevention of injuries in youth baseball. JAMA 2003;289(5):568–74.
99. Crisco JJ, Hendee SP, Greenwald RM. The influence of baseball modulus and mass on head and chest impacts: a theoretical study. Med Sci Sports Exerc 1997;29(1):26–36.
100. Viano DC, McCleary JD, Andrzejak DV, et al. Analysis and comparison of head impacts using baseballs of various hardness and a hybrid III dummy. Clin J Sport Med 1993;4:217–28.
101. Janda DH. The prevention of baseball and softball injuries. Clin Orthop Relat Res 2003;409:20–8.
102. Norton K, Schwerdt S, Lange K. Evidence for the aetiology of injuries in Australian football. Br J Sports Med 2001;35(6):418–23.
103. Naunheim R, McGurren M, Standeven J, et al. Does the use of artificial turf contribute to head injuries? J Trauma 2002;53(4):691–4.

104. Durkin MS, Laraque D, Lubman I, et al. Epidemiology and prevention of traffic injuries to urban children and adolescents. Pediatrics 1999;103(6):e74.
105. Berg P, Westerling R. A decrease in both mild and severe bicycle-related head injuries in helmet wearing ages–trend analyses in Sweden. Health Promot Int 2007;22(3):191–7.
106. Abu-Zidan FM, Nagelkerke N, Rao S. Factors affecting severity of bicycle-related injuries: the role of helmets in preventing head injuries. Emerg Med Australas 2007;19(4):366–71.
107. Hagel B, Meeuwisse W. Risk compensation: a "side effect" of sport injury prevention? Clin J Sport Med 2004;14(4):193–6.
108. Finch CF, McIntosh AS, McCrory P, et al. A pilot study of the attitudes of Australian Rules footballers towards protective headgear. J Sci Med Sport 2003;6(4): 505–11.
109. Mihalik JP, McCaffrey MA, Rivera EM, et al. Effectiveness of mouthguards in reducing neurocognitive deficits following sports-related cerebral concussion. Dent Traumatol 2007;23(1):14–20.

Long-term Neurocognitive Dysfunction in Sports: What Is the Evidence?

Gary S. Solomon, PhD[a],*, Summer D. Ott, PsyD[b],
Mark R. Lovell, PhD[c]

KEYWORDS

- Neurocognitive dysfunction • Computerized assessment
- Athletes • Concussive injury

Perhaps no issue in sports medicine has attracted so much attention in the media and popular press as the issue of potential long-term consequences of sports-related mild traumatic brain injury (mTBI or concussion). This issue resulted in several congressional hearings in 2009 and 2010 and has led to changes in management policies at the professional, collegiate, and high-school sports levels. For the 2010 football season, no athlete at any level of competition (ie, high school, collegiate, or professional) was allowed to return to play in the same game (or practice) once a concussion had been diagnosed. Similarly, no athlete who sustained a concussion was allowed to return to play before being cleared by a health care professional. At the time of the writing of this article, 6 states in the United States had passed laws mandating medical evaluation and clearance of concussed high-school athletes before their return to play.

Although it can be argued that many of the changes in rules of play and in the management of concussive injuries are long overdue and may lead to a reduction in disability in athletes at all levels of play, the state of scientific investigation regarding the long-term consequences of brain injury in athletes is still in its infancy and the state of affairs is far from clear. Despite public opinion to the contrary, many questions have yet to be answered regarding the actual risk of long-term disability caused by repeated concussion, factors that may influence outcome, and why some athletes seem to develop trauma-related difficulties and others do not. This issue is of significant

[a] Departments of Neurological Surgery and Psychiatry, Vanderbilt University School of Medicine, T-4224 MCN, Nashville, TN 37232-2380, USA
[b] Methodist Hospital Neurological Institute Concussion Center, 3100 Timmons Lane, Houston, TX 77027, USA
[c] Department of Orthopaedic Surgery, University of Pittsburgh Medical Center, 3200 South Water Street, Pittsburgh, PA 15203, USA
* Corresponding author.
E-mail address: gssolomon1@yahoo.com

Clin Sports Med 30 (2011) 165–177
doi:10.1016/j.csm.2010.09.002
0278-5919/11/$ – see front matter © 2011 Elsevier Inc. All rights reserved.

importance to athletes of all ages as we certainly want to better understand and limit the potential for chronic brain-related dysfunction in athletes. However, on the other side of the issue, the notion that repeated concussions lead to irreversible brain dysfunction could have the unfortunate consequence of limiting participation in contact or collision sports for generations of children for whom participation in athletics provides the basis for personal, physical, and social growth.

The purpose of this article is to summarize the published data on the long-term effects of sports concussive injuries, with a focus on high-school/collegiate athletes, professional boxers, and (American) football players. The systematic study of the potential long-term effects of concussive injury on younger/amateur athletes is in its infancy, and little long-term data are available. Thus, the available data on amateur high-school and collegiate athletes is referred to as intermediate effects, and the available data on professional boxing and (American) football players is referred to as long-term effects. The immediate neurocognitive effects of sports-related concussion have been well documented (see Belanger and Vanderploeg[1] for a meta-analysis of studies).

The current state of knowledge regarding intermediate and long-term disability in athletes is summarized and reviewed, and the available scientific evidence is reviewed. More specifically, recent neuropsychological studies on high-school and collegiate athletes as well as survey and neuropathologic research of older boxers and football athletes are reviewed. Future lines of scientific inquiry that may help to increase our knowledge base in the not so distant future are also discussed.

AMATEUR HIGH-SCHOOL AND COLLEGIATE ATHLETES

Several studies have addressed the issue of potential cumulative effects of concussion on neurocognitive test performance in high-school and collegiate athletes. Macciocchi and colleagues[2] matched a group of college football players with a history of 1 grade 1 concussion (according to American Association of Neurology guidelines) with a group of players with 2 grade 1 concussions. This study was part of a larger study of 2300 division 1-A collegiate football players who were retrospectively examined and followed for 4 years in an effort to investigate the neuropsychological effects of concussive injuries. Participants in this study were matched by age, education, and years in competitive football. All athletes underwent preseason baseline assessment of neurocognitive function by completing several traditional paper-pencil cognitive tests. Baseline assessment also included a history questionnaire and a symptom checklist. Following concussion, players were assessed at 24 h, 5 days, and 10 days after injury. Performance on neuropsychological tests and self-reported symptoms of players who sustained 2 concussions were compared with those players who only sustained 1 concussion. There were no statistically significant differences in test scores between players who sustained 2 concussive injuries versus those with 1 concussive injury. Although there was an expected increase in postconcussive symptoms compared with baseline symptom endorsement, symptoms returned to baseline levels within 10 days for both groups. The investigators also examined within-group differences for players with 2 concussions and found no difference in neurocognitive test performance in players who sustained concussions in close proximity (mean = 33 days) or in subsequent seasons (mean = 532 days). In addition, there was no significant difference found in the number of symptoms endorsed after the first or second concussion in players who sustained 2 injuries.

In the prospective cohort National Collegiate Athletic Association study that evaluated duration of symptoms of collegiate football players after recurrent concussion,

Guskiewicz and colleagues[3] found that players with a history of previous concussions were more likely to sustain subsequent concussions than counterparts who did not have any history of concussion. A total of 2905 football players from 25 US colleges (including athletes from Division I, II, and III schools) were followed during their college careers.

All players underwent baseline measures that included a Graded Symptom Checklist (GCS) and an extensive health questionnaire. However, the athletes did not seem to undergo any objective baseline neuropsychological assessment. The GCS was again administered 1, 2, 3, 5, and 7 days after injury. Out of the 2905 college football players who were followed for 3 football seasons, 196 concussions were reported in 184 players. Twelve players sustained repeated concussions within the same season, with 11 players experiencing a second concussion within 10 days of the first injury and 9 concussions occurred within 7 days of the first injury. The rate of concussions occurred with greater frequency in Division III athletes than in Divisions I and II. Many of the concussions that occurred in the sample of athletes could not be retrospectively graded because of insufficient or missing data. The investigators reported that, on average, most athletes who suffered a concussion indicated they were symptom free within 1 week after their injury.

The investigators found that athletes with a history of 3 or more concussions appeared 3 times more likely to sustain a subsequent concussion than those without prior history of concussion. In addition, athletes with a history of multiple concussions experienced a longer duration of symptoms as assessed by athletic trainers. The investigators concluded that college football players with a history of concussion seem more likely to experience another concussive injury. Results from the study also led investigators to conclude that a history of concussion was not only associated with a greater likelihood of future concussive injury but also a slower recovery as indicated by self-report of symptoms.

Iverson and colleagues[4] matched a group of 19 high-school and collegiate athletes with a history of 3 or more concussions with a group of nonconcussed athletes. Subjects were matched by gender, age, education, and sport. All athletes completed a preseason computerized neuropsychological (ImPACT) baseline and were retested within 5 days after concussion (mean = 1.7 days). Baseline differences in symptom scores were noted, with athletes having a positive 3+ history of concussion reporting more symptoms than nonconcussed athletes. There were no statistically significant differences in baseline scores, although a trend toward lower baseline memory test scores was noted in the concussed group. The investigators speculated that the small sample size (and subsequently limited statistical power) precluded the attainment of statistical significance. There was a significant difference on ImPACT memory scores after concussion for the athletes with a history of multiple concussions. The investigators reported that athletes with a history of multiple concussions were 7.7 times more likely to show a major decline in postconcussion memory test performance than athletes with no history of concussion. Iverson and colleagues[4] interpreted this finding as preliminary evidence suggestive of a cumulative effect of multiple concussions.

Moser and colleagues[5] studied 223 high-school athletes who had undergone baseline testing with a symptom checklist and paper-pencil neuropsychological tests. Cumulative grade point averages (GPA) were also available fors all students. Athletes were grouped into those with a recent concussion (1 week before testing; n = 40), athletes with no history of concussion (n = 82), and asymptomatic athletes who had experienced 1 (n = 56), 2, or more (n = 45) prior concussions. The results indicated that asymptomatic athletes with a history of 2 or more concussions performed similarly to athletes with a recent concussive injury. Athletes with a rich history of concussion had lower GPAs than athletes with no history of concussion. The investigators concluded that multiple concussions may have enduring neuropsychological effects in this age group.

Three studies appeared in the *British Journal of Sports Medicine* in 2006 addressing the issue of cumulative effects of concussion on neurocognitive test performance. The first study published was by Iverson and colleagues.[6] Subjects were 867 high-school and collegiate athletes who had completed preseason baseline neuropsychological testing (ImPACT). Athletes were grouped according to self-reported history of concussion. There were 664 athletes with no prior concussions, 149 athletes with 1 prior concussion, and 54 athletes with 2 prior concussions. A multivariate analysis of variance revealed no significant effect, leading the investigators to conclude that if there was indeed a cumulative effect for multiple concussions, it was small and undetectable using computerized neurocognitive test methodology.

The second study was published by Collie and colleagues,[7] who studied 521 Australian Rules footballers. Athletes were divided into groups based on self-reported history of concussion: no concussion (n = 244), 1 concussion (n = 95), 2 concussions (n = 72), 3 concussions (n = 48), and 4 or more concussions (n = 62). All athletes completed baseline neurocognitive measures (CogSport) for 2 consecutive seasons. There were no statistically significant differences in reaction time and total error rates among the groups, leading the investigators to conclude that there was no association between number of previous concussions and current neurocognitive test performance.

The third study was reported by Broglio and colleagues.[8] They retrospectively studied 235 university athletes with a HeadMinder CRI neurocognitive baseline test, and 264 university athletes with a baseline ImPACT test. The athletes were divided into groups based on self-reported history of concussion. No history of concussion was reported by 336 athletes, 105 reported a history of 1 concussion, 36 reported 2 concussions, and 22 reported having had 3 concussions. A multivariate analysis of variance revealed no effect for history of concussion on neurocognitive test performance on either HeadMinder or ImPACT. The investigators concluded that there is either no effect of multiple concussions on neurocognitive test performance or that the decrements may be so subtle that they are undetectable by these neurocognitive measures.

In a more recent study, Bruce and Echemendia[9] investigated the relationship between self-reported history of concussion and performance on neurocognitive tests in a multisport (eg, ice hockey, soccer, lacrosse, football basketball, and so forth) sample of college athletes. The researchers conducted 3 studies as part of their project. First, the association between self-reported history of concussion and performance on computerized neuropsychological tests (ImPACT) was examined. A second study included examination of the association between self-reported history of concussion and performance on traditional paper-pencil neurocognitive tests. The paper-pencil battery of neuropsychological assessment tools included Digit Symbol, Symbol Modalities Test, Stroop Test, Controlled Oral Word Association Test, Trail Making Test A & B, and the Hopkins Verbal Learning Test. As part of the third study, a separate group of athletes were administered both traditional neuropsychological tests and computerized neuropsychological tests (ImPACT) and the relationship between performance on both of these measures and reported history of concussion was examined. The results from the studies did not find an association between a history of self-reported concussion and performance on ImPACT or paper-pencil neuropsychological tests. Based on their findings, the investigators concluded that a history of multiple concussive injuries did not result in clear neurocognitive deficits in their sample of athletes.

In summary, 5 of the 8 studies reviewed revealed no evidence for cumulative adverse effects on neurocognitive function in sports-related concussion. Two studies raised the possibility of a cumulative effect, and another suggested a protracted recovery period following multiple concussions. Our informal analysis is consistent with the results of a recent meta-analysis of athletes reporting multiple concussions.[10] In this study of 614 multiply concussed athletes culled from 8 published studies meeting the investigators' inclusion criteria (6 of which have been reviewed earlier), the overall effect of multiple concussions was determined to be minimal. However, the investigators reported that follow-up analyses indicated that multiple concussions were associated with poorer neurocognitive performance on tests of delayed memory and executive functioning.

PROFESSIONAL ATHLETES

In this section, the available data on professional boxers and professional (American) football players are reviewed.

Boxing

Perhaps in no other area of sports is the evidence more compelling for long-term adverse neurocognitive effects than in professional boxing. One stated objective in boxing is to inflict a concussion on one's opponent, preferably with loss of consciousness for longer than a count of 10. In 1928 Martland[11] coined the term punch drunk to refer to the long-term neurocognitive effects of boxing. The term dementia pugilistica was introduced by Millspaugh[12] in 1937 and in 1962 Courville[13] referred to the "psychopathic deterioration of pugilists." Jordan and colleagues[14] referred to this disorder as "chronic traumatic brain injury" in boxers. The most recent iteration of this diagnostic classification has been termed chronic traumatic encephalopathy (CTE).[15]

In any discussion of possible long-term cognitive effects from boxing, it is important to distinguish between amateur and professional boxers. A recent meta-analysis of neurocognitive studies of amateur boxers revealed little or no evidence of chronic neurocognitive effects.[16] Conversely, in 1969[17] Roberts reported that 17% of retired professional boxers who had active careers in the earlier part of the twentieth century developed CTE. Clausen and colleagues[18] pointed out that the incidence of CTE in professional boxers was likely on the decline, given that the average duration of a boxer's career in the 1930s was 19 years (currently at 5 years), and that the average number of bouts has been reduced from 336 to 13.

A comprehensive review of studies related to dementia pugilistica was published by Erlanger and colleagues.[19] They estimated the prevalence of moderate to severe dementia in boxers at 20%.

The study by Jordan and colleagues[14] published in *JAMA* is particularly remarkable and worthy of review. Jordan and colleagues[14] studied 30 professional boxers, aged 23 to 76 years, assessing genetic typing (apolipoprotein E4 alleles, a known risk factor for late onset Alzheimer dementia) and neurobehavioral functioning (a combination of motor, cognitive, and neuropsychiatric symptoms). The results indicated that the boxers with the highest exposure (defined as 12 or more professional bouts) had lower neurobehavioral scores than those with less than 12 bouts. The ApoE E4 genotype frequencies among the boxers were reported to parallel the typical distribution in the general population. High-exposure boxers who were positive for at least 1 ApoE allele had the worst neurobehavioral functioning of any subgroup assessed. Jordan and colleagues[14] concluded that boxing exposure and possession of an ApoE E4 allele interacted to result in greater impairment in neurobehavioral functioning.

Survey Research with National Football League Athletes

Several major survey studies of National Football League (NFL) retirees' cognitive and biopsychosocial characteristics have been conducted and published in the past decade. These studies have been cited as evidence of long-term adverse effects on mood and/or cerebral functioning in professional athletes. The data presented in these surveys merit a detailed review.

The first study was conducted by a multidisciplinary group associated with the Center for the Study of Retired Athletes at the University of North Carolina at Chapel Hill.[20] In the spring and summer of 2001 and in early 2002, the investigators sent out a general health questionnaire to 3683 living members of the National Football League's Retired Player's Association. A total of 2552 players responded, yielding a response rate of 69.3%. History of concussion was assessed through self-reports, and a concussion was defined as "… an injury resulting from a blow to the head that caused an alteration in mental status and one or more of the following symptoms: headache, nausea, vomiting, dizziness/balance problems, fatigue, trouble sleeping, drowsiness, sensitivity to light or noise, blurred vision, difficulty remembering, and difficulty concentrating" [(p720)].

The results regarding concussion indicated that 1513 retirees (60.8%) reported having sustained at least 1 concussion during their professional playing career, and 597 (24%) reported sustaining 3 or more concussions. About half of those athletes sustaining concussions experienced either loss of consciousness or memory loss. Subjectively, about 17.6% of those athletes sustaining a concussion believed that the concussion had a permanent effect on their thinking and memory skills as they aged.

The health questionnaire also included the SF-36 Measurement Model for Functional Assessment of Health and Well-Being, an index of health, well-being, and activities of daily living. The investigators derived a "… mental health component score, which includes scores of vitality, social functioning, role emotional, and mental health" [(p720)], and compared the scores of the retired athletes with age- and gender-matched norms provided by prior research.[21] A review of the SF-36 reveals that the vitality domain includes 4 items, the social functioning domain includes 2 items, the role-emotional domain includes 3 items, and the mental health domain includes 5 items. The respondent answers each item with a frequency score, with 6 response options available in the original version of the SF-36, and 5 response options available in version 2 of the test.

The Mental Component Scale (MCS) scores on the SF-36 for the NFL retirees aged 50 years and older were similar to those of the general population for all age groups. However, when players were grouped according to the number of reported concussions sustained while playing professional football, the MCS scores of the retired players with 3 or more concussions were worse than those retirees with 0, 1, or 2 concussions at a statistical probability level of less than .001. Inspection of the group means, however, reveals that the average score of the normative group was 52.42 (SD not reported), and the average score of the NFL retirees with 3 or more concussions was 50.31 (SD = 11.26), a mean difference of roughly 2 points. The standard deviations of the MCS scores of the concussion groups ranged from 8.50 to 11.26. Although the mean difference between the groups was statistically significant (with subject numbers ranging from 374 to 814 per group), the question arises as to whether this 2-point mean difference between groups is of any clinical, functional, or practical significance. In 2005, Guskiewicz and colleagues[22] interpreted this finding as evidence of a "… progressive decline in mental health functioning …" [(p722)]. This conclusion may be debatable.

The potential relationship between a history of concussions in professional football and the emergence of late-life depression was discussed in greater detail in a paper published by Guskiewicz and colleagues,[22] in 2007. However, as pointed out by Casson,[23] the data presented in the 2007 paper was based on the same data presented in the 2005 publication; those findings have been addressed earlier in this article.

Approximately 4 months later a second survey focusing on memory and issues related to mild cognitive impairment (MCI) was sent to a subset of 1754 NFL retirees aged 50 years or older, with a copy sent to the player's informant, defined as a spouse or close relative. MCI is a diagnostic classification believed to represent the intermediate domain or transitional phase between normal aging and dementia.[24] Generally speaking, MCI involves the presence of subjectively reported and objectively assessed impairment in at least 1 area of cognitive functioning (typically memory) with preservation of basic activities of daily living.

MCI and memory questionnaire data were available for 758 players and from 641 retired players' spouses/informants. There were 22 cases of physician-diagnosed MCI among the retirees (3 cases involving cerebrovascular accident) and 77 cases of retirees who had significant memory impairment based on informant data. Although percentages are not reported by the investigators, we calculate a rate of physician-diagnosed MCI at 2.9% among retiree-reported data (22/758), and a rate of 12.01% (77/641) based on the informant data.

Plassman and colleagues[25] assessed the prevalence of cognitive impairment without dementia (a functional diagnostic equivalent of MCI) in the US population in a longitudinal study conducted from 2001 to 2005. Overall, they found a 22.2% prevalence rate for cognitive impairment without dementia. They found a 16% prevalence rate in the 71- to 79-year-old cohort (the youngest cohort reported), which is closest to the older NFL retirees in age (mean age of 62.4 years). For the NFL retirees, the physician-based diagnosis rate of MCI (2.9%) and the informant-based rate (12.01%) are less than those reported by Plassman and colleagues[25] for the general population (16%).

Age is a critical variable in the prevalence of MCI, as it is the greatest single risk factor for this diagnosis.[26] The authors were unable to locate a study of prevalence rates of MCI in the Unites States among the 60- to 69-year age range, as most studies use age 70 years as the lower limit for inclusion. Thus, the rates reported earlier based on the Plassman data may not be ideally comparable with the NFL retirees, because the Plassman cohort is, on average, a decade older than the NFL cohort. However, if the rates reported by the NFL retirees were increased by 50% in an inelegant attempt to make age-appropriate prevalence estimates, the NFL retirees' prevalence data remain consistent with (and certainly do not exceed) the general US population data reported by Plassman and colleagues.[25]

In assessing the relationship between number of concussions reported and the presence of Alzheimer disease (AD), the investigators reported that there was no association between the number of concussions sustained as a professional football player and a diagnosis of AD. Thirty-three retirees (1.3%) reported a physician's diagnosis of AD, and about half of those were receiving nootropic (memory-enhancing) therapy. However, the investigators reported that there was a higher prevalence of AD in the retiree cohort than in the corresponding general population, leading the investigators to conclude that "... this group may have an earlier onset of AD than the general American male population" [(p721)]. Plassman and colleagues[25] reported a 5.5% prevalence rate for prodromal AD in the general population. The term prodromal AD is said to be the equivalent of the clinical criteria for a diagnosis of AD, but lacks biopsy or autopsy confirmation. The 1.3% prevalence rate of AD among NFL retirees reported by Guskiewicz and colleagues[20] is less than the age-matched population rate of 5.5% reported by Plassman and colleagues.[25] Again, however, the age variable must be kept in mind, as the retirees were on average, younger than those in the Plassman study.

The second study was conducted in November and December 2008 by the University of Michigan Institute for Social Research.[27] The investigators presented a stratified random survey of 1063 retired NFL players. A wide array of demographic, health, religious, financial, and psychosocial data were collected, including information on depression, intermittent explosive disorder, and dementia. The researchers split the NFL retirees into younger (age 30–49 years) and older (age 50+ years) groups. The data are reported in terms of percentages, and the NFL retirees' data are compared with all US men in similar age brackets (30–49 years and 50+ years). No statistical analyses were conducted to determine if any group differences were statistically significant.

Depression was assessed using a combination of 4 screener items from the National Study of American Life along with items from the Patient Health Questionnaire. There was a higher rate of endorsement of all 4 screener questions for depression among the younger retired players (37.6%) versus the comparable group from all US men (20.7%). Among older retirees, 23% endorsed all 4 screener questions in the positive direction versus 15% in the age-matched all US men group. Current major depression was reported by 3.9% and 3.6% of the younger and older retirees, respectively. The corresponding rates for all US men were 3.0% for the younger group and 3.9% for the older group. The investigators suggested that younger retirees may have a higher rate of depression than age-matched counterparts. This was not the case for the older retirees.

The investigators also screened for intermittent explosive disorder (IED), defined as "episodes of unpremeditated and uncontrollable anger" [(p32)]. A 3-question screening test was used. Irrespective of age, the NFL retirees scored lower on any of the 3 screening items than their age-matched counterparts from the general population. More than half (54.8%) of the younger men from the general population endorsed at least 1 of the screening questions, whereas the corresponding figure for younger NFL retirees was 30.7%). Among older individuals, NFL retirees endorsed at least 1 of the screening questions 29.3% of the time, whereas the corresponding figure for the general male population was 47.2%. The investigators concluded that "... NFL retirees are much less likely to report symptoms of anger than the general population" [(p32)].

The investigators acknowledged that individuals with dementia were more difficult to diagnose than those with depression or IED because dementia directly affects an individual's ability to participate in such a survey. The investigators also acknowledge that they did not administer cognitive tests, neurologic examinations, or review medical records. Weir and colleagues[27] interviewed a proxy reporter (generally the wife) of the retired player. The respondent was asked if a diagnosis of dementia, AD, or other memory-related disease had ever been made. In the younger age group, 0.1% of the general population and 1.9% of the NFL retirees reported these diagnoses. The corresponding figures for the older groups were 1.2% for the general male population and 6.1% for the NFL retirees. The 6.1% rate of dementia diagnoses is similar to the 5.5% rate reported by Plassman and colleagues.[25]

From a research methodological perspective, there are many limitations to survey research. A partial list of the limitations (as pointed out by Guskiewicz and colleagues[20]) include retrospective analysis, the self-reporting nature of responses (often without objective verification), response bias (including socially desirable responding), and sampling error. The authors view survey data as quite useful in the exploratory aspects of a field of inquiry. However, survey data do not typically allow for cause and effect scientific analysis. Although we applaud the investigators of these surveys for making scientific inquiries, we do not believe that survey results allow for cause and effect statements of an evidence-based sort. Our goal is not to criticize the investigators of these surveys for their research; our goal is to clarify the justifiable conclusions from their data.

NEUROPATHOLOGIC STUDIES OF ATHLETES

In the past several years, neuropathologic studies of retired athletes have appeared in the literature, and significant media attention has been focused on these reports. More specifically, the tragic deaths and subsequent autopsies of 3 retired NFL athletes fueled speculation that NFL athletes were at an increased risk for premature dementia, presumably secondary to multiple blows to the head (concussive or subconcussive) throughout their playing careers. The first reports were individual autopsy studies of 3 NFL athletes.[28–30] The first published report generated a heated rebuttal by Casson and colleagues,[31] criticizing the study on definitional and methodological grounds. These autopsy studies pointed toward CTE as the neuropathologic substrate of premature dementia and death in these athletes. A fourth case involving an NFL athlete was reported in 2007,[32] and a fifth NFL case was reported by McKee and her colleagues[15] in 2009.

The most comprehensive article on CTE was published by McKee and colleagues,[15] who reviewed data from 48 previously published and autopsy-verified cases of CTE and presented data on 3 additional athletes. McKee and colleagues[15] described CTE as a "... neuropathologically distinct slowly progressive tauopathy with a clear environmental etiology" [(p709)]. They described the neurobehavioral manifestations of CTE as changes in memory, behavior, personality, gait, and speech, along with parkinsonism. Neuropathologically, atrophic changes are noted in the cerebral hemispheres, mamillary bodies, medial temporal lobe, and brainstem, with ventricular dilatation and a fenestrated cavum septum pellucidum. Microscopically, CTE involves extensive tau-immunoreactive neurofibrillary and astrocytic tangles along with spindle and thread-like neurites throughout the brain. Beta-amyloid deposition (plaques), 1 of the hallmark features of AD, are said to occur in less than half the cases.

The autopsy-verified cases of CTE reviewed by McKee and colleagues[15] included 39 boxers, 5 NFL players (4 previously published cases and 1 new case), and 1 case each from the sports of wrestling and soccer. Two of the cases reviewed from the literature were head bangers (1 autistic), 1 case died of physical abuse, 1 case had epilepsy, and 1 case was a circus clown with alcoholism who had a history of repeatedly being shot out of a cannon. McKee and colleagues[15] present a detailed comprehensive review of the clinical manifestations in each of the previously published and the 3 newly presented cases. Thus, of the 51 autopsy-verified cases of CTE reviewed by McKee and colleagues,[15] 46 (90%) were athletes, and 39 of the 46 athletes (85%) were boxers.

These initial NFL cases have led to the more systematic recruitment of athletes for eventual postmortem study. This effort has been gaining momentum steadily in the past 5 years and has resulted in the establishment of 2 formal programs at West Virginia University and at Boston University (the latter in conjunction with the Sports Legacy Institute of Boston). These programs have been structured to recruit living athletes for inclusion in the postmortem studies on their deaths.

LIMITATIONS OF OUR REVIEW

Our review has several limitations. First, our review is restricted to the sports concussion literature, and we have not reviewed the published studies of the intermediate and long-term neurocognitive effects of concussion in nonathletes (civilian and military). Second, not all of the available studies of the effects of concussive injury have been reviewed; studies based on the sport and quality of the research were chosen. Third, a formal meta-analysis of available studies was not done (see Ref.[10] for a recent meta-analysis), as our goal was simply to provide an overview of the research in this area. The emerging data on intermediate neurophysiologic changes in sports-related concussion have not been discussed, as several studies have emerged recently documenting persistent changes in cortical electrophysiologic functions after concussion.[33–35]

FUTURE DIRECTIONS

As we reviewed the sports concussion literature, we found several moderator variables that could affect the state of the knowledge base regarding the potential adverse long-term effects of multiple concussions. First, many studies contain mixed groups of athletes. For example, published studies have an admixture of men and women, various sports, different ages, and multiple comorbid medical and psychiatric conditions (eg, migraine headaches, attention deficit hyperactivity disorder, learning disabilities). It has been shown in several studies that these biopsychosocial variables may have systematic effects on response to concussive injury, and ultimately may be relevant in determining long-term outcome. For example, gender differences in incidence and response to concussive injury are emerging and it seems that women may have a more protracted outcome.[36,37] Age has been posited to be a significant factor in determining response to sports concussive injury, as some empiric studies[38] and consensus clinical experience[39] have suggested that younger (child and adolescent) athletes may have a lengthier course of recovery than older athletes. Collins and colleagues[40] reported that collegiate athletes with learning disabilities and/or attention deficit spectrum disorders who sustained multiple concussions may have poorer neurocognitive test performances. Mihalik and colleagues[41] found that concussed high-school and collegiate athletes classified as having posttraumatic migraine headache had significantly poorer neurocognitive performances after concussion than those with uncomplicated headache or no headache. The most recent position paper from the Concussion in Sport Group[39] indicated that depression or other psychiatric or sleep disorders may be considered significant modifiers of response to concussive injury. A history of emotional disturbance or psychological illness that predates concussion may also influence the recovery process. In some cases, the athlete's emotional issues may have been fairly controlled until the injury and associated stress results in reemergence of previous emotional difficulties. The elucidation of the role of genetic factors in the incidence and response to concussive injury is another area in need of further study. For example, Terrell and colleagues[42] reported that collegiate athletes with an APOE promoter G-219T TT genotype may be at increased risk for sustaining concussion, and raised the question of the role of tau Ser-50-Pro polymorphism as a risk factor for concussive injury.

Further prospective studies on the intermediate and long-term effects of concussive injuries in various athletic populations are awaited, and it is to be hoped that researchers will include and assess the biopsychosocial factors discussed earlier as potential moderator variables in these studies. In the interim, it is our conclusion based on the literature reviewed that adverse long-term neurocognitive effects of concussive injury have been demonstrated empirically in professional boxers only.

REFERENCES

1. Belanger HG, Vanderploeg RD. The neuropsychological impact of sports-related concussion: a meta-analysis. J Int Neuropsychol Soc 2005;11:345–57.
2. Macciocchi S, Barth J, Littlefield L, et al. Multiple concussions and neuropsychological functioning in collegiate football players. J Athl Train 2001;36: 303–6.
3. Guskiewicz K, McCrea M, Marshall S, et al. Cumulative effects associated with recurrent concussion in collegiate football players. JAMA 2003;290:2549–55.
4. Iverson GL, Gaetz M, Lovell MR, et al. Cumulative effects of concussion in amateur athletes. Brain Inj 2004;18:433–43.
5. Moser RS, Schatz P, Jordan BD. Prolonged effects of concussion in high school athletes. Neurosurgery 2005;57:300–6.
6. Iverson GL, Brooks BL, Lovell MR, et al. No cumulative effects for one or two previous concussions. Br J Sports Med 2006;40:72–5.
7. Collie A, McCrory P, Makdissi M. Does history of concussion affect current cognitive status? Br J Sports Med 2006;40:550–1.
8. Broglio SP, Ferrara MS, Piland SG, et al. Concussion history is not a predictor of computerized neurocognitive performance. Br J Sports Med 2006;40:802–5.
9. Bruce J, Echemendia R. History of multiple self-reported concussions is not associated with reduced cognitive abilities. Neurosurgery 2009;64:100–6.
10. Belanger HG, Spiegel E, Vanderploeg RD. Neuropsychological performance following a history of multiple self-reported concussions: a meta-analysis. J Int Neuropsychol Soc 2010;16:262–7.
11. Martland HS. Punch drunk. JAMA 1928;91:1103–7.
12. Millspaugh JA. Dementia pugilistica. U S Nav Med Bull 1937;35:297–303.
13. Courville CB. Punch drunk. Its pathogenesis and pathology on the basis of a verified case. Bull Los Angel Neuro Soc 1962;27:160–8.
14. Jordan BD, Relkin NR, Ravdin LD, et al. Alipoprotein E e4 associated with chronic traumatic brain injury in boxing. JAMA 1997;278:136–40.
15. McKee AC, Cantu RC, Nowinski CJ, et al. Chronic traumatic encephalopathy in athletes: progressive tauopathy after repetitive head injury. J Neuropathol Exp Neurol 2009;68:709–35.
16. Loosemore M, Knowles CH, Whyte GP. Amateur boxing and risk of chronic traumatic brain injury: systematic review of observational studies. BMJ 2007;335:809–17.
17. Roberts AH. Brain damage in boxers. London: Pitman Publishing; 1969.
18. Clausen H, McCrory P, Anderson V. The risk of chronic traumatic brain injury in professional boxing: change in exposure variables over the past century. Br J Sports Med 2005;39:661–4.
19. Erlanger DM, Kutner KC, Barth JT, et al. Neuropsychology of sports-related head injury: dementia pugilistica to post concussion syndrome. Clin Neuropsychol 1999;13:193–209.
20. Guzkiewicz KM, Marshall SW, Bailes J, et al. Association between recurrent concussion and late-life cognitive impairment in professional football players. Neurosurgery 2005;57:719–26.
21. Ware JE, Gandek B, Kosinski M, et al. The equivalence of SF-36 summary health scores estimated using standard and country-specific algorithms in 10 countries:

results from the IQOLA Project International Quality of Life Project. J Clin Epidemiol 1998;51:1167–70.

22. Guskiewicz KM, Marshall SM, Bailes J, et al. Recurrent concussion and risk of depression in retired professional football players. Med Sci Sports Exerc 2007; 39:903–9.

23. Casson IR. Do the "facts" really support an association between NFL players' concussions, dementia, and depression? Neurology Today 2010;3:6–7.

24. Peterson RC, Stevens JC, Ganguli M, et al. Practice parameter: early detection of dementia-MCI (an evidence-based review). Report of the Quality Standards Subcommittee of the American Academy of Neurology. Neurology 2001;56: 1133–44.

25. Plassman BL, Langa KM, Fisher GG, et al. Prevalence of cognitive impairment without dementia in the United States. Ann Intern Med 2008;148:427–34.

26. DeCarli C. Mild cognitive impairment: prevalence, prognosis, etiology, and treatment. Lancet Neurol 2003;2:15–21.

27. Weir DR, Jackson JS, Sonnega A. National Football League Player Care Foundation study of retired NFL players. 2009. Available at: www.ns.umich.edu/Releases/2009/Sep09/Finalreport.pdf. Accessed June 15, 2010.

28. Omalu BI, DeKosky ST, Minster RL, et al. Chronic traumatic encephalopathy in a National Football League player. Neurosurgery 2006;57:128–33.

29. Omalu BI, DeKosky ST, Minster RL, et al. Chronic traumatic encephalopathy in a national football league player: part II. Neurosurgery 2006;59: 1086–92.

30. Omalu BI, Hamilton RL, Kamboh MI, et al. Chronic traumatic encephalopathy (CTE) in a National Football League player: case report and emerging medicolegal practice questions. J Forensic Nurs 2010;6:40–6.

31. Casson IR, Pellman EJ, Viano DC. Chronic traumatic encephalopathy in a National Football League player (letter). Neurosurgery 2006;58:1003–7.

32. Cajigal S. Fourth case of chronic traumatic encephalopathy reported in former NFL player. Neurology Today 2007;7(14):6–8.

33. DeBeaumont L, Brisson B, Lassonde M, et al. Long term electrophysiologic changes in athletes with a history of multiple concussions. Brain Inj 2010;21: 631–44.

34. DeBeaumont L, Theoret H, Mongeon D, et al. Brain function decline in healthy retired athletes who sustained their last sports concussion in early adulthood. Brain 2009;132:695–703.

35. Theirault M, DeBeaumont L, Tremblay S. Cumulative effects of concussions in athletes revealed by electrophysiological abnormalities on visual working memory. J Clin Exp Neuropsychol 2010;17:1–12.

36. Farace E, Alves W. Do women fare worse? A meta-analysis of gender differences in traumatic brain injury outcome. J Neurosurg 2000;93:539–45.

37. Broshek DK, Kaushik T, Freeman JR, et al. Sex differences in outcome following sports-related concussion. J Neurosurg 2005;102:856–63.

38. Field M, Collins M, Lovell M, et al. Does age play a role in recovery from sport-related concussion? A comparison of high school athletes and collegiate athletes. J Pediatr 2003;142:546–53.

39. McCrory P, Meeuwisse W, Johnston K, et al. Consensus statement on Concussion in Sport: The 3rd International Conference on Concussion in Sport held in Zurich, November 2008. Br J Sports Med 2009;43(Suppl 1):76–84.

40. Collins MW, Grindel SH, Lovell MR, et al. Relationship between concussion and neuropsychological performance in college football players. JAMA 1999;282: 964–70.
41. Mihalik JP, Stump JE, Collins MW, et al. Posttraumatic migraine characteristics in athletes following sports-related concussion. J Neurosurg 2005;102:850–5.
42. Terrell TR, Bostick RM, Abramson R, et al. APOE, APOE promoter, and tau genotypes and risk for concussion in college athletes. Clin J Sport Med 2008;18:10–7.

Chronic Traumatic Encephalopathy: A Potential Late Effect of Sport-Related Concussive and Subconcussive Head Trauma

Brandon E. Gavett, PhD[a,b], Robert A. Stern, PhD[a,b],
Ann C. McKee, MD[a,b,c,d],*

KEYWORDS

- Encephalopathy, Post-traumatic
- Neurodegenerative disorders • Concussion • Athletic injuries
- Dementia • Motor neuron disease

It has been understood for decades that certain sporting activities may increase an athlete's risk of developing a neurodegenerative disease later in life. Not surprisingly, this association was originally noted in boxers, athletes who receive numerous blows to the head during training and competition. In 1928, Harrison Martland, a New Jersey pathologist and medical examiner, first described the clinical spectrum of abnormalities found in "nearly one half of the fighters who have stayed in the game long enough."[1]

This work was supported by NIA P30AG13846, Supplement 0572063345-5, National Operating Committee on Standards for Athletic Equipment, and by the Department of Veterans Affairs. This work was also supported by an unrestricted gift from the National Football League. The funding sources were not involved in the preparation, review, or approval of this article.

a Center for the Study of Traumatic Encephalopathy and Alzheimer's Disease Center, Boston University School of Medicine, 72 East Concord Street, B-7800, Boston, MA 02118, USA
b Department of Neurology, Boston University School of Medicine, 72 East Concord Street, B-7800, Boston, MA 02118, USA
c Department of Pathology, Boston University School of Medicine, 72 East Concord Street, B-7800, Boston, MA 02118, USA
d Bedford Veterans Affairs Medical Center, 200 Springs Road, Building 18, Room 118, Bedford, MA 01730, USA
* Corresponding author. Bedford Veterans Affairs Medical Center, 200 Springs Road, Building 18, Room 118, Bedford, MA 01730.
E-mail address: amckee@bu.edu

Clin Sports Med 30 (2011) 179–188
doi:10.1016/j.csm.2010.09.007
0278-5919/11/$ – see front matter. Published by Elsevier Inc.

sportsmed.theclinics.com

Boxers exhibiting cognitive, behavioral, or motor abnormalities were well known to lay persons, sportswriters, and others within the boxing community and were referred to by various terms, such as "punch drunk," "goofy," and "slug-nutty"[2,3]; later, the more formal term *dementia pugilistica* was introduced to lend medical validity to the condition.[4] By the 1970s, a sufficient number of boxers with dementia pugilistica had been studied pathologically to support the conclusion that this form of neurodegeneration was similar to, but distinguishable from, other causes of neurodegenerative disease.[5] As evidence of the clinical and neuropathologic consequences of repeated mild head trauma grew, it became clear that this pattern of neurodegeneration was not restricted to boxers, and the term chronic traumatic encephalopathy (CTE), originally coined by Miller[6] became most widely used.

Over the last several decades, clinical and neuropathologic evidence of CTE has emerged in association with various sports, including American football, professional wrestling, professional hockey, and soccer, as well as other activities associated with repetitive mild head trauma, such as physical abuse, epileptic seizures, and head banging.[7–13] Although the incidence and prevalence of CTE is currently unclear, it probably varies by sport, position, duration of exposure, and age at the time of initial or subsequent head trauma, and with additional variables, such as genetic predisposition. To date, there have been no randomized neuropathologic studies of CTE in deceased athletes, and as such, there is a selection bias in the cases that have come to autopsy. If one considers the prevalence in deceased professional American football players who died between February 2008 and June 2010, there were 321 known player deaths[14] and the brains of 12 of the 321 underwent postmortem neuropathologic examination at Boston University Center for the Study of Traumatic Encephalopathy (BU CSTE). All 12 examined neuropathologically showed evidence of CTE, suggesting an estimated lifetime prevalence of at least 3.7%. If one assumes that all deceased players who did not come to autopsy did not have CTE and that the amount of head trauma in professional football has remained fairly constant over the past 5 decades, a prevalence of 3.7% would result. Although this represents a conservative estimate, it suggests a significant public-health risk for persons who suffer repetitive mild traumatic brain injury (TBI).

CLINICAL SIGNS AND SYMPTOMS OF CTE

Whereas concussion and postconcussion syndrome represent temporary states of neuronal and axonal derangement, CTE is a neurodegenerative disease that occurs years or decades after recovery from the acute or postacute effects of head trauma. The exact relationship between concussion and CTE is not entirely clear, although repetitive axonal perturbation may initiate a series of metabolic, ionic, membrane, and cytoskeletal disturbances, which trigger the pathologic cascade that leads to CTE in susceptible individuals.[15,16] The onset of CTE is often in midlife, usually after athletes have retired from their sport. In some individuals, the early manifestations of CTE affect behavior; in particular, individuals with neuropathologically documented CTE have been described by family and friends as being more irritable, angry, or apathetic or as having a shorter fuse. Increased suicidality seems to be a particularly salient symptom of CTE.[17] In other cases, cognitive difficulties may be the first signs to emerge, with poor episodic memory and executive functioning being two of the most common cognitive dysfunctions reported. Later in the disease, movement (eg, parkinsonism), speech, and ocular abnormalities may emerge in the context of declining cognition and worsening comportment. A minority of cases with neuropathologically documented CTE developed dementia before death; the relative infrequency of dementia in individuals with CTE may be due in part to many individuals with CTE having committed suicide or died from accidents or drug overdose at an early age.[11,17]

NEUROPATHOLOGY OF CTE
Gross Pathology

Neuropathologic studies of athletes with a history of repeated mild head injuries have produced several consistent findings that, together, make CTE a distinctive disorder. On gross examination, there is often anterior cavum septi pellucidi and, usually, posterior fenestrations. These changes may be caused by the force of the head impact being transmitted through the ventricular system, thereby affecting the integrity of the intervening tissue. Enlargement of the lateral and third ventricles is also commonly seen in CTE; the third ventricle may be disproportionately widened. Additional gross features include atrophy of the frontal and temporal cortices and of the medial temporal lobe, thinning of the hypothalamic floor, shrinkage of the mammillary bodies, pallor of the substantia nigra, and hippocampal sclerosis. Atrophy of the cerebrum, diencephalon, basal ganglia, brainstem, and cerebellum may result in an overall reduction in brain mass.[11]

Microscopic Neuropathology

Tau

Microscopically, CTE is characterized by an abundance of neurofibrillary inclusions in the form of neurofibrillary tangles (NFTs), neuropil threads (NTs), and glial tangles (GTs). The main protein composing NFTs is the microtubule-associated protein tau, and NFTs are aggregates of filamentous tau polymers. Although CTE shares many microscopic similarities with Alzheimer disease (AD) and other tauopathies, it has several distinguishing features. First, the distribution of tau pathology is unique; it is most commonly found in the more superficial cortical laminae (II and III), whereas tau NFTs in AD are preferentially distributed in large projection neurons in layers III and V. Further, the regional tau pathology is extremely irregular, largely confined to uneven foci in the frontal, temporal, and insular cortices, unlike the more uniform cortical NFT distribution seen in AD. Tau NFTs, NTs, and GTs are found throughout the medial temporal lobe, often in densities greater than those found in severe AD, and are also prominent in the diencephalon, basal ganglia, and brainstem. NTs and GTs are also found in the subcortical white matter. Finally, NFTs in CTE are most dense at the depths of cortical sulci, and are typically perivascular, which might indicate that disruptions of the cerebral microvasculature and the blood brain barrier that occur at the time of the traumatic injury play a critical role in the formation of NFTs.[11]

Although the precise pathologic mechanisms that tie repeated mild head injuries to NFT formation are not known, they may involve a series of diffuse axonal injuries (DAI) set in motion by the initial trauma and aggravated by subsequent mild traumatic injuries. During a TBI, the brain and spinal cord undergo shear deformation producing a transient elongation or stretch of axons. Traumatic axonal injury results in alterations in axonal membrane permeability, ionic shifts including massive influx of calcium, and release of caspases and calpains that might trigger tau phosphorylation, misfolding, truncation, and aggregation, as well as breakdown of the cytoskeleton with dissolution of microtubules and neurofilaments.[15,18,19]

Increasing evidence indicates that tau phosphorylation, truncation, aggregation, and polymerization into filaments represents a toxic gain of function, and continued accumulation of tau leads to neurodegeneration. This is supported by tau's involvement in some genetic forms of frontotemporal degeneration[20] and by work that shows that plasmids containing human tau complementary DNA constructs microinjected into lamprey neurons in situ produce tau filaments that accumulate and lead to neuronal degeneration.[21,22] However, it is also possible that the intracellular NFTs, by themselves, are the byproducts rather than the cause of cellular injury and that NFT formation indicates neurons that survived the initial injury and sequestered the abnormally phosphorylated, truncated, and folded tau.[23] A possible tau toxic factor or transcellular propagation by the misfolded tau protein may explain how a neurodegeneration that starts multifocally around small blood vessels or in the depths of cortical sulci ultimately spreads to involve large regions of brain as a systemic degeneration, such as CTE.[24]

Beta-amyloid

Beta-amyloid (Aβ) deposits are found in 40% to 45% of individuals with CTE, in contrast to the extensive Aβ deposits that characterize nearly all cases of AD. Although neuritic plaques are typically abundant in AD and are essential to the diagnosis, Aβ plaques in CTE, when they occur, are less dense and predominantly diffuse.[11] Despite the fairly minor role Aβ plaques seem to play in the neuropathologic manifestation of CTE, the role of Aβ in the pathogenesis of CTE has yet to be elucidated. It is known that acute head injuries cause an upregulation of amyloid precursor protein (APP) production and that Aβ plaques may be found in up to 30% of patients who die within hours of TBI.[25–27] DAI, often a consequence of mild TBI, is thought to influence changes in Aβ after head injury. Interruption of axonal transport causes an accumulation of multiple proteins in the axon, including APP, in varicosities along the length of the axon or at disconnected axon terminals, termed axonal bulbs.[28] Although the axonal pathology in TBI is diffuse in that it affects widespread regions of the brain, typically, the axonal swellings are found in multifocal regions of the subcortical and deep white matter, including the brainstem. Because of the rapid and abundant accumulation of APP in damaged axons after TBI, APP immunostaining is used for the pathologic assessment of DAI in humans. Accordingly, this large reservoir of APP in injured axons might be aberrantly cleaved to rapidly form Aβ after TBI.[25,29,30] However, it remains unclear whether the large quantities of APP and Aβ found in damaged axons after TBI play any mechanistic role in neurodegeneration or neuroprotection.[28,31,32] Moreover, it is unknown how long the increased APP and Aβ lasts or what mechanisms may result in variable clearance.

TDP-43

Recently, in addition to severe tau neurofibrillary pathology, the authors found a widespread TDP-43 proteinopathy in more than 80% of their cases of CTE.[13] Moreover, in 3 athletes with CTE who developed a progressive motor neuron disease several years before death, there were extensive TDP-43 immunoreactive inclusions in the anterior horns of the spinal cord, along with tau-immunoreactive GTs, neurites, and, occasionally, extensive NFTs. These findings suggest that a distinctive, widespread TDP-43 proteinopathy is also associated with CTE and that, in some individuals, the TDP-43 proteinopathy extends to involve the spinal cord and is clinically manifest as motor neuron disease with a presentation that may appear similar to amyotrophic lateral sclerosis (ALS).[13] The shared presence of 2 aggregated phosphorylated proteins associated with neurodegeneration in the great majority of cases of CTE suggests that a common stimulus, such as repetitive axonal injury, provokes the pathologic accumulation of both proteins.[33] Recent studies in vitro and in vivo suggest that overexpression of wild-type human TDP-43 and its dislocation from the neuronal nucleus to the cytoplasm are associated with neurodegeneration and cell death.[34–36] By virtue of its capacity to bind to neurofilament messenger RNA (mRNA) and stabilize the mRNA transcript, TDP-43 plays a critical role in mediating the response of the neuronal cytoskeleton to axonal injury. TDP-43 is intrinsically prone to aggregation, and its expression is upregulated after experimental axotomy in spinal motor neurons of the mouse.[37] Traumatic axonal injury may also accelerate TDP-43 accumulation, aggregation, and dislocation to the cytoplasm, thereby enhancing its neurotoxicity.

CLINICAL IMPLICATIONS
CTE is a Potential Late Effect of Repeated Head Injuries

CTE is not thought to be a long-term sequela after a specific head trauma. Rather, its clinical symptoms emerge later in life, usually after athletes retire from their sport. Like most other neurodegenerative diseases that cause dementia, CTE has an insidious onset and gradual course. Based on a recent review of neuropathologically confirmed CTE in athletes[11], the mean age at onset is 42.8 years (SD = 12.7; range = 25–76 years). On average, onset occurs approximately 8 years after retirement (SD = 10.7), although approximately one-third of athletes were reportedly symptomatic at the time of retirement. In athletes, the course seems to be considerably protracted (mean duration = 17.5 years, SD = 12.1), especially in boxers. The average duration of the disease in boxers is 20 years (SD = 11.7) and 6 years in American football players (SD = 2.9).[11] If the affected individual does not die of other causes, full-blown clinical dementia may occur late in the course of the disease.

Diagnosis of CTE

Currently, the clinical diagnosis of CTE is difficult because there are no consensus diagnostic criteria or large-scale longitudinal clinicopathologic correlation studies. The differential diagnosis of CTE often includes AD[38] and frontotemporal dementia (FTD)[39], depending on the age at onset and the presenting problem. Older individuals with memory difficulties may seem to have AD, and, in fact, may have evidence of AD and CTE neuropathologically.[11] When the age at onset is earlier (eg, 40s or 50s) and the patient presents with behavioral dysregulation or apathy, it may be difficult to rule out FTD. Although a history of remote head trauma may be suggestive of CTE, head trauma has been implicated as a risk factor of AD, Parkinson disease, ALS, and other neurodegenerative diseases.[40–42] Therefore, without neuropathologic confirmation, currently, a clinical diagnosis of CTE cannot be made with a high degree of confidence. Furthermore, the clinical phenotype of CTE may be confounded by alcohol or other drug abuse. Several individuals with neuropathologically confirmed CTE are thought to have developed problems with drug abuse as a consequence of the loss of inhibitory control caused by the neurodegenerative disease. From a clinical perspective, however, it can be difficult to determine whether the drug abuse problems are a cause of symptoms or simply one of many ways in which CTE is manifested.

Although the neuropathologic features of CTE seem to be distinct from other neurodegenerative diseases, no currently agreed neuropathologic criteria exist for the diagnosis of CTE. Once established, these criteria can be applied at autopsy in large-scale, prospective longitudinal studies of athletes with a history of repetitive head injuries. Establishing neuropathologic diagnostic criteria would allow for the identification of clinical criteria and biomarkers to improve the accuracy of CTE diagnosis in the living.

Several biomarkers are believed to have the potential to contribute to identifying CTE in vivo. For instance, the changes to white-matter integrity caused by repeated head trauma may be amenable to detection using diffusion tensor magnetic resonance imaging.[43] Magnetic resonance spectroscopy may be capable of detecting changes in glutamate/glutamine, N-acetyl aspartate, and myo-inositol, molecular abnormalities that may serve as markers of brain damage caused by head injuries.[44] Further, measuring tau and phospho-tau in cerebrospinal fluid may yield diagnostically useful markers of CTE.[45]

Risk and Protective Factors

CTE research is in its infancy, and decades of research are probably necessary to achieve CTE diagnosis early in its course using a combination of clinical tools and biomarkers. However, the research already conducted has profound implications for current practice by medical professionals, athletic trainers, and related specialists, as well as policy makers in government and athletic organizations. CTE is the only known neurodegenerative dementia with a specific identifiable cause; in this case, head trauma. It is unknown whether a single blow to the head is sufficient to initiate the metabolic cascade that precedes the clinical and neuropathologic changes characteristic of CTE, because all confirmed cases of CTE to date have had a history of multiple head injuries. Therefore, the most obvious way to prevent CTE is, in theory, to prevent repetitive head injuries from occurring. In some sports, such as boxing and American football, it may be impossible to prevent repetitive head injuries, especially the repeated subconcussive blows that are characteristic of the impacts felt by offensive and defensive linemen in football on nearly every play. For sports in which repeated blows to the head are unavoidable, proper concussion assessment and management may be paramount for preventing long-term consequences. Currently, it is unknown whether returning to play while symptomatic from a previous concussion or sustaining a second concussion while symptomatic is a risk factor of developing CTE. However, other strategies to reduce the number and severity of head traumas are possible, such as limiting full-contact practices, implementing rules of play that diminish the likelihood of repeated head trauma (eg, removing the 3-point stance in football), or increasing the use of newer protective headgear aimed at absorbing force, thus diminishing the impact to the brain.

Along these lines, many potential variables surrounding head trauma in athletes may be important for preventing CTE later in life. The sport played and the position played within each sport may be relevant; for instance, boxers receive a greater proportion of rotational forces to the head, whereas American football players receive a greater proportion of linear forces to the head.[46] Even within the same sport, athlete exposure to head injuries can differ considerably. In American football, some positions, such as wide receiver, may receive occasional severe blows with the potential to cause unconsciousness, whereas other players, such as linemen, may take hundreds of small impacts per season, most of which are not, by themselves, forceful enough to cause symptoms.[47] It is unknown whether CTE is more likely to occur after a small number of severe head injuries, a large number of subconcussive injuries, or other forms of head trauma. Currently, investigations are ongoing that attempt to quantify the force of head impacts across different sports and positions.[48] These findings will play an important role in understanding the specific head injury variables that influence CTE risk.

The age at which athletes suffer their head injuries may also influence CTE risk. At younger ages, the brain may be more vulnerable to injury.[49] Conversely, the increased plasticity of the young brain may be better able to compensate for specific difficulties, such as behavioral dysfunction.[50] It is also not clear whether particular lifestyle factors may be protective against CTE in the context of repetitive head injuries. In other neurodegenerative diseases such as AD, the neuropathology is thought to precede the clinical symptoms, possibly by several decades.[51] The same may be true of CTE, as evidenced by the presence of CTE neuropathology in asymptomatic individuals studied at autopsy. Conceivably, health and medical factors that are absent or present during this preclinical stage may influence the extent of neurodegeneration or the brain's ability to compensate for any neurodegeneration. For instance, the presence of chronic inflammation, as in that which accompanies medical conditions such as obesity, hypertension, diabetes mellitus, atherosclerosis, and heart disease, may facilitate neurodegeneration and NFT formation.[52–55] Also, as with other neurodegenerative diseases like AD, some individuals may have greater *cognitive reserve*, thus increasing the threshold for the clinical manifestation of the underlying neuropathologic condition.

Genetic variations may also play an important role in moderating the relationships between head trauma, neuropathologic changes, and disordered cognition and behavior. One of the genes thought to influence CTE risk is the apolipoprotein E (APOE) gene. The APOE ε4 allele, important in the genetics of AD, may also increase the risk of CTE. Based on genetic testing conducted in conjunction with neuropathologic examinations of individuals with a history of repeated head injuries, approximately 57% of individuals with neuropathologically confirmed CTE possessed at least one APOE ε4 allele. When contrasted with the estimated 28% of the population possessing at least one APOE ε4 allele,[56] the frequency of this allele in those with CTE seems higher than expected. This genetic link is currently speculative, because formal epidemiologic studies have yet to be conducted. However, individuals carrying the APOE ε4 allele may be more likely to have a poor outcome after TBI, especially in individuals younger than 15 years.[57–59] Epidemiologic data have also implicated the APOE ε4 genotype as a risk factor for the development of AD after TBI,[60,61] and carriers of the APOE ε4 allele were found to be at increased risk of Aβ deposition after TBI.[62]

SUMMARY

CTE is a neurodegenerative disease that occurs later in the lives of some individuals with a history of repeated head trauma. The exact relationship between repetitive mild TBI, with or without symptomatic concussion, and CTE is not entirely clear, although it is possible that repetitive axonal injury sets up a series of metabolic, ionic, and cytoskeletal disturbances that trigger a pathologic cascade, leading to CTE in susceptible individuals. CTE has been reported in association with American football, professional wrestling, soccer, and hockey, as well as in association with physical abuse, epilepsy, and head banging behaviors, suggesting that mild TBI of diverse origin is capable of instigating CTE. CTE often manifests in midlife and produces clinical symptoms of disordered cognition, memory loss and executive dysfunction, depression, apathy, disinhibition, and irritability, as well as parkinsonian signs. The characteristic neuropathologic features of CTE include extensive tau-immunoreactive inclusions scattered throughout the cerebral cortex in a patchy, superficial distribution, with focal epicenters at the depths of sulci and around the cerebral vasculature and widespread TDP-43-immunoreactive inclusions that may occasionally be associated with symptoms of motor neuron disease. Currently, neuropathologic examination of brain tissue is the only way to diagnose CTE, although intense research efforts are underway to identify biomarkers to detect the disease and monitor its progression and to develop therapies to slow or reverse its course. Longitudinal research efforts are underway to shed additional light on the specific variables related to head trauma, neuropathology, and clinical presentation of CTE that remain in question.

REFERENCES

1. Martland HS. Punch drunk. JAMA 1928;91:1103–7.
2. Critchley M. Medical aspects of boxing, particularly from a neurological standpoint. Br Med J 1957;1:357–62.
3. Parker H. Traumatic encephalopathy ('punch drunk') of professional pugilists. J Neurol Psychopathol 1934;15:20–8.
4. Millspaugh JA. Dementia pugilistica. U S Nav Med Bull 1937;35:297–303.
5. Corsellis JA, Bruton CJ, Freeman-Browne D. The aftermath of boxing. Psychol Med 1973;3:270–303.
6. Miller H. Mental after-effects of head injury. Proc R Soc Med 1966;59:257–61.
7. Geddes JF, Vowles GH, Nicoll JA, et al. Neuronal cytoskeletal changes are an early consequence of repetitive head injury. Acta Neuropathol 1999;98:171–8.
8. Omalu BI, DeKosky ST, Hamilton RL, et al. Chronic traumatic encephalopathy in a national football league player: part II. Neurosurgery 2006;59:1086–92.
9. Omalu BI, DeKosky ST, Minster RL, et al. Chronic traumatic encephalopathy in a national football league player. Neurosurgery 2005;57:128–34.
10. Cajigal S. Brain damage may have contributed to former wrestler's violent demise. Neurology Today 2007;7:1–16.
11. McKee A, Cantu R, Nowinski C, et al. Chronic traumatic encephalopathy in athletes: progressive tauopathy after repetitive head injury. J Neuropathol Exp Neurol 2009;68:709–35.
12. Omalu BI, Bailes J, Hammers JL, et al. Chronic traumatic encephalopathy, suicides and parasuicides in professional American athletes: the role of the forensic pathologist. Am J Forensic Med Pathol 2010;31:130–2.
13. McKee AC, Gavett BE, Stern RA, et al. TDP-43 proteinopathy and motor neuron disease in chronic traumatic encephalopathy. J Neurol Exp Neuropathol 2010;69: 918–29.
14. Oldest living pro football players. 2009–2000 Necrology. Available at: http://www.freewebs.com/oldestlivingnfl/20092000necrology.htm. Accessed May 15, 2010.
15. Giza C, Hovda D. The neurometabolic cascade of concussion. J Athl Train 2001; 36:228–35.
16. Yuen TJ, Browne KD, Iwata A, et al. Sodium channelopathy induced by mild axonal trauma worsens outcome after a repeat injury. J Neurosci Res 2009;87:3620–5.
17. Omalu BI, Hamilton RL, Kamboh MI, et al. Chronic traumatic encephalopathy (CTE) in a national football league player: case report and emerging medicolegal practice questions. J Forensic Nurs 2010;6:40–6.
18. Binder LI, Guillozet-Bongaarts AL, Garcia-Sierra F, et al. Tau, tangles, and Alzheimer's disease. Biochim Biophys Acta 2005;1739:216–23.
19. Serbest G, Burkhardt MF, Siman R, et al. Temporal profiles of cytoskeletal protein loss following traumatic axonal injury in mice. Neurochem Res 2007;32:2006–14.
20. Spillantini MG, Bird TD, Ghetti B. Frontotemporal dementia and Parkinsonism linked to chromosome 17: a new group of tauopathies. Brain Pathol 1998;8:387–402.
21. Hall GF, Chu B, Lee G, et al. Human tau filaments induce microtubule and synapse loss in an in vivo model of neurofibrillary degenerative disease. J Cell Sci 2000;113:1373–87.
22. Hall GF, Yao J, Lee G. Human tau becomes phosphorylated and forms filamentous deposits when overexpressed in lamprey central neurons in situ. Proc Natl Acad Sci U S A 1997;94:4733–8.
23. de Calignon A, Fox LM, Pitstick R, et al. Caspase activation precedes and leads to tangles. Nature 2010;464:1201–4.

24. Frost B, Jacks RL, Diamond MI. Propagation of tau misfolding from the outside to the inside of a cell. J Biol Chem 2009;284:12845–52.
25. Gentleman SM, Nash MJ, Sweeting CJ, et al. Beta-amyloid precursor protein (beta APP) as a marker for axonal injury after head injury. Neurosci Lett 1993;160:139–44.
26. Roberts GW, Gentleman SM, Lynch A, et al. Beta amyloid protein deposition in the brain after severe head injury: implications for the pathogenesis of Alzheimer's disease. J Neurol Neurosurg Psychiatry 1994;57:419–25.
27. Roberts GW, Gentleman SM, Lynch A, et al. beta A4 amyloid protein deposition in brain after head trauma. Lancet 1991;338:1422–3.
28. Johnson VE, Stewart W, Smith DH. Traumatic brain injury and amyloid-beta pathology: a link to Alzheimer's disease? Nat Rev Neurosci 2010;11:361–70.
29. Gorrie C, Oakes S, Duflou J, et al. Axonal injury in children after motor vehicle crashes: extent, distribution, and size of axonal swellings using beta-APP immunohistochemistry. J Neurotrauma 2002;19:1171–82.
30. Sherriff FE, Bridges LR, Sivaloganathan S. Early detection of axonal injury after human head trauma using immunocytochemistry for beta-amyloid precursor protein. Acta Neuropathol 1994;87:55–62.
31. Smith DH, Chen XH, Iwata A, et al. Amyloid beta accumulation in axons after traumatic brain injury in humans. J Neurosurg 2003;98:1072–7.
32. Chen XH, Johnson VE, Uryu K, et al. A lack of amyloid beta plaques despite persistent accumulation of amyloid beta in axons of long-term survivors of traumatic brain injury. Brain Pathol 2009;19:214–23.
33. Uryu K, Chen XH, Martinez D, et al. Multiple proteins implicated in neurodegenerative diseases accumulate in axons after brain trauma in humans. Exp Neurol 2007;208:185–92.
34. Barmada SJ, Skibinski G, Korb E, et al. Cytoplasmic mislocalization of TDP-43 is toxic to neurons and enhanced by a mutation associated with familial amyotrophic lateral sclerosis. J Neurosci 2010;30:639–49.
35. Tatom JB, Wang DB, Dayton RD, et al. Mimicking aspects of frontotemporal lobar degeneration and Lou Gehrig's disease in rats via TDP-43 overexpression. Mol Ther 2009;17:607–13.
36. Wils H, Kleinberger G, Janssens J, et al. TDP-43 transgenic mice develop spastic paralysis and neuronal inclusions characteristic of ALS and frontotemporal lobar degeneration. Proc Natl Acad Sci U S A 2010;107:3858–63.
37. Moisse K, Mepham J, Volkening K, et al. Cytosolic TDP-43 expression following axotomy is associated with caspase 3 activation in NFL-/- mice: support for a role for TDP-43 in the physiological response to neuronal injury. Brain Res 2009;1296:176–86.
38. McKhann G, Drachman D, Folstein M, et al. Clinical diagnosis of Alzheimer's disease: report of the NINCDS-ADRDA work group under the auspices of department of health and human services task force on Alzheimer's disease. Neurology 1984;34:939–44.
39. Neary D, Snowden JS, Gustafson L, et al. Frontotemporal lobar degeneration: a consensus on clinical diagnostic criteria. Neurology 1998;51:1546–54.
40. Mortimer JA, van Duijn CM, Chandra V, et al. Head trauma as a risk factor for Alzheimer's disease: a collaborative re-analysis of case-control studies. EURODEM risk factors research group. Int J Epidemiol 1991;20:S28–35.
41. Goldman SM, Tanner CM, Oakes D, et al. Head injury and Parkinson's disease risk in twins. Ann Neurol 2006;60:65–72.
42. Chen H, Richard M, Sandler DP, et al. Head injury and amyotrophic lateral sclerosis. Am J Epidemiol 2007;166:810–6.

43. Jones DK, Dardis R, Ervine M, et al. Cluster analysis of diffusion tensor magnetic resonance images in human head injury. Neurosurgery 2000;47:306–13.

44. Ross BD, Ernst T, Kreis R, et al. 1H MRS in acute traumatic brain injury. J Magn Reson Imaging 1998;8:829–40.

45. Shaw LM, Vanderstichele H, Knapik-Czajka M, et al. Cerebrospinal fluid biomarker signature in Alzheimer's disease neuroimaging initiative subjects. Ann Neurol 2009;65:403–13.

46. Viano DC, Casson IR, Pellman EJ, et al. Concussion in professional football: comparison with boxing head impacts–part 10. Neurosurgery 2005;57:1154–72.

47. Rowson S, Brolinson G, Goforth M, et al. Linear and angular head acceleration measurements in collegiate football. J Biomech Eng 2009;131:061016.

48. Brolinson PG, Manoogian S, McNeely D, et al. Analysis of linear head accelerations from collegiate football impacts. Curr Sports Med Rep 2006;5:23–8.

49. Field M, Collins MW, Lovell MR, et al. Does age play a role in recovery from sports-related concussion? A comparison of high school and collegiate athletes. J Pediatr 2003;142:546–53.

50. Anderson V, Spencer-Smith M, Leventer R, et al. Childhood brain insult: can age at insult help us predict outcome? Brain 2009;132:45–56.

51. Näslund J, Haroutunian V, Mohs R, et al. Correlation between elevated levels of amyloid beta-peptide in the brain and cognitive decline. JAMA 2000;283:1571–7.

52. Arnaud LT, Myeku N, Figueiredo-Pereira ME. Proteasome-caspase-cathepsin sequence leading to tau pathology induced by prostaglandin J2 in neuronal cells. J Neurochem 2009;110:328–42.

53. Ke YD, Delerue F, Gladbach A, et al. Experimental diabetes mellitus exacerbates tau pathology in a transgenic mouse model of alzheimer's disease. PLoS One 2009;4:e7917.

54. Duong T, Nikolaeva M, Acton PJ. C-reactive protein-like immunoreactivity in the neurofibrillary tangles of alzheimer's disease. Brain Res 1997;749:152–6.

55. Arnaud L, Robakis NK, Figueiredo-Pereira ME. It may take inflammation, phosphorylation and ubiquitination to 'tangle' in alzheimer's disease. Neurodegener Dis 2006;3:313–9.

56. Hill JM, Bhattacharjee PS, Neumann DM. Apolipoprotein E alleles can contribute to the pathogenesis of numerous clinical conditions including HSV-1 corneal disease. Exp Eye Res 2007;84:801–11.

57. Teasdale GM, Murray GD, Nicoll JAR. The association between APOE epsilon4, age and outcome after head injury: a prospective cohort study. Brain 2005;128:2556–61.

58. Friedman G, Froom P, Sazbon L, et al. Apolipoprotein E-epsilon4 genotype predicts a poor outcome in survivors of traumatic brain injury. Neurology 1999;52:244–8.

59. Sundström A, Marklund P, Nilsson LG, et al. APOE influences on neuropsychological function after mild head injury: within-person comparisons. Neurology 2004;62:1963–6.

60. Mayeux R, Ottman R, Maestre G, et al. Synergistic effects of traumatic head injury and apolipoprotein-epsilon 4 in patients with alzheimer's disease. Neurology 1995;45:555–7.

61. Mayeux R, Ottman R, Tang MX, et al. Genetic susceptibility and head injury as risk factors for Alzheimer's disease among community-dwelling elderly persons and their first-degree relatives. Ann Neurol 1993;33:494–501.

62. Nicoll JA, Roberts GW, Graham DI. Apolipoprotein E epsilon 4 allele is associated with deposition of amyloid beta-protein following head injury. Nat Med 1995;1:135–7.

When to Consider Retiring an Athlete After Sports-Related Concussion

Cara L. Sedney, MD[a],*, John Orphanos, MD[b], Julian E. Bailes, MD[b]

KEYWORDS

• Concussion • Mild traumatic brain injury • Athletes

The decision to retire an athlete due to sports-related concussion is often a controversial one, fraught with conflicting pressures from the athlete and others involved in the sport. Postconcussion syndrome has long been recognized as resulting from participating in sports and is discussed in sports medicine texts.[1,2] The retirement of several National Football League (NFL) players in the 1990s from chronic postconcussive effects has recently brought this issue into the public eye. Currently, the decision to retire an athlete after concussion is based on several basic principles of neurology, sports medicine, and concussion management. This knowledge in turn stems from the biology of concussion and traumatic brain injury and from increasing understanding of the effect of chronic brain trauma. Although concussion guidelines continue to play an important role in acute management of concussion, the decision to retire an athlete is a more complex one, dependent on myriad factors.

SOCIAL AND LEGAL IMPLICATIONS IN THE DECISION TO RETIRE

Concussive injury has been observed to manifest in four stages (**Table 1**) with a distinct temporal association. In the acute concussive stage lasting up to 1 week after injury, physical symptoms, cognitive deficits, and emotional disturbances may be evident. This may be followed by a postconcussive stage consisting of persistent acute phase symptoms, which are nevertheless self-limited to approximately 6 weeks after mild traumatic brain injury (MTBI). A prolonged postconcussion syndrome lasting up to 6 months may be experienced and may be manifested by declining athletic, work, or school performance. Finally, a severe and rare form of chronic concussive injury,

[a] Department of Neurosurgery, West Virginia University, PO Box 9183, Robert C. Byrd Health Sciences Center, Morgantown, WV 26506, USA
[b] Department of Neurosurgery, West Virginia University, PO Box 9183, Robert C. Byrd Health Sciences Center, Morgantown, WV 26505, USA
* Corresponding author.
E-mail address: csedney@hsc.wvu.edu

Clin Sports Med 30 (2011) 189–200
doi:10.1016/j.csm.2010.08.005
0278-5919/11/$ – see front matter © 2011 Elsevier Inc. All rights reserved.

Table 1
Stages of concussive injury

Acute Concussion	Postconcussion Syndrome	Prolonged Postconcussion Syndrome	Chronic Traumatic Encephalopathy
Physical symptoms (headache, dizziness, hearing loss, balance difficulty, insomnia, nausea/vomiting, sensitivity to light or noise, diminished athletic performance) Cognitive deficits (loss of short-term memory, difficulty with focus or concentration, decreased attention, diminished work or school performance) Emotional disturbances (irritability, anger, fear, mood swings, decreased libido)	Persistent concussion symptoms Usually lasting 1–6 weeks after MTBI Self-limiting	Symptoms lasting over 6 months Lowered concussion threshold Diminished athletic performance Diminished work or school performance	Latency period (usually 6–10 years) Personality disturbances Emotional lability Marriage/ personal relationship failures Depression Alcohol/ substance abuse Suicide attempt/ completion

chronic traumatic encephalopathy (CTE), may manifest after a variable latency period and demonstrates profound personality changes and dysfunction in many areas of life.

CONCUSSION PATHOPHYSIOLOGY

There is a greater understanding of concussion now than ever before. The pathophysiology of concussion is characterized by a variety of metabolic mechanisms, which are both acute and subacute in nature. On initial insult, a hypermetabolic state is created with excessive release of excitatory neurotransmitters, despite a decrease in cerebral blood flow.[3] This is characterized by ion movements, such as influx of calcium and efflux of potassium, causing extensive depolarization of neurons, along with decreased intracellular magnesium. Glycolysis is accelerated and lactate accumulates, causing neuronal membrane damage and resulting in altered blood-brain barrier permeability.[3] This initial hypermetabolic state is followed by a hypometabolic state of widespread neuronal suppression, called a spreading depression,[3] possibly due to the relative decrease in cerebral blood flow. Increased intracellular calcium leads to mitochondrial dysfunction but rarely leads to cell death in experimental concussion.[3] Neuronal dysfunction results from the decrease in magnesium, accumulation of lactate, and relative hypoxia. In addition, mechanical factors, such as stretching or tearing of neuronal axons, may further result in membrane disruption and ion fluxes.

These pathophysiologic changes usually occur over a specific time frame and in a specific sequence, accounting for the stepwise progression of symptoms after sports-related concussion, and also relate to the susceptibility of more severe injury after an initial insult. Although new pathologic methods have shown an anatomic basis for chronic concussive changes, overall, these effects have classically been thought of as physiologic rather than structural in nature and account for the majority of symptoms-based guidelines in the management of concussion. Ordinarily, brain imaging studies are normal, although postconcussive positron emission tomography may reflect the decreased glucose metabolism, and certain immunohistochemical stains may demonstrate neuronal damage (**Fig. 1**).

LONG-TERM EFFECTS OF CONCUSSION

The long-term pathophysiology of repeated head trauma is particularly important to the decision to retire an athlete after sports-related concussion. Despite the early recognition of symptomatology in retired boxers with early neurodegenerative changes, many chronic concussive effects are still being explored and are incompletely understood. The first report of chronic, permanent neurologic sequelae in career boxers was by Martland[4] in 1928, which he termed, *dementia pugilistica* (DP). This introduced the possibility of long-term effects from sport in the form of advanced parkinsonism, pyramidal tract dysfunction, ataxia, and behavioral abnormalities in a 38-year-old man. It is believed that DP is present in approximately 20% of retired boxers. Since then, persistent concussive symptoms, such as memory problems; decreased attention, focus, or concentration; and mood swings or personality changes have been recognized as having long-term effects on athletic, work or school, and interpersonal functioning. These consequences may present at any age and any level of sporting competition (**Fig. 2**).

More recently, the discovery of specific pathologic findings during the autopsies of several well-publicized deaths among retired athletes has solidified the association of repeated head trauma with another rare condition, CTE, which causes severe cognitive and behavioral disturbances.[5,6] Much of research on chronic effects of head injury is based on clinical and autopsy observations rather than laboratory investigation. Both macro- and microscopic pathologic changes have been described. Corsellis and colleagues[7] describe gross pathologic findings in the brains of men who had been boxers, including cavum septum pellucidum, scarring of cerebellar folia, and degeneration of the substantia nigra. Microstructural changes may be more pertinent to the pathophysiology of chronic concussion, however, and include accumulation of tau protein in the form of neurofibrillary tangles (NFTs) and neuritic threads (NTs) (**Fig. 3**).

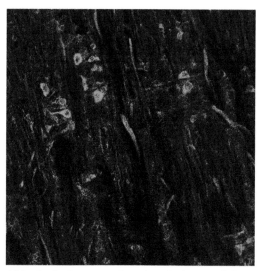

Fig. 1. Torn axons within the brainstem and corticospinal tract of the rat, shown via immunohistochemical staining of β-amyloid precursor protein after traumatic brain injury.

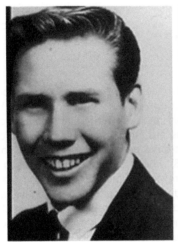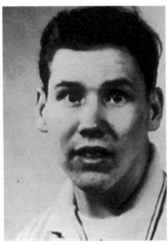

Fig. 2. Consecutive photographs of a high school football player before and after concussive injury sustained in sport. (*From* Schieder R. Head and neck injuries in football. 1st edition. Baltimore [MD]: Williams and Wilkins; 1973; with permission.)

Corsellis and colleagues[7] reported the first neurohistologic evidence of CTE on postmortem examination of boxers. Furthermore, recent case reports by Omalu and colleagues[5,6] illustrate histopathologic changes comprising a diffuse accumulation of tau proteins (NFTs and NTs) in patients after chronic, repeated exposure to brain impact during a sporting career. Their series of patients, including seven professional football players, two professional wrestlers, and one boxer, exhibited "diffuse, sparse to frequent" and "sparse to moderate" tau-immunoreactive NFTs and NTs.[6] The NFTs may take a variety of forms, including band-shaped, flame-shaped, and large and small perikaryal tangles. Both the NFTs and NTs are made up of helical, paired tau proteins.[8] Neuritic plaques may be found but were absent in several cases in Omalu and colleagues'[5] series, bearing resemblance to a rare type of dementia, known as tangle-only dementia.[9] The only direct confirmation of CTE remains direct postmortem examination of the brain with immunohistochemistry, because no neuroimaging study is capable of visualizing these changes.

CTE seems to affect the brain's emotional function, as reflected in the Papez circuit described by James Papez[10] in 1937. This limbic pathway plays a role in memory and emotion by connecting primitive areas of the brain, such as the hippocampal formation, mammillary bodies, entorhinal cortex, thalamus, and brainstem nuclei, and structures, such as the locus ceruleus.

The pathophysiology of CTE is believed due to microstructural changes within neurons because of the effects discussed previously, especially hyperphosphorylation of microtubule-associated tau protein.[11] It is found that the abnormal metabolism of injured neurons leads to accumulation of neuronal cytoskeletal and transmembrane proteins[12–14] and likely altered function of these neuronal elements. Further theories on the effect of protein accumulation include decreased efficacy of neuronal repair or increased susceptibility to reactive oxygen species.

DECISION-MAKING PROCESS

The basic principles of sports medicine and acute concussion management deal with the implications of the pathophysiology (discussed previously), specifically, the

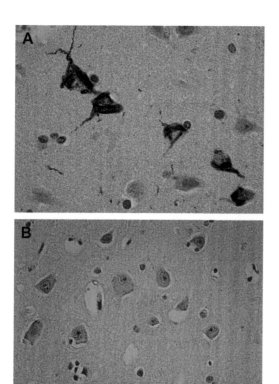

Fig. 3. (*A*) Tau antibody stain from the cerebral cortex of a professional football player showing typical changes of CTE: NFTs (large, globular intracellular inclusions) and NTs (whispy). (*B*) Normal control.

predictable, stepwise nature of symptoms, the susceptibility to further injury after initial insult, and the prevalence of physiologic rather than structural abnormalities. The statement of the First International Conference on Concussion in Sport, held in Vienna in 2001, succinctly outlined these principles.[15] These basic principles have led to the establishment of a variety of guidelines on concussion management. The Colorado Medical Society system, the Cantu grading system, and the American Academy of Neurology system are all currently in use. The Colorado and Cantu systems both include the recommendation that retirement should be considered after three or more concussions.

The decision to retire an athlete, however, is rarely due to one, or even several, incidents, but rather multiple concussions and subconcussive injuries over an extended period of time, many of which may not be diagnosed or recognized. Often the concussion guidelines do not apply in these cases. Furthermore, current research suggests that the effects of concussion may be cumulative, with new manifestations of this being seen in research and in emerging cases. Therefore, the decision to retire an athlete due to concussion must be made after extensive study of the patient's history and neurologic examination as well as advanced methods, such as neuropsychological testing and neuroimaging. **Box 1** lists several decisive factors for retirement, either from the season or from contact sports entirely.

Box 1
Decisive factors for retirement[a]

Season Ending

  Prolonged post concussion syndrome

  3 or more concussions in single season

  2 or more major concussions[b] in single season

  Diminished academic performance

  Diminished athletic performance

  CT or MRI brain scan abnormality

Career Ending

  Chiari malformation

  Intracranial hemorrhage

  Diminished academic performance or cognitive abilities

  Persistent prolonged post concussion syndrome

  Lowering of threshold for concussion (as judged by physicians, athletes, coaches, certified athletic trainers)

  3 or more major concussions

  CT or MRI scan documentation of structural brain injury

  Nonresolving functional MRI scan deficits

  CTE symptoms

[a] All return to play and retirement decisions are individualized. Some features are relative contraindications for return to play.
[b] Major concussion: symptomatic for greater than 1 week.

The basis for retirement from contact sports is complex, and the many factors may be encountered in any stage of an athlete's career, from high school to professional levels. Retirement after concussion generally reflects the underlying brain injury and falls into one of the four categories (discussed previously) (see **Table 1**), depending on the timing of concussion. Some athletes may choose to retire due to intractable acute symptoms after concussion. This may include symptoms that interfere with play or acute catastrophic injury. Others may choose to retire due to postconcussive syndrome, which usually consists of self-limited sequelae of concussion, such as dizziness, headaches, and declining academic or athletic performance. Thirdly, more prolonged postconcussive effects are evident thereafter and may result in a decision to retire due to changes in performance, motivation, or personality, which again may manifest in declining athletic or academic abilities. Finally, in unique subsets of patients, displaying signs or symptoms of CTE may prompt a decision to retire.

History

Exposure to MTBI is the primary historical information used in a decision to retire an athlete. The number, symptoms, and time to recovery after concussion are all important factors, as is a history of returning to play while still symptomatic. Although rare, a history of postconcussive seizures should be sought. The mechanism of concussion, if known, as well as the type of protective equipment, if any, being worn is also important. Information regarding current postconcussive symptomatology is important, and this is best gleaned from the patient, family, athletic trainers, and others. The frequency and severity of headaches should be recorded. Mood swings, irritability, insomnia, lack of concentration, or impaired memory are pertinent. Personality changes may be pervasive. Any persistent postconcussive symptoms or permanent neurologic symptoms from a concussion, such as organic dementia, hemiplegia, and homonymous hemianopsia, should prompt investigation into retiring an athlete.[16] A history of declining school or athletic performance may be a sensitive indicator of both early and chronic changes after concussion and this is particularly important to elicit if present.

For a subset of patients with a long history of exposure, symptoms suggestive of CTE should be sought, such as explosive behavior, excessive jealousy, mood disorders, and paranoia. These symptoms often demonstrate latency from initial exposure and are progressive. Omalu and colleagues[5] performed an extensive postmortem psychological history during their series of 5 patients and unearthed a variety of common historical clues pointing to chronic cognitive and neuropsychological decline. These included drug and alcohol abuse, increasing religiosity, suicidal ideations or attempts, insomnia, hyperactivity, breakdown of intimate or family relationships, exaggerated responses to stressors, poor business or financial management, bankruptcy, and others.[5] Although the latency period of symptoms in CTE is not known, these should be investigated when interviewing an athlete and family for possible retirement after concussion.

Documented Brain Injury

Specific, potentially catastrophic events after concussion, such as second impact syndrome and surgically treated brain injuries (eg, subdural hematoma), would ordinarily disqualify an athlete from further participation in contact sports. As discussed by Cantu,[16] any athlete surviving a second impact syndrome should retire from contact sports. In addition, any athlete requiring surgery for evacuation of an intracranial hemorrhage should be considered for retirement, due to multiple factors, including changes in cerebrospinal fluid dynamics[16] and the decrease in structural integrity of the skull, although some investigators have reported that, rarely, an athlete may be considered to return to play after craniotomy after healing of bony defect.[17] Non–sports-related concussions during an athlete's life, including childhood injuries, may also contribute to the magnitude of injury and these must be documented and considered.

Outcome of Examinations

The proper management of an athlete after acute concussion requires accurate examination and testing to guide decision making regarding play. Several guidelines have been proposed to assist caregivers in determining an initial grade of concussion followed by a delayed concussion grading to improve accuracy in diagnosis and management. These principles assist in making a decision to retire an athlete.

The physical examination should center on any abnormal neurologic findings. A complete and detailed neurologic examination should be performed, searching for any focal abnormalities. Visual field testing should be completed. Tests of balance and coordination should be performed to assess for ataxia. Examination of reflexes for hyperreflexia as well as other long-tract findings should be documented. Patients should be observed for signs of parkinsonism. Mental status examination is an important clinical prelude to further neuropsychological testing. Even with extensive neurologic examination, findings may be normal in a large percentage of patients with recurrent concussion.

Neuropsychological testing has undergone an evolution in its sports applications, and the neurocognitive and neuropsychological features may be measured with current methods. Neuropsychological impairment has been related to concussive and subconcussive injury in boxing, football, and soccer players, and neuropsychological testing is crucial in the determining the consequences of concussive injury. The number of concussive events has been shown by Guskiewicz and colleagues[18,19] to be significantly related to lifetime risk of depression as well as late-life cognitive impairment, with a suggestion that increasing number of concussions leads to higher prevalence. Several recent studies show the subtle cognitive effects of concussive injury and suggest that specialized testing of attention and information processing be used for assessment of postconcussive effects.[20] These discoveries have lead to a consensus statement among the participants of the most recent International Conference on Concussion in Sport held in Zurich, which emphasizes the importance of neuropsychological testing.[21] It has been recommended by Echemendia and colleagues[22] that clinical neuropsychologists, rather than athletic trainers or others, administer the complex psychometric tests to evaluate for these subtle abnormalities. Furthermore, it has been suggested that specifically developed computer-based tests be used, such as ImPACT, Cogsport, ANAM, and others.[23]

The advent of these computerized platforms, with access to the Internet and qualified neuropsychological opinion, make neuropsychological testing all the more practical and available for a larger population. For accurate assessment of effects of concussive injury on athletes before making a decision to end an athlete's career, it is imperative that these tests be administered. It has been shown by multiple sources that simple tests of intellectual and mental function do not reveal the true extent of cognitive decline. Furthermore, baseline neuropsychological examinations are important and preferred for comparison and more sensitive detection of decline. Although there are many nuances of correctly applying neuropsychological testing and interpreting their results, both traditional and computer-based instruments have proved invaluable in athletic concussion management. Therefore, neuropsychological testing, either in consultation with a neuropsychologist or computer based, is objective data that greatly aid sports medicine clinicians when deciding if retirement from sport should be pursued.

Imaging studies are integral for a full evaluation and should be performed. Although a CT scan may be performed to rule out any obvious abnormalities (eg, intracranial hemorrhage), the standard imaging method is MRI of the brain for further anatomic signs of trauma. Diffuse cerebral atrophy or ventriculomegaly may be encountered as well as other signs of chronic injury (**Fig. 4**). Imaging studies may reveal further, nontraumatic anatomic abnormalities and although these aspects may not be directly related to concussion, they too may prompt decision to retire an athlete. Discovery of any symptomatic abnormalities of the foramen magnum, such as a Chiari I malformation (**Fig. 5**), should prompt consideration of retirement, especially when combined with syringomyelia, obliteration of subarachnoid space, or indentation of the anterior medulla.[24] This has also been suggested for discovery of hydrocephalus or the incidence of spontaneous subarachnoid hemorrhage from any cause although no guidelines are currently in place.[16] More recently, MRI diffusion tensor imaging has demonstrated a correlation of increased fractional anisotropy and decreased radial diffusivity with increasing severity of postconcussive symptoms in adolescents after concussion.[25] This is currently increasing the ability to visualize and characterize postconcussive effects.

A Role for Future Genetic Testing

Early research in CTE and other neurodegenerative diseases has found a trend of developing these diseases with certain genetic traits. Specifically, the ApoE4 and the ApoE3 alleles, in both homozygous and heterozygous forms, have been implicated

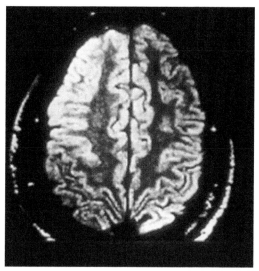

Fig. 4. MRI of a 24-year-old professional football player with career-ending postconcussion syndrome and a high-intensity lesion of the centrum semiovale.

in developing Alzheimer disease and CTE after brain trauma.[26,27] This was first discovered in a population of 30 career boxers and has since been confirmed in other populations with neurotrauma.[28] These proteins are various alleles of the apolipoprotein E, which is important for lipid transport and widely produced in the brain. Although this clinical science is still in its infancy, it may be possible to someday predict who will develop long-term problems from repeated head trauma in sports. Genetic testing, although raising ethical questions, may be a valuable tool for athletes who wish to know their risk for sustaining repeated concussive injury and may play a role in the decision to retire athletes in the future. Furthermore, although presence of hetero- or homozygous ApoE4 or ApoE3 confers a three- to ninefold increased risk of developing various forms of dementia after traumatic brain injury, the etiology is most likely multifactorial.

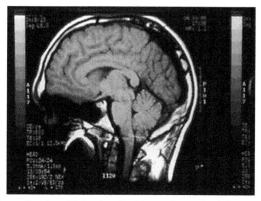

Fig. 5. Chiari malformation in a high school athlete who retired due to persistent postconcussion syndrome; a relative contraindication to continued contact sports participation.

Social and Legal Implications in the Decision to Retire

One of the difficulties in a decision to retire an athlete based on concussive injury is noted by Bailes and Cantu,[29] who recognize that athletes generally desire to continue play, and thus continue their exposure to potential concussions. Although the decision to retire an athlete is a difficult one because of the many factors to be considered, it is made further contentious because of the many social factors involved. Not only the athlete but also the coach, team members, agents, and athlete's family have considerable stake in the decision to retire. Often athletes are under considerable financial stress to continue in their sport; and this can extend to all levels of competition, from high school athletes hoping for a college scholarship to professional athletes who may have limited other marketable skills and are supporting a family. These aspects are further confirmed by Gerberich and colleagues,[30] who noted that athletes are often reticent to describe their full symptomatology after concussive injury. This phenomenon may have less of an impact during a decision to retire an athlete compared with a return to play decision, because these debates are often initiated only after firm evidence of postconcussive injury is apparent to all involved. Nevertheless, social and financial factors may have a significant impact on this decision.

Despite the many complexities of a retirement decision, clearly the athlete must be involved in this life-changing decision. Ideally, this decision should be made with the athlete and family in agreement. At times, however, the very cognitive and neuropsychological decline that may prompt a decision to retire interferes with the executive functioning and judgment of the athlete. In this case, neuropsychological testing must be performed and documented regarding the extent of a patient's ability to participate in the retirement decision.

The decision to retire an athlete after concussion may be compounded by complicating factors. Goldberg[31] notes that frequently team-employed physicians have been cited as downplaying injury and encouraging return to play. He makes the case that sports-related health decisions should be made by independent physicians as in workers compensation claims. To avoid this complicating factor, some have advised for retirement assessments to be performed by an independent physician or to encourage a second opinion from one. This is currently being implemented by the NFL to provide local neurosurgeons and neurologists for "second opinion" consultations of concussion.

Finally, the decision to allow or disallow return to play when a question of retirement arises has several legal implications for treating physicians. The decision to retire is usually symptom driven. Furthermore, much has still to be learned about the potential for chronic brain injury and CTE. In spite of the uncertainty of the impact of concussive injury on long-term functioning, however, physicians nevertheless must weigh carefully the benefits and risks of return to play and counsel athletes accordingly; some have advocated a conservative approach.[32] Furthermore, physicians have a responsibility to provide athletes with full information about their medical condition and possible consequences of return to play so that their own decision is informed. In making this decision, the duty of a physician is to protect the health and safety of the athlete, regardless if he or she wants to return to play.

In summary, the effects of concussion may lead to a variety of short- and long-term effects, which may lead to the decision to retire from contact sports. These effects follow a recognizable progression and may cause an athlete to opt out of play at any point along this progression. To elucidate the effect of concussion or MTBI and weigh in on a decision to retire, the treating physician needs to take into account the history, neurologic examination, brain imaging, and neuropsychological testing.

In addition, myriad social factors surrounding play must be taken into consideration. As always, neurologic sports medicine requires an individualized approach.

REFERENCES

1. Schneider R. Head and neck injuries in football. 1st edition. Baltimore (MD): Williams and Wilkins; 1973.
2. Torg J. Athletic injuries to the head, neck, and face. 2nd edition. St Louis (MO): Mosby; 1991.
3. Giza C, Hovda D. The neurometabolic cascade of concussion. J Athl Train 2001; 36:228–35.
4. Martland H. Punch drunk. J Am Med Assoc 1928;91:1103–7.
5. Omalu B, Bailes J, Hammers J, et al. Chronic traumatic encephalopathy, suicides, and parasuicides in professional American athletes: the role of the forensic pathologist. Am J Forensic Med Pathol 2010;31:130–2.
6. Omalu B, Bailes J, Hamilton R, et al. Emerging histomophologic subtypes of Chronic Traumatic Encephalopathy (CTE) in American athletes. J Neurosurg, in press.
7. Corsellis J, Bruton C, Freeman-Browne C. The aftermath of boxing. Psychol Med 1973;3:270–303.
8. Omalu B, Fitzsimmons R, Hammers J, et al. Chronic traumatic encephalopathy in a professional American wrestler. J Forensic Nurs 2010;6:130–6.
9. Omalu B, Hamilton R, Kamboh M, et al. Chronic Traumatic Encephalopathy (CTE) in a National Football League Player: case report and emerging medicolegal practice questions. J Forensic Nurs 2010;6:40–6.
10. Papez J. A proposed mechanism of emotion. Arch Neurol Psychiatry 1937;38: 725–43.
11. Smith D, Chen X, Nonaka M, et al. Accumulation of amyloid beta and tau in the formation of neurofilament inclusions following diffuse brain injury in the pig. J Neuropathol Exp Neurol 1999;58:982–92.
12. DeKosky S, Abrahamson E, Ciallella J, et al. Association of increased cortical soluble abeta42 levels with diffuse plaques after severe brain injury in humans. Arch Neurol 2007;64:541–4.
13. Gabbita S, Scheff S, Menard R, et al. Cleaved-tau: a biomarker of neuronal damage after traumatic brain injury. J Neurotrauma 2005;22:83–94.
14. Ilkonomovic M, Uryu K, Abrahamson E, et al. Alzheimer's pathology in human temporal cortex surgically excised after severe brain injury. Exp Neurol 2004; 190:192–203.
15. Aubry M, Cantu R, Dvorak J, et al. Summary and agreement statement of the first International Conference on Concussion in Sport, Vienna 2001. Br J Sports Med 2002;36:6–10.
16. Cantu R. Head injuries in sport. Br J Sports Med 1996;30:289–96.
17. Miele V, Bailes J, Martin N. Participation in contact or collision sports in athletes with epilepsy, genetic risk factors, structural brain lesions, or history of craniotomy. Neurosurg Focus 2006;21:E9.
18. Guskiewicz K, Marshall S, Bailes J, et al. Recurrent concussion and risk of depression in retired professional football players. Med Sci Sports Exerc 2007; 39:903–9.
19. Guskiewicz K, Marshal S, Bailes J, et al. Association between recurrent concussion and late-life cognitive impairment in retired professional football players. Neurosurgery 2005;57:719–26.

20. Collins M, Grindel S, Lovell M, et al. Relationship between concussion and neuro-psychological performance in college football players. JAMA 1999;282:964–70.
21. McCrory P, Meeuwisse W, Johnston K, et al. Consensus statement on concussion in Sport: the 3rd international conference on concussion in sport held in Zurich in November 2008. Br J Sports Med 2009;43(Suppl 1):i76–90.
22. Echemendia R, Herring S, Bailes J. Who should conduct and interpret the neuro-psycholocial assessment in sports-related concussion? Br J Sports Med 2009; 43(Suppl 1):i32–5.
23. Cantu R. An overview of concussion consensus statements since 2000. Neuro-surg Focus 2006;21:E3.
24. Callaway G, O'Brien S, Tehrany A. Chiari I malformation and spinal cord injury: cause for concern in contact athletes? Med Sci Sports Exerc 1996;28:1218–20.
25. Wilde E, McCauley S, Hunter J, et al. Diffusion tensor imaging of acute mild trau-matic brain injury in adolescents. Neurology 2008;70:948–55.
26. Omalu B, Dekosky S, Minster R, et al. Chronic Traumatic Encephalopathy in a national football league player. Neurosurgery 2005;57:128–34.
27. Geddes J, vowles G, Robinson S, et al. Neurofibrillary tangles, but not Alzheimer-type pathology, in a young boxer. Neuropathol Appl Neurobiol 1996;22:12–6.
28. Jordan B, Relkin N, Ravdin L, et al. Apolipoprotein E4 associated with chronic traumatic brain injury in boxing. JAMA 1997;278:136–40.
29. Bailes J, Cantu R. Head injury in athletes. Neurosurgery 2001;48:26–45.
30. Gerberich S, Priest J, Boen J, et al. Concussion incidences and severity in secondary school varsity football players. Am J Public Health 1983;73:1370–5.
31. Goldberg D. Concussions, professional sports, and conflicts of interest: why the national football league's current policies are bad for its (players') health. HEC Forum 2008;20:337–55.
32. Osborne B. Principles of liability for athletic trainers: managing sport-related concussion. J Athl Train 2001;36:316–21.

Future Advances and Areas of Future Focus in the Treatment of Sport-Related Concussion

Paul McCrory, MBBS, PhD, FRACP, FACSP, FFSEM, GradDipEpidBiostats

> **KEYWORDS**
> - Sports concussion • Athletic injuries
> - Chronic traumatic encephalopathy • Traumatic brain injury

THE END OF THE BEGINNING

The critical issues in the clinical management of sports concussion include confirming the diagnosis, differentiating concussion from other pathologies (particularly structural head injury), and determining when players have recovered so that they can be safely returned to competition. When expressed in this fashion, the management process seems simple. Yet the occurrence and management of this injury provokes more debate and concern than virtually all other sports injuries combined.

In the past 3 decades, clinicians have gone from mostly anecdotal strategies to an international consensus–based approach and the early evolution of evidence-based practice, particularly in the area of injury prevention.[1–5] We have come far, but the situation in 2011 should be seen as the end of the beginning, not the beginning of the end.

The past 2 to 3 years have seen increasing engagement by mainstream neuroscientists in this field, which had previously been dominated by sports team physicians. This change has been useful in bringing a range of expertise (eg, neuropathology, neuroradiology) to the debate. However, it has been disappointing because the interchange has largely taken place in the media rather than through scientific journals. The

Financial disclosure: the author has received research funding and conference support from the National Health & Medical Research Council of Australia, the Australian Research Council, the International Rugby Board, Victorian Department of Health, Australian Sports Commission, the International Olympic Commission, Fédération Internationale de Football Association, and CogState Inc.
No reprints will be available.
Centre for Health, Exercise & Sports Medicine & Brain Research Institute, University of Melbourne, Parkville, Victoria 3010, Australia
E-mail address: paulmccr@bigpond.net.au

resultant media interest has caused significant alarm in the minds of the public about putative long-term risks and concern about how an acute injury should be managed, particularly in communities that currently lack access to quality medical resources.

Tragic stories of athletes who have not been managed according to current guidelines, or who have failed to fully disclose their injury to team medical staff, resulting in catastrophic outcomes, are regularly aired in the media and, at least in the United States, have caused legislators to propose regulatory measures that restrict medical management of concussion in ways that apply to no other medical condition. When last checked in 2009, 13 US states had bills either before their legislatures or passed related to sports concussion in addition to proposed national legislation. In many cases, the principle of the bills is primarily educative. However, in some states, mandatory preseason cognitive testing and other paradigms are included. The tragedy in this area is the replacement of scientific management by media anecdote. This is ironic given that the focus in sports concussion in the past 3 decades has been the opposite.

This paper examines some of the key areas that are likely to be the focus of research in the next few years. From the media perspective, the risk of long-term injury is paramount. However, from the sports perspectives globally, the major concern is how community athletes who may lack the resources available for elite athletes can safely be managed.

OPENING THE CHAMBER OF SECRETS

In many ways, elite sport has been its own worst enemy in this field. The sight of concussed professional athletes returning to play on the day of injury in many sports globally[6] gives the public the wrong perception of the seriousness of this injury. Although it is broadly accepted that all athletes, regardless of their level of participation, should be managed using the same return-to-play paradigm, elite teams have far greater resources such as access to emergent neuroimaging, immediate neuropsychological assessment, as well as high-level expertise in concussion evaluation, which in turn means that the accurate assessment of recovery can occur in shorter time frames. However, the public never sees the back-office assessment, simply the rapid return of a concussed athlete to the field of play. The public assumes that similar rapid return is possible at lesser levels of competition. This lack of understanding makes the need for community education much more urgent, so that athletes, coaches, parents, trainers, and others involved in athlete care become aware of the significance of the injury and its appropriate management.

SAME-DAY RETURN TO PLAY

The basic management principles, namely full clinical and cognitive recovery before consideration of return to play, should be followed. This approach is supported by the major published guidelines such as the American Academy of Neurology, US Team Physician Consensus Statement, US National Athletic Trainers Association Position Statement, and the Zurich Consensus statement.[1,3–5]

There is published evidence that some professional American football players are able to return to play on the same day without a risk of concussion recurrence or sequelae.[6] However, there are also data showing that, at the collegiate and high school level, some athletes allowed to return to play on the same day show neuropsychological deficits that may not be evident on the sidelines, and are more likely to have delayed onset of symptoms.[7,8]

This disparity in outcomes between elite and college/high school athletes highlights a key area in the debate, namely that any concussion management strategy needs to be tailored by age and possibly level of performance. A 'one-size-fits-all strategy may not be possible unless one takes the ultraconservative view and simply has a policy of no return to play on the same day. Increasingly, research and clinical focus will be directed at managing different age groups with safe and appropriate guidelines. In many cases, this may involve no return on the day of injury, a strategy that may create concern, particularly at US collegiate levels.

THE BLACK DOG OF DEPRESSION

Mental health issues (such as depression) have been reported as a long-term consequence of sports-related concussion, occurring in approximately 11%, with a possible association with recurrent concussion.[9] It is important to examine the wider perspective, because depression and anxiety symptoms occur in 15% to 60% of patients following traumatic brain injury from any cause.[10–13] Neuroimaging studies using functional magnetic resonance imaging and other neuroimaging modalities suggest that a depressed mood following brain injury may reflect an underlying pathophysiologic abnormality consistent with a limbic-frontal model of depression.[14,15]

Although this issue highlights the need to be vigilant for all mental health problems in all current and retired athletes, it seems that sport per se is not the concern here, but rather the presence of a traumatic brain injury, which in itself carries an inherent risk of depression, suicide, and other mental health issues. In addition to awareness, psychological approaches may have potential applications in this injury and remain an underused resource in sports medicine.[16,17] Caregivers are also encouraged to evaluate for affective symptoms such as depression, not only in the concussed athlete but also in healthy athletes during preparticipation screenings to prevent future problems.[18]

PUNCH-DRUNK ATHLETES?

Recent cross-sectional descriptive epidemiologic studies have suggested an association between repeated sports concussions during a career and late-life cognitive impairment.[19] Similarly, case reports have noted anecdotal cases in which possible neuropathologic evidence of chronic traumatic encephalopathy was observed in retired football players as well as other sportsmen, such as boxers.[20–24]

Major methodological flaws exist in these observational studies, and the putative associations may be spurious. Much of the debate in this regard has been in the media rather than in the scientific literature, and many of the cases proposed are easily explained by mechanisms other than participation in sport, with or without recognized head injury. Even the recent cases reported with neuropathologic features (such as tau positive neurofibrillary tangles) have other possible causes and, of more concern, differ in their microscopic features from the older cases of punch-drunk syndrome (which also have β amyloid deposition) in boxers, which were the basis for the current understanding of this condition.[25–27] At the present time, the classification and neuropathologic understanding of this condition still needs resolution.

One particular concern is raised by clinicians is that, if this condition is a potential risk for all athletes (even reported in footballers never diagnosed with concussion during their career), then why are there not more cases of retired footballers with dementia? Sports such as Australian football have a risk of concussion 15 times that of American football, yet long-term follow-up studies do not show similar findings.[28,29] More importantly, prospective cohort studies using neuropsychological assessment in athletes have been available since the late 1980s, and these published studies do not conclusively support evidence of deteriorating cognitive function during an athletic career following recurrent concussions. However, they do suggest that having 1 concussion may increase the risk and/or severity of subsequent concussions.[30–32]

In many ways, this parallels the debate about the small percentage of boxers who seem disproportionately affected by chronic traumatic encephalopathy. However, most boxers, many of whom have had substantial head trauma during their careers, remain unaffected.[33] The data from the original work by Corsellis and Roberts[25,26] suggest that extremes of head injury exposure are a risk factor for chronic traumatic encephalopathy in boxers. However, such levels are simply not seen in other sports. It seems that there is likely to be an alternative explanation, such as a particular genetic factor that puts these athletes at greater risk. The significance of apolipoprotein (Apo) E ε4, ApoE promoter gene, tau polymerase, and other genetic markers in the risk of sports concussion or injury outcome is unclear at this time.[34–36] Additional concerns are the role of risk-taking behavior, alcohol use, and drug use by elite athletes, which in turn may have adverse neuropathologic consequences.[37,38]

At this time, the frequency or risk, if any, of long-term consequences of sports concussion are unknown. However, ongoing monitoring during and after an athletic career is a reasonable approach. Clinicians need to be mindful of the potential for long-term problems in the management of all athletes.

LITTLE ADULTS OR DIFFERENT MANAGEMENT STRATEGIES FOR CHILDREN?

It was accepted by the Zurich international consensus group that the adult athlete evaluation and management recommendations could be applied to children and adolescents down to the age of 10 years with a few important differences.[1] Younger than that age, children report different concussion symptoms than adults and require age-appropriate symptom checklists as a part of the assessment. When assessing the child or adolescent athlete with a concussion, the health care professional needs to consider input from parents, teachers, and other school personnel.[39–42]

Although neuropsychological assessment is widely used following symptom resolution in adult concussion, its timing differs in children, because it may be used to assist planning for school and home management while the patient is still symptomatic. If cognitive testing is performed, then it must be developmentally sensitive through the late teen years. It is particularly important to consider the use of trained neuropsychologists to interpret data, particularly in children with learning disorders and/or attention-deficit hyperactivity disorder who may need more sophisticated assessment strategies.[39,43,44]

Because of the different physiologic response, longer recovery after concussion, and specific risks (eg, diffuse cerebral swelling) related to head impact during childhood and adolescence, a more conservative return-to-play approach is usually recommended for children and adolescents. It is not appropriate for a child or adolescent athlete with concussion to return to play on the same day as the injury, regardless of the level of athletic performance.

PREVENTION IS BETTER THAN CURE

Consideration of rule changes to reduce the head injury risk may be appropriate if a specific mechanism is implicated. An example of this is in football (soccer), for which published studies show that upper limb to head contact in heading contests accounted for approximately 50% of concussions.[45] By penalizing such contact and enforcing the rules, the risk of injury has been substantially reduced.[46,47]

There is no good clinical evidence that currently available protective equipment (especially soft-shell helmets) prevents concussion. However, mouthguards have a definite role in preventing dental and orofacial injury.[48,49] For skiing and snowboarding, there are several studies to suggest that helmets provide protection against soft tissue head (not brain) and facial injury. Hence, they may be recommended for participants in alpine sports.[50–52] In specific sports such as cycling, motor sports, and equestrian sports, protective helmets may prevent other forms of head injury (eg, skull fracture) that are related to falling on hard surfaces. These may be important injury prevention issues for those sports.[53–59]

EDUCATING THE MASSES

Because the ability to reduce the effects of concussive injury after the event is minimal, the education of athletes, colleagues, and the general public is a mainstay of progress in this field. All people involved in athlete care, including referees, administrators, parents, coaches, as well as the athletes themselves, must be educated regarding the importance of injury and the principles of safe return to play. However, in spite of the efforts by sports to promulgate such information, evidence that these educational strategies are effectively reaching their target groups is lacking.[60–63]

Methods to improve education, including Web-based resources, are important in delivering the message and providing peer support.[64,65] In addition, enlightened bodies, such as Fédération Internationale de Football Association (FIFA), the International Olympic Committee, the International Rugby Board, and the International Ice Hockey Federation, are to be congratulated for their support because their efforts reach a global audience.

WHERE TO NOW?

There are several areas of focus at the present time that require resolution. The role of the Concussion in Sport group as an international forum for research exchange and in the development of consensus guidelines cannot be underestimated. In specific countries, such as the US, local guidelines have had a similarly important role in educating medical staff but have yet to translate into mainstream community education. The engagement of mainstream neuroscience is important, but, rather than conducting the debate through the media, the issues raised need to be tested by scientific peer review. We must remember that the plural of anecdotes is not data.

REFERENCES

1. McCrory P, Meeuwisse W, Johnston K, et al. Consensus statement on concussion in sport: the 3rd International Conference on Concussion in Sport held in Zurich, November 2008. Br J Sports Med 2009;43(Suppl 1):i76–90.
2. Cantu RC, Aubry M, Dvorak J, et al. Overview of concussion consensus statements since 2000. Neurosurg Focus 2006;21(4):E3.
3. Guskiewicz KM, Bruce SL, Cantu RC, et al. National Athletic Trainers' Association position statement: management of sport-related concussion. J Athl Train 2004; 39(3):280–97.
4. Herring S, Bergfeld J, Boland A, et al. Concussion (mild traumatic brain injury) and the team physician: a consensus statement. Med Sci Sports Exerc 2006; 38(2):395–9.
5. Kelly JP, Rosenberg JH. The development of guidelines for the management of concussion in sports. J Head Trauma Rehabil 1998;13(2):53–65.

6. Pellman EJ, Viano DC, Casson IR, et al. Concussion in professional football: players returning to the same game–part 7. Neurosurgery 2005;56(1):79–90 [discussion: 90–2].

7. Guskiewicz KM, McCrea M, Marshall SW, et al. Cumulative effects associated with recurrent concussion in collegiate football players. JAMA 2003;290(19):2549–55.

8. Lovell M, Collins M, Bradley J. Return to play following sports-related concussion. Clin Sports Med 2004;23(3):421–41, ix.

9. Guskiewicz KM, Marshall SW, Bailes J, et al. Recurrent concussion and risk of depression in retired professional football players. Med Sci Sports Exerc 2007; 39(6):903–9.

10. Rao V, Bertrand M, Rosenberg P, et al. Predictors of new-onset depression after mild traumatic brain injury. J Neuropsychiatry Clin Neurosci 2010;22(1):100–4 Winter.

11. Fann JR, Hart T, Schomer KG. Treatment for depression after traumatic brain injury: a systematic review. J Neurotrauma 2009;26(12):2383–402.

12. Silver JM, McAllister TW, Arciniegas DB. Depression and cognitive complaints following mild traumatic brain injury. Am J Psychiatry 2009;166(6):653–61.

13. Menzel JC. Depression in the elderly after traumatic brain injury: a systematic review. Brain Inj 2008;22(5):375–80.

14. Fleminger S. Long-term psychiatric disorders after traumatic brain injury. Eur J Anaesthesiol Suppl 2008;42:123–30.

15. Chen JK, Johnston KM, Petrides M, et al. Neural substrates of symptoms of depression following concussion in male athletes with persisting postconcussion symptoms. Arch Gen Psychiatry 2008;65(1):81–9.

16. Bloom G, Horton A, McCrory P, et al. Sport psychology and concussion: new impacts to explore. Br J Sports Med 2004;38(5):519–21.

17. Weiss MR, Gill DL. What goes around comes around: re-emerging themes in sport and exercise psychology. Res Q Exerc Sport 2005;76(Suppl 2):S71–87.

18. Johnston K, Bloom G, Ramsay J, et al. Current concepts in concussion rehabilitation. Curr Sports Med Rep 2004;3:316–23.

19. Guskiewicz KM, Marshall SW, Bailes J, et al. Association between recurrent concussion and late-life cognitive impairment in retired professional football players. Neurosurgery 2005;57(4):719–26 [discussion: 726].

20. Omalu BI, DeKosky ST, Hamilton RL, et al. Chronic traumatic encephalopathy in a national football league player: part II. Neurosurgery 2006;59(5):1086–92 [discussion: 1092–3].

21. Omalu BI, DeKosky ST, Minster RL, et al. Chronic traumatic encephalopathy in a National Football League player. Neurosurgery 2005;57(1):128–34 [discussion: 134].

22. Cantu RC. Chronic traumatic encephalopathy in the National Football League. Neurosurgery 2007;61(2):223–5.

23. Casson IR, Pellman EJ, Viano DC. Chronic traumatic encephalopathy in a National Football League player. Neurosurgery 2006;59(5):E1152.

24. McKee AC, Cantu RC, Nowinski CJ, et al. Chronic traumatic encephalopathy in athletes: progressive tauopathy after repetitive head injury. J Neuropathol Exp Neurol 2009;68(7):709–35.

25. Corsellis JA, Bruton CJ, Freeman-Browne D. The aftermath of boxing. Psychol Med 1973;3:270–303.

26. Roberts AH. Brain damage in boxers: a study of the prevalence of traumatic encephalopathy among ex-professional boxers. London: Pitman; 1969.

27. Roberts GW, Allsop D, Bruton C. The occult aftermath of boxing. J Neurol Neurosurg Psychiatr 1990;53(5):373–8.

28. McCrory P. 2002 Refshauge Lecture. When to retire after concussion? J Sci Med Sport 2002;5(3):169–82.
29. McCrory PR, Berkovic SF, Cordner SM. Deaths due to brain injury among footballers in Victoria, 1968-1999. Med J Aust 2000;172(5):217–9.
30. Iverson GL, Brooks BL, Lovell MR, et al. No cumulative effects for one or two previous concussions. Br J Sports Med 2006;40(1):72–5.
31. Collins MW, Lovell MR, Iverson GL, et al. Cumulative effects of concussion in high school athletes. Neurosurgery 2002;51(5):1175–9 [discussion: 1180–1].
32. Guskiewicz KM, McCrea M, Marshall SW, et al. Cumulative effects associated with recurrent concussion in collegiate football players: the NCAA Concussion Study. JAMA 2003;290(19):2549–55.
33. McCrory P, Zazryn T, Cameron P. The evidence for chronic traumatic encephalopathy in boxing. Sports Med 2007;37(6):467–76.
34. Kristman VL, Tator CH, Kreiger N, et al. Does the apolipoprotein epsilon 4 allele predispose varsity athletes to concussion? A prospective cohort study. Clin J Sport Med 2008;18(4):322–8.
35. Terrell TR, Bostick RM, Abramson R, et al. APOE, APOE promoter, and Tau genotypes and risk for concussion in college athletes. Clin J Sport Med 2008;18(1):10–7.
36. Jordan B, Relkin N, Ravdin L. Apolipoprotein E epsilon 4 associated with chronic traumatic brain injury in boxing. J Am Med Assoc 1997;278:136–40.
37. Peretti-Watel P, Guagliardo V, Verger P, et al. Sporting activity and drug use: alcohol, cigarette and cannabis use among elite student athletes. Addiction 2003;98(9):1249–56.
38. Dietze PM, Fitzgerald JL, Jenkinson RA. Drinking by professional Australian Football League (AFL) players: prevalence and correlates of risk. Med J Aust 2008;189(9):479–83.
39. Purcell L, Carson J. Sport-related concussion in pediatric athletes. Clin Pediatr (Phila) 2008;47(2):106–13.
40. Lee LK. Controversies in the sequelae of pediatric mild traumatic brain injury. Pediatr Emerg Care 2007;23(8):580–3 [quiz: 584–6].
41. Schnadower D, Vazquez H, Lee J, et al. Controversies in the evaluation and management of minor blunt head trauma in children. Curr Opin Pediatr 2007;19(3):258–64.
42. Wozniak JR, Krach L, Ward E, et al. Neurocognitive and neuroimaging correlates of pediatric traumatic brain injury: a diffusion tensor imaging (DTI) study. Arch Clin Neuropsychol 2007;22(5):555–68.
43. Gioia G, Janusz J, Gilstein K, et al. Neuropsychological management of concussion in children and adolescents: effects of age and gender on ImPACT [abstract]. Br J Sports Med 2004;38:657.
44. McCrory P, Collie A, Anderson V, et al. Can the authors manage sport related concussion in children the same as in adults? Br J Sports Med 2004;38(5):516–9.
45. Andersen T, Arnason A, Engebretsen L, et al. Mechanism of head injuries in elite football. Br J Sports Med 2004;38:690–6.
46. Dvorak J. Give Hippocrates a jersey: promoting health through football/sport. Br J Sports Med 2009;43(5):317–22.
47. Blatter JS, Dvorak J. Football for health - prevention is better than cure. Scand J Med Sci Sports 2010;20(Suppl 1):v.
48. Benson BW, Hamilton GM, Meeuwisse WH, et al. Is protective equipment useful in preventing concussion? A systematic review of the literature. Br J Sports Med 2009;43(Suppl 1):i56–67.

49. McIntosh AS, McCrory P, Finch CF, et al. Does padded headgear prevent head injury in rugby union football? Med Sci Sports Exerc 2009;41(2):306–13.
50. Hagel BE, Pless IB, Goulet C, et al. Effectiveness of helmets in skiers and snowboarders: case-control and case crossover study. BMJ 2005;330(7486):281.
51. McCrory P. The role of helmets in skiing and snowboarding. Br J Sports Med 2002;36(5):314.
52. Sulheim S, Holme I, Ekeland A, et al. Helmet use and risk of head injuries in alpine skiers and snowboarders. JAMA 2006;295(8):919–24.
53. Delaney JS, Al-Kashmiri A, Drummond R, et al. The effect of protective headgear on head injuries and concussions in adolescent football (soccer) players. Br J Sports Med 2008;42(2):110–5 [discussion: 115].
54. Viano DC, Pellman EJ, Withnall C, et al. Concussion in professional football: performance of newer helmets in reconstructed game impacts–part 13. Neurosurgery 2006;59(3):591–606 [discussion: 591–606].
55. Finch C, Braham R, McIntosh A, et al. Should football players wear custom fitted mouthguards? Results from a group randomised controlled trial. Inj Prev 2005; 11(4):242–6.
56. McIntosh A, McCrory P. The dynamics of concussive head impacts in rugby and Australian Rules football. Med Sci Sports Exerc 2000;32:1980–5.
57. McIntosh A, McCrory P. Impact energy attenuation performance of football headgear. Br J Sports Med 2000;34:337–42.
58. McIntosh A, McCrory P. Effectiveness of headgear in a pilot study of under 15 rugby union football. Br J Sports Med 2001;35:167–70.
59. McIntosh A, McCrory P, Finch C, et al. Rugby headgear study. Sydney: The University of New South Wales; 2005.
60. Sullivan SJ, Bourne L, Choie S, et al. Understanding of sport concussion by the parents of young rugby players: a pilot study. Clin J Sport Med 2009;19(3): 228–30.
61. Sullivan SJ, Schneiders AG, McCrory P, et al. Physiotherapists' use of information in identifying a concussion: an extended Delphi approach. Br J Sports Med 2008; 42(3):175–7 [discussion: 177].
62. Sye G, Sullivan SJ, McCrory P. High school rugby players' understanding of concussion and return to play guidelines. Br J Sports Med 2006;40(12):1003–5.
63. Valovich McLeod TC, Schwartz C, Bay RC. Sport-related concussion misunderstandings among youth coaches. Clin J Sport Med 2007;17(2):140–2.
64. Ahmed OH, Sullivan SJ, Schneiders AG, et al. iSupport: do social networking sites have a role to play in concussion awareness? Disabil Rehabil 2010; 32(22):1877–83.
65. Provvidenza CF, Johnston KM. Knowledge transfer principles as applied to sport concussion education. Br J Sports Med 2009;43(Suppl 1):i68–75.

Index

Note: Page numbers of article titles are in **boldface** type.

Clin Sports Med 30 (2011) 209–215
doi:10.1016/S0278-5919(10)00096-7
0278-5919/11/$ – see front matter © 2011 Elsevier Inc. All rights reserved.

sportsmed.theclinics.com

Moving?

Make sure your subscription moves with you!

To notify us of your new address, find your **Clinics Account Number** (located on your mailing label above your name), and contact customer service at:

Email: journalscustomerservice-usa@elsevier.com

800-654-2452 (subscribers in the U.S. & Canada)
314-447-8871 (subscribers outside of the U.S. & Canada)

Fax number: 314-447-8029

Elsevier Health Sciences Division
Subscription Customer Service
3251 Riverport Lane
Maryland Heights, MO 63043

*To ensure uninterrupted delivery of your subscription, please notify us at least 4 weeks in advance of move.

Printed and bound by CPI Group (UK) Ltd, Croydon, CR0 4YY

14/10/2024

01773690-0001